MCQs for the Primary FRCA

KHALED ELFITURI
Consultant Anaesthetist

GRAHAM ARTHURS
Consultant Anaesthetist

LES GEMMELL
Consultant Anaesthetist
Anaesthetic Department
Maelor Hospital, Wrexham

RICHARD SHILLITO
Specialist Anaesthetist, New Zealand MCQ Tutor

TONY BAILEY
Illustrations

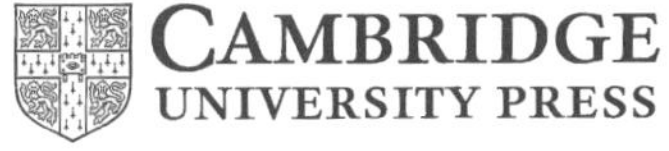
CAMBRIDGE
UNIVERSITY PRESS

CAMBRIDGE UNIVERSITY PRESS
Cambridge, New York, Melbourne, Madrid, Cape Town, Singapore, São Paulo

Cambridge University Press
The Edinburgh Building, Cambridge CB2 8RU, UK

Published in the United States of America by Cambridge University Press, New York

www.cambridge.org
Information on this title: www.cambridge.org/9780521705097

First published 2008

Printed in the United Kingdom at the University Press, Cambridge

A catalogue record for this publication is available from the British Library

ISBN 978-0-521-70509-7 paperback

Contents

Acknowledgements

The authors are very grateful to Richard Shillito for all his efforts in writing the MCQ tutor program and to Tony Bailey for providing the fine illustrations.

Introduction

This book contains 540 questions in 6 papers as they might appear in the examination. Each paper has 90 questions, each with 5 parts. There are 30 physiological questions, 30 pharmacology questions and 30 physics, clinical measurement and statistics questions.

The questions have been constructed using information remembered by candidates sitting the London college examination in recent years. These may not be the exact questions as they appeared in the examination but will be of the same degree of difficulty and cover the same topics.

In order to pass the primary anaesthesia examination, knowledge is required and it is essential to learn about all the topics that might be examined. These questions are a guide to the syllabus and the subjects that should be covered before appearing in the examination.

It is probably not realistic to try to learn by just reading an MCQ book. But once the trainee has studied for 6 months or more then a book such as this is one way of testing whether enough of the topics have been covered and then the level of knowledge and understanding that has been achieved.

It is important to practise a technique for answering MCQ questions. In the examination hall it is a good idea not to record the answers on the answer sheet during the first 15 minutes as that is when mistakes of entering the answers under the wrong question number occur. But it is important that, every time a question is read, a decision is made about the answer and that decision should be recorded on the question sheet, before transferring anything to the answer sheet. Use a code that allows you to record a decision every time you read a question. Place a mark against each question on the question paper such as T (true), F (false) or X (do not know). Start to transfer your certain answers to the answer sheet only once the adrenaline is settling down. Go back again and re-read the questions you were not certain about. Look at what you thought the answer was the first time and if you think it is the same on a second reading it may be worth transferring that answer. Use the suggested answers in the book to check if you are guessing too much and getting it wrong too often or not transferring some of your hunches which are proving to be correct.

It is always difficult to be certain of the pass mark, but below 50% will not be a pass, between 50% and 55% will sometimes be a pass, between 55% and 60% should be a pass, but it will vary between each sitting of the examination.

If the examination changes to one correct answer for every five questions the answering technique will remain the same. Record your answer on the question paper to start with and only transfer answers when you are certain and when your adrenaline has settled. Then go back and check the ones you have not transferred. If there is no negative marking you should answer all the questions with your best guess but you want to avoid making too many changes on the answer sheet.

Read each question carefully. Some common problems include seeing a question on a familiar topic but not checking the decimal point, the units used or the negative phrasing. The words 'may' and 'can' are usually true but not always and 'always' will usually be false in medical matters.

MCQ tutor program

To complement this book, but separate from the book, the MCQ Tutor program has been developed by Dr Richard Shillito, who is an anaesthetist. The aim of the program is to specifically help candidates to work out if they are too cautious and do not answer questions that they would probably get right or are inclined the other way and guess too much and so score a lot of negative points.

For details of the program visit the Cambridge University Press website www.cambridge.org/9780521705097.

You will need Microsoft 2000 or XP in order to run this program. The program uses the same test papers that are in this book. The reader is asked to enter their answers – true/false – or if you are uncertain mark true/false and possible or do not know.

When the test paper is finished two scores will be calculated. One for all the answers given and a second score for the answers only marked as certain. From the two scores it will be possible to determine whether all the certain answers by themselves would have been enough to pass, or whether the 'possible' answers should be included.

This is the first program that we are aware of that allows the candidate to find out if their guesses are good guesses that should be used to add to their total score or bad guesses that are reducing their overall score. The authors are very grateful to Richard Shillito for all his efforts in writing this program.

Abbreviations

2,3-DPG	2,3-diphosphoglycerate
AA	amino acids
ACEI	angiotensin converting enzyme inhibitor
ACTH	adrenocorticotropic hormone
ADH	antidiuretic hormone
ADP	adenosine diphosphate
ALT	alanine aminotransferase
ANP	atrial natriuretic peptide
aPTT	activated partial thromboplastin time
ARDS	acute respiratory distress syndrome
AST	aspartate aminotransferase
ATP	adenosine triphosphate
AUC	area under the curve
AV	atrioventricular
AVP	arginine vasopressin
BBB	blood–brain barrier
BiS	bispectral analysis
cAMP	cyclic adenosine monophosphate
CBF	cerebral blood flow
CMRR	common mode rejection ratio
CoHb	carboxyhaemoglobin
CPAP	continuous positive airways pressure
CPP	coronary perfusion pressure
CSF	cerebrospinal fluid
CTZ	chemoreceptor trigger zone
CV	closing volume
DCT	distal convoluted tubule
DINAMAP	devices for indirect non-invasive automated mean arterial pressure measurement
DPPC	dipalmitoylphosphatidylcholine
DRA	dosage regimen adjustment
ECFV	extracellular fluid volume

EDP	end-diastolic pressure
EF	ejection fraction
EPSP	excitatory postsynaptic potential
FFA	free fatty acids
FRC	functional residual capacity
GFR	glomerular filtration rate
GIP	gastric inhibitory peptide
HbA	adult haemoglobin
HbF	fetal haemoglobin
ICFV	intracellular fluid volume
IOP	intraocular pressure
IP_3	inositol trisphosphate
IPPV	intermittent positive-pressure ventilation
IPSP	inhibitory postsynaptic potential
ISFV	interstitial fluid volume
IVC	inferior vena cava
LOH	loop of Henle
LOS	lower oesophageal sphincter
LVEDP	left ventricular end-diastolic pressure
MAO	monoamine oxidase
MAC	minimum alveolar concentration
MAP	mean arterial pressure
MetHb	methaemoglobin
MRI	magnetic resonance imaging
NANC	non-adrenergic, non-cholinergic
NIDDM	non-insulin-dependent diabetes mellitus
NIST	non-interchangeable screw thread
NMDA	N-methyl-D-aspartate
NSAIDs	non-steroidal anti-inflammatory drugs
ODC	oxyhaemoglobin dissociation curve
P_{50}	oxygen tension of 50% saturation
PA	pulmonary artery
PAH	para-aminohippuric acid
PCT	proximal convoluted tubule
PCV	packed cell volume
PDE	phosphodiesterase
PEEP	positive end-expiratory pressure
PEFR	peak expiratory flow rate
PONV	postoperative nausea and vomiting

PT	prothrombin time
PTH	parathyroid hormone
PV	plasma volume
PVR	pulmonary vascular resistance
RAM	random access memory
REM	rapid eye movement
ROM	read only memory
RPF	renal plasma flow
RQ	respiratory quotient
RV	residual volume
SA	sinoatrial
SD	standard deviation
SELV	safety extra low-voltage
SEM	standard error of the mean
SIADH	syndrome of inappropriate ADH secretion
SLE	systemic lupus erythematosus
SVP	saturated vapour pressure
SVT	supraventricular tachyarrhythmias
TBG	thyroxine-binding globulin
TBPA	thyroxine binding pre-albumin
TBW	total body water
TENS	transcutaneous electrical nerve stimulation
TLC	total lung capacity
TmG	tubular maximum
TMP	transmembrane pressure
TOE	transoesophageal echocardiography
TSH	thyroid-stimulating hormone
UF	ultrafiltrate
V/Q	ventilation/perfusion
VIC	vaporiser inside the circle

Note: Certain drug names used are known by alternatives:

- adrenaline–epinephrine
- noradrenaline–norepinephrine
- lidocaine–lignocaine
- amitriptyline–amitriptiline

Paper 1 Questions

Physiology

1 Pulse pressure

(a) is the median value between the systolic and the diastolic blood pressures
(b) is reduced during tachycardia
(c) is determined by the compliance of the arterial tree
(d) decreases in old age
(e) at a given time is the same throughout the arterial tree

2 Myocardial work increases when there is an increase in

(a) stroke volume
(b) ventricular systolic pressure
(c) contractility
(d) heart rate
(e) systemic vascular resistance

3 Fetal haemoglobin

(a) forms 60% of circulating haemoglobin at birth
(b) is normally replaced by haemoglobin A (HbA) within 6–9 months
(c) has a sigmoid-shaped dissociation curve
(d) has a greater oxygen content at any given PO_2 than adult haemoglobin
(e) binds 2,3-DPG more avidly than HbA

4 In the normal ECG the

(a) Q wave is normally present in lead V6
(b) T wave is normally inverted in aVR
(c) Q wave is normally present in V1
(d) R wave is larger than the S wave in V1
(e) QRS duration depends on the recording electrode

5 Pulmonary vascular resistance is

(a) increased when the haematocrit is abnormally high
(b) decreased when breathing 21% oxygen in 79% helium
(c) increased by the application of 5 cmH_2O positive end-expiratory pressure
(d) increased by hypercapnia
(e) decreased by moderate exercise

6 Concerning baroreceptors

(a) they are located in the carotid sinus and aortic arch
(b) they are stretch receptors
(c) the neuronal discharge decreases as the mean arterial pressure increases
(d) the neuronal firing increases as the heart rate increases
(e) baroreceptors in the carotid sinus are more sensitive than aortic receptors to changes in blood pressure

7 Lung compliance

(a) describes the relationship between pressure and flow
(b) decreases with age
(c) is reduced in the supine position
(d) is normally 1.5–2.0 l/kPa
(e) is related to body size

8 During normal inspiration there is an increase in

(a) intrapleural pressure
(b) alveolar pressure
(c) intra-abdominal pressure
(d) the relative humidity of air in the trachea
(e) the partial pressure of oxygen in the trachea

9 Alveolar dead space is increased in

(a) pulmonary embolism
(b) haemorrhage
(c) increased tidal volumes
(d) changing from the supine to the erect posture
(e) intermittent positive-pressure ventilation

10 Functional residual capacity (FRC)

(a) measurement by the helium dilution technique gives a higher value than that given by body plethysmography
(b) is equal to total lung capacity minus the reserve volume
(c) is increased by changing from the erect to the supine posture
(d) is reduced during pregnancy
(e) is decreased in old age

11 The ascending limb of the loop of Henle

(a) is impermeable to sodium
(b) is involved in the active transport of potassium ions into the lumen
(c) is involved in the transport of chloride out of the lumen
(d) actively transports water
(e) contains hypotonic urine at the distal end

12 In an awake, healthy individual assuming the lateral position the

(a) dependent lung has less ventilation
(b) dependent lung has more perfusion
(c) $\dot{V}/\dot{Q}$ ratio is higher in the dependent lung
(d) PO_2 is higher in the lower lung
(e) P_aCO_2 is lower in the lower lung

13 A pressure volume curve can be used for measuring

(a) the work of breathing
(b) compliance
(c) functional residual capacity (FRC)
(d) respiratory quotient
(e) anatomical dead space

14 Cerebrospinal fluid

(a) is formed by the choroid plexus
(b) has a specific gravity of 1030 at body temperature
(c) total volume in a 70-kg adult is 500 ml
(d) normal pressure in the lateral position is 70–150 kPa
(e) total protein content is more than that of serum proteins

15 Concerning the transport process in the proximal convoluted tubules (PCT)

(a) about 50% of the normal filtered load of HCO_3 ion is absorbed in the proximal tubule
(b) absorption of glucose is linked to sodium reabsorption
(c) normally most of the phosphate filtered is excreted
(d) there are active secretory mechanisms for penicillin and *para*-aminohippuric acid (PAH)
(e) amino acid absorption is independent of sodium reabsorption

16 The stretch reflex

(a) consists of only one synapse within the central nervous system
(b) involves gamma motor fibres as the efferent link
(c) causes jerkiness of body movements
(d) involves glutamate as a neurotransmitter at the central synapse
(e) is highly facilitated in a decerebrate animal

17 Following major surgery a young fit 70-kg man will normally excrete, in 24 h

(a) 500 ml water
(b) 30 mmol Na^+
(c) 10 mmol K^+
(d) 20 mmol urea
(e) 10 mmol Cl^-

18 During periods of starvation in humans

(a) glycogen stores are depleted in 24 h
(b) amino acids are converted to glucose
(c) tissue breakdown initially provides 900 calories per day
(d) urinary nitrogen loss progressively increases
(e) a loss of 40% body cell mass is compatible with survival

19 In the fetal circulation the

(a) foramen ovale closes due to pressure change
(b) ductus venosus carries mixed venous blood
(c) blood can reach the aorta from the superior vena cava without passing through the left atrium or the left ventricle
(d) saturation of fetal haemoglobin (Hb F) in the descending aorta is more than in the aortic arch
(e) oxygen saturation in the umbilical vein is 45%

20 Delta waves on the EEG are associated with

(a) hypoxia
(b) hypercarbia
(c) sleep
(d) closing eyes
(e) deep general anaesthesia

21 Erythropoietin

(a) is a circulating hormone without which hypoxia has little or no effect on red cell production
(b) is formed in the kidney and in the liver
(c) production is stimulated by epinephrine and norepinephrine
(d) production is increased within minutes of the development of hypoxia
(e) activity is decreased when the red cell volume is increased

22 The following receptors are present in the chemoreceptor trigger zone (CTZ)

(a) opioid
(b) dopaminergic D_1 receptors
(c) muscarinic M3 receptors
(d) adrenergic $\alpha 1$ and $\alpha 2$
(e) serotogenic $5HT_3$

23 With regard to the vomiting reflex the

(a) diaphragm relaxes
(b) glottis opens
(c) epiglottis closes
(d) oesophageal sphincter closes
(e) respiration stops

24 Aldosterone

(a) does not directly affect renal blood flow
(b) increases the acidity of urine
(c) reduces the sodium content of sweat
(d) potentiates the effects of vasopressin in hypovolaemia
(e) is excreted in response to angiotensin

25 The respiratory quotient (RQ)

(a) is the ratio of CO_2 to O_2 at any given time
(b) is the ratio in the steady-state of the volume of CO_2 produced to the volume of O_2 consumed per unit of time
(c) is 0.7 with a diet of carbohydrate
(d) is decreased during hyperventilation
(e) increases during severe exercise

26 Compensatory reactions activated by haemorrhage include

(a) decreased movement of interstitial fluid into the capillaries
(b) decreased plasma protein synthesis
(c) increased secretion of ADH
(d) decreased glomerular filtration rate
(e) decreased filtration fraction

27 In the renal tubule

(a) hydrogen ions are excreted in combination with ammonia
(b) hydrogen ions are excreted mostly as phosphate
(c) aldosterone increases sodium absorption in the distal convoluted tubule (DCT) and collecting duct
(d) ADH increases water permeability in the DCT
(e) almost 99% of the glomerular filtrate is reabsorbed

28 When compared to normal people athletes have

(a) a larger stroke volume at rest
(b) a lower heart rate at any given level of exercise
(c) a decreased maximal oxygen consumption ($\dot{V}O_{2\ max}$)
(d) a smaller increase in blood lactate production with exercise
(e) a higher muscle blood flow

29 Plasma proteins

(a) exert an osmotic pressure of approximately 5.3 kPa (40 mmHg)
(b) provide one-half of the buffering capacity of the blood
(c) include plasminogen
(d) are mostly in the anionic form
(e) are the main source of carbamino groups

30 The motility of the gastrointestinal tract is increased by

(a) vagotomy
(b) complete transection of the spinal cord at T3

(c) stellate ganglion block
(d) mechanical bowel obstruction
(e) neostigmine

Pharmacology

31 The following statements are true regarding drug receptors
(a) they are found only in cell membranes
(b) drug receptor activity is always G-protein-coupled
(c) the concentration of receptors in the cell membranes is dynamic
(d) GABA receptors are ligand-gated ion channels
(e) competitive antagonists bind reversibly to the receptors

32 The following drugs are extensively metabolised
(a) prilocaine
(b) digoxin
(c) chlorpromazine
(d) diazepam
(e) paracetamol

33 The following drugs are well absorbed from the stomach
(a) morphine
(b) diamorphine
(c) midazolam
(d) loperamide
(e) propranolol

34 The following factors enhance the diffusion of a drug across the blood-brain barrier
(a) high plasma protein binding
(b) high degree of ionisation at physiological pH
(c) high molecular weight
(d) high lipid solubility
(e) high plasma–brain concentration gradient

35 pH alters the structure of the following drugs
(a) diazepam
(b) midazolam
(c) lidocaine

(d) atracurium
(e) suxamethonium

36 The following drugs induce the enzyme cytochrome P450
(a) carbamazepine
(b) nitrazepam
(c) metronidazole
(d) ranitidine
(e) rifampicin

37 The following anaesthetic agents cause direct sympathetic stimulation
(a) enflurane
(b) sevoflurane
(c) desflurane
(d) halothane
(e) isoflurane

38 The following speed up the induction of anaesthesia with volatile anaesthetics
(a) use of CO_2
(b) increased cardiac output
(c) agents with a high blood/gas solubility coefficient
(d) increased alveolar ventilation
(e) hypotension

39 The following cause dystonic reactions
(a) ondansetron
(b) metoclopramide
(c) cyclizine
(d) prochlorperazine
(e) domperidone

40 Etomidate
(a) reduces intraocular pressure
(b) is solubilised in propylene glycol
(c) causes a higher incidence of venous sequelae than thiopentone

(d) reduces plasma cortisol concentrations by an action on the pituitary gland
(e) is excreted unchanged in the kidney

41 Prilocaine

(a) has a p*K*a of 5.0
(b) has a longer duration of action than lidocaine
(c) is metabolised by plasma cholinesterase
(d) has a higher p*K*a than bupivacaine
(e) is more protein bound than bupivacaine

42 Lidocaine (lignocaine)

(a) prolongs the duration of action of the cardiac action potential
(b) inhibits plasma cholinesterase
(c) causes sedation
(d) causes atrioventricular block
(e) has a high hepatic extraction ratio

43 Which of the following are true of the mechanisms of opioid action?

(a) there are currently five separate opioid receptors
(b) the mu (μ) receptor has been classified as the op1 receptor
(c) opioid receptors are found at peripheral sites
(d) buprenorphine is a partial agonist at the mu (μ) receptor
(e) nalbuphine is an effective mu (μ) receptor antagonist

44 Naloxone

(a) is a kappa receptor agonist
(b) has a high oral bioavailability
(c) has an elimination half-life of 1–2 h
(d) causes pulmonary oedema
(e) prevents conversion of angiotensin I to angiotensin II

45 The following are $5HT_3$ blockers

(a) octreotide
(b) methysergide
(c) cyproheptadine
(d) ketanserine
(e) ondansetron

Paper 1 Questions

46 Flumazenil

(a) is a competitive benzodiazepine antagonist
(b) is an inverse agonist at the benzodiazepine receptor
(c) has a relatively short half-life
(d) is useful in treating hepatic encephalopathy
(e) is indicated in status epilepticus

47 Midazolam when compared with diazepam

(a) is more lipid soluble
(b) produces longer-acting active metabolites
(c) causes less discomfort on injection
(d) has a significantly lower volume of distribution
(e) has a shorter elimination half-life

48 Neostigmine

(a) is a tertiary amine
(b) is metabolised in the liver
(c) may prolong the action of suxamethonium
(d) inhibits both cholinesterase and pseudocholinesterase
(e) if given during pregnancy can cause fetal muscle weakness

49 Potentiation of neuromuscular block by neomycin is

(a) more likely with a non-depolarising block than with a depolarising block
(b) intensified by enflurane
(c) lessened by the administration of calcium
(d) antagonised by the administration of neostigmine
(e) increased by simultaneously administering trimethoprim

50 Class 1a anti-arrhythmic drugs usually

(a) slow depolarisation
(b) increase the threshold potential
(c) increase the action potential
(d) are indicated for atrial arrhythmias
(e) have local anaesthetic activity

51 The following drugs increase the gastric emptying time
- (a) ranitidine
- (b) domperidone
- (c) morphine
- (d) neostigmine
- (e) glycopyrrolate

52 Angiotensin converting enzyme inhibitors (ACEI)
- (a) reduce arteriolar tone more than venous tone
- (b) cause renal impairment in patients with renal artery stenosis
- (c) cause troublesome cough
- (d) are used to treat pregnancy-induced hypertension
- (e) cause hypokalaemia

53 Injection of intramuscular or intravenous epinephrine causes
- (a) increased pulmonary artery systolic pressure
- (b) increased pulmonary blood flow
- (c) increased pulmonary artery wedge pressure
- (d) no change in pulmonary artery pressure
- (e) an increase in diastolic blood pressure

54 Adenosine
- (a) is used to reduce atrioventricular conduction in the treatment of supraventricular tachyarrhythmias
- (b) may cause bronchospasm
- (c) has a long elimination half-time
- (d) is a potent coronary vasodilator
- (e) is contraindicated in heart block

55 Intravenous mannitol
- (a) is a polyhydric alcohol
- (b) is used as a fuel substrate for most cells in the body
- (c) extravasations can cause tissue necrosis
- (d) causes haemolysis
- (e) can cause a delayed increase in cranial pressure

56 Doxapram
- (a) acts by stimulating peripheral chemoreceptors
- (b) is contraindicated in epilepsy
- (c) interacts with aminophylline

(d) reduces systolic arterial blood pressure
(e) is a competitive antagonist at the mu receptor

57 Omeprazole
(a) is a pro-drug
(b) acts by blocking histamine (H2) receptors
(c) is longer acting than cimetidine
(d) has a rapid onset of action
(e) is effective in Zollinger–Ellison syndrome

58 Drugs which have a context-sensitive half-time which increases with time include
(a) remifentanil
(b) alfentanil
(c) fentanyl
(d) propofol
(e) morphine

59 The following are side-effects of heparin
(a) thrombocytopenia
(b) urticaria
(c) intrauterine fetal haemorrhage
(d) osteoporosis
(e) alopecia

60 Glibenclamide
(a) may cause hypoglycaemia
(b) increases secretion of insulin
(c) increases the peripheral action of insulin
(d) causes lactic acidosis
(e) is excreted by the kidney

Physics, measurement and statistics

61 Laminar flow through a horizontal tube has the following characteristics
(a) flow rate is proportional to the viscosity
(b) flow rate is inversely proportional to the density

(c) flow rate is inversely related to the length of the tube
(d) flow rate is turbulent when the Reynolds number is larger than 4000
(e) velocity at the centre of the tube is greater than at the sides

62 The critical temperature of a gas

(a) is the temperature above which a gas cannot be liquefied
(b) is the temperature below which it requires a lower pressure to liquefy a gas
(c) varies with pressure
(d) is the temperature at which a gas exists simultaneously in the gaseous and liquid states at atmospheric pressure
(e) is the temperature at which oxygen is liquefied by a pressure of 50 bar

63 The following are properties of a capacitor

(a) a capacitor consists of two conductor plates separated by an insulator
(b) the size of a capacitor depends on the number of turns of wire around the coil
(c) the size of a capacitor depends on the surface area of the plates
(d) the unit of capacitance is the joule
(e) AC current flow ceases through a capacitor when fully charged

64 The ease with which a liquid will vaporise is related to

(a) the latent heat of vaporisation of the liquid
(b) the latent heat of crystallisation of the liquid
(c) the blood/gas solubility coefficient
(d) the density of the liquid
(e) the specific gravity of the liquid

65 The following statements apply to the classification of electrical medical devices

(a) class I is represented by the symbol □
(b) class III can be connected to the mains
(c) type CF must have a leakage current of $<25\ \mu A$
(d) type B can be class I, II or III
(e) class I requires a single fuse

66 The correct SI unit for

(a) time is the second
(b) mass is the gram
(c) force is the pascal
(d) energy is the watt
(e) length is the metre

67 Regarding surgical diathermy

(a) the degree of burning at the tip of an active electrode is dependent on the current density
(b) bipolar diathermy operates at a higher power output than unipolar diathermy
(c) if the plate is detached the current will not flow
(d) the current frequency is the same at the active electrode and at the patient's plate
(e) isolating capacitors are used because they have low impedance to a low-frequency current

68 Regarding statistical tests

(a) the middle observation in an ordered series is the median
(b) the mean is the most frequently occurring observation in a series
(c) the standard deviation gives an indication of the scatter of the observations
(d) 95% of all values lie within ±2 SD
(e) the standard deviation is a measure of the significance of observations

69 Pressure gauges

(a) reduce high pressures to low pressures
(b) regulate flow from a cylinder
(c) are calibrated in pascals
(d) form part of a device for measuring gas flow
(e) utilise the principle of the Burdon gauge

70 Principles involved in oxygen analysis intraoperatively include

(a) the volumetric method
(b) Graham's law

(c) oxygen extraction
(d) paramagnetism
(e) absorption of oxidative energy

71 Transoesophageal Doppler

(a) requires a probe of 50–60 cm length
(b) gives information about stoke volume
(c) readings are affected by temperature
(d) measures the blood velocity in the ascending aorta
(e) uses acceleration and peak velocity to indicate myocardial performance

72 Oxygen for medical use

(a) is prepared by the fractional distillation of air
(b) for pipelines contains 0.3% nitrogen
(c) forms an inflammable mixture with oil
(d) from concentrators provides an F_iO_2 of over 80%
(e) has similar magnetic properties to nitrous oxide

73 The pneumotachograph

(a) directly measures change across a resistance
(b) must have a resistance of sufficient diameter to ensure laminar gas flow
(c) is not suitable for accurate breath-by-breath monitoring
(d) possesses accuracy affected by temperature change
(e) possesses accuracy unaffected by alterations in gas composition

74 The following are true of nerve stimulators

(a) the applied electrical potential can be as high as 150 V
(b) the apparatus uses a square-wave electrical signal
(c) the pulse current should be 0.5–5.0 mA when skin electrodes are used
(d) when the resistance increases the current must decrease, at a constant voltage
(e) stimulation at a constant current is preferable to stimulation at constant voltage

Paper 1 Questions

75 Serum osmolarity is

(a) a measure of the number of particles in solution
(b) usually expressed in milliosmoles per litre
(c) commonly determined by the temperature at which a solution freezes
(d) proportional to the valency of the particles in solution
(e) dependent on the serum albumin concentration

76 The gas volume can be measured accurately using a

(a) Wright's respirometer
(b) vitalograph
(c) Benedict Roth spirometer
(d) dry gas meter
(e) pneumotachograph

77 The following are agent specific

(a) mass spectrometry
(b) ultraviolet analyser
(c) infrared analyser
(d) piezoelectric analysis
(e) refractometer

78 Transcutaneous electrical nerve stimulation

(a) uses a current up to 90 mA
(b) uses a frequency of 0–100 Hz
(c) pulse duration is 0.1–0.5 ms
(d) at low frequency acts by closing the gate
(e) at high frequency acts by releasing endorphin

79 The following are true of the transfer of heat

(a) an adiabatic change retains the heat of the reaction within the system
(b) boiling involves transferring heat without a change in temperature
(c) a body with a high heat capacity will transfer heat to one with a lower heat capacity at the same temperature
(d) radiation is proportional to the fourth power of the absolute temperature
(e) the response time of a thermometer increases with its heat capacity

80 Linear regression analysis

(a) applies a technique of minimising squared differences
(b) can be used to analyse variables that are not distributed normally
(c) gives a regression coefficient
(d) yields an intercept that defines the position of the line
(e) finds the line that best predicts *X* from *Y*

81 Surface tension

(a) is measured in newtons per metre
(b) in the wall of a sphere, is directly proportional to the diameter of the sphere
(c) is due to attraction between molecules in a liquid (molecular cohesion)
(d) leads to a water manometer under-reading
(e) leads to a mercury manometer over-reading

82 Plethysmography is used to measure

(a) total lung capacity
(b) functional residual capacity
(c) residual volume
(d) forearm blood flow
(e) coronary blood flow

83 A pressure of 1 bar is equal to

(a) 1 kg/cm
(b) 14.5 lb/in
(c) 7.5 torr
(d) 1006.2 cmH_2O
(e) 101.01 pascal

84 With regard to a substance

(a) 1 mol equals 0.012 g carbon-12
(b) 1 mol occupies 2.24 l at s.t.p.
(c) In 1 mol of any substance are 6.022×10^{23} molecules
(d) mole is the SI unit of volume
(e) one gram molecular weight of any gas occupies the same volume

85 With regard to medical piped gases

(a) the nitrous oxide pressure is 4 bar (4×10^5 Pa)
(b) after maintenance of O_2 pipes the O_2 analyser is used to test the integrity of the system
(c) the non-interchangeable screw thread (NIST) has one diameter in the shaft which is specific for each gas
(d) the Schrader probe has a non-return valve
(e) the pipeline oxygen supply pressure enters the machine at 420 kPa (60 psi) pressure

86 Regarding the physiological principles underlying haemofiltration

(a) the pore size of the membrane allows molecules up to 50,000 daltons to pass through
(b) an ultrafiltrate of up to 1000 ml per hour can be formed
(c) plasma water is removed by convective flow
(d) the buffer of choice is bicarbonate in very low concentrations
(e) transmembrane potential equals hydrostatic pressure – oncotic pressure

87 Student's *t*-test

(a) is used to analyse normally distributed data
(b) is used for comparing a single small sample
(c) should be used as a one-tailed test whenever possible
(d) deals with the problems associated with inference based on 'small' samples
(e) is typically used to compare the means of two populations

88 Regarding electrical safety

(a) an electrical current of 5 mA passing through the body will cause a tingle
(b) class II electrical equipment must be double insulated
(c) class III equipment can only work with a low voltage ($<$24 V)
(d) the leakage current from any equipment that can come in contact with the heart must be less than 50 mA
(e) anaesthetic proof (AP) may be used in the zone of risk 5–25 cm from an enclosed medical gas system

89 A strain gauge can be used to measure

(a) gas flow
(b) intensity of light
(c) arterial blood pressure
(d) forearm blood flow
(e) force of muscle contraction

90 Concerning trans-oesophageal echocardiography

(a) the Doppler probe employs high-frequency sound waves
(b) the Doppler effect is due to a change in frequency of the ultrasound waves
(c) ultrasound gives a precise measure of cardiac output
(d) the speed of medical ultrasound is 1540 m/s
(e) medical ultrasound passes better through air than blood

Table for answers for primary paper 1

	(a)	(b)	(c)	(d)	(e)
1					
2					
3					
4					
5					
6					
7					
8					
9					
10					
11					
12					
13					
14					
15					
16					
17					
18					
19					
20					
21					
22					
23					
24					
25					
26					
27					
28					
29					

	(a)	(b)	(c)	(d)	(e)
30					
31					
32					
33					
34					
35					
36					
37					
38					
39					
40					
41					
42					
43					
44					
45					
46					
47					
48					
49					
50					
51					
52					
53					
54					
55					
56					
57					
58					
59					
60					

	(a)	(b)	(c)	(d)	(e)
61					
62					
63					
64					
65					
66					
67					
68					
69					
70					
71					
72					
73					
74					
75					
76					
77					
78					
79					
80					
81					
82					
83					
84					
85					
86					
87					
88					
89					
90					

Paper 2 Questions

Physiology

1 Coronary blood flow

(a) occurs only during diastole
(b) is reduced during tachycardia
(c) is determined by the pressure difference between the aorta and the left ventricular end-diastolic pressure
(d) is reduced in hypovolaemia
(e) is reduced when the central venous pressure rises

2 Parathyroid hormone

(a) is a mucopolysaccharide
(b) inhibits osteolytic action
(c) activates vitamin D
(d) increases urinary excretion of phosphate
(e) is released in response to a low extracellular concentration of free calcium

3 Concerning the absolute refractory period of the cardiac muscle

(a) it is the period immediately following the discharge of a nerve impulse
(b) it is the period when no further action potential can be generated
(c) it is shorter for pacemaker tissue than for normal cardiac muscle
(d) it is twice the length of the S-T segment
(e) stronger than normal stimuli can cause excitation

4 The following vessels are important in physiological shunt

(a) bronchial veins
(b) thebesian veins

(c) coronary sinus
(d) ductus venosus
(e) azygos veins

5 Pulmonary surfactant

(a) production can be increased by a reduction in pulmonary blood flow
(b) synthesis is stimulated by thyroxine
(c) maturation is inhibited by glucocorticoids
(d) deficiency in babies born to diabetic mothers is due to fetal hyperinsulinism
(e) concentration per unit area is directly proportional to the surface tension

6 The calibre of the bronchi decreases

(a) in response to stimulation of their parasympathetic nerve supply
(b) during inspiration
(c) in response to stimulation of beta receptors in their smooth muscle
(d) during coughing
(e) in response to histamine

7 The oxygen content of arterial blood with the same PO_2 is raised by

(a) increased haematocrit
(b) temperature
(c) anaemia
(d) increased 2,3-DPG
(e) increased PCO_2

8 On ascending to an altitude of 3500 m the physiological changes include

(a) an increase in cerebral blood flow
(b) an initial increase in plasma pH
(c) a fall in arterial PO_2
(d) an increase in minute volume
(e) a rise in urine pH

9 P_{50} on the oxygen dissociation curve is increased by

(a) increased PH
(b) fetal haemoglobin (HbF)
(c) decreased 2,3-DPG
(d) carboxyhaemoglobin
(e) increased temperature

10 The following are associated with hyperventilation

(a) decrease in $PaCO_2$
(b) increase in PaO_2
(c) increase in ionised calcium
(d) decrease in CSF bicarbonate
(e) increase in plasma bicarbonate

11 Regarding glucose handling in the kidney

(a) re-uptake is passive
(b) it is filtered at the rate of approximately 100 mg per minute
(c) tubular maximum (TmG) is the same for all nephrons
(d) reabsorption is inversely proportional to lipid solubility
(e) tubular maximum in the nephrons is 375 mg/min

12 With regard to glomerular filtration rate (GFR)

(a) *para*-aminohippuric acid (PAH) is used to measure GFR
(b) the normal ratio of the GFR to renal plasma flow is about 0.3
(c) the hydrostatic pressure in the glomerular capillary remains at 45 mmHg throughput its entire length
(d) the oncotic pressure (π) in the glomerulus rises as blood flows through it
(e) creatinine clearance underestimates GFR

13 Liver function can be assessed by

(a) plasma electrophoresis
(b) acid phosphatase
(c) prothrombin levels
(d) urea levels
(e) alkaline phosphatase

14 The blood–brain barrier

(a) is composed mainly of endothelial cells
(b) is functionally affected by infections of the central nervous system
(c) restricts passive diffusion of glucose from blood to brain
(d) is less permeable in neonates than adults
(e) is freely permeable to hydrogen ions

15 Stimulation of the parasympathetic nervous system

(a) dilates the pupil
(b) increases heart rate
(c) causes vasoconstriction
(d) decreases the rate of gastric emptying
(e) causes contraction of the detrusor muscle in the bladder

16 During a nerve action potential

(a) intracellular sodium and potassium ion concentrations become equal
(b) sodium ions move into the cell
(c) the sodium pump is inhibited
(d) calcium slow channels are blocked
(e) repolarisation results from increased potassium permeability

17 Active transport system includes

(a) movements of sodium out of nerve cells
(b) thyroxine release
(c) H^+ ion secretion at gastric mucosa
(d) reabsorption of H_2O at proximal convoluted tubules
(e) H_2O reabsorption at collecting ducts

18 A reflex action

(a) can be monosynaptic or polysynaptic
(b) may involve simultaneous contraction of some skeletal muscles and relaxation of others
(c) may be carried out by skeletal, smooth or cardiac muscle or by glands
(d) is not influenced by higher centres in the brain
(e) results from stimulation of two synapses in series

19 The ventilatory response to inhaled CO_2

(a) can be abolished by complete section of the ninth and tenth cranial nerves
(b) becomes more effective during hypoxia
(c) is increased by 0.1 l/min for every 0.75 kPa increase in $PaCO_2$
(d) is more prominent in peripheral chemoreceptors
(e) is shifted to the right by sleep and morphine

20 The following enzymes are responsible for protein digestion

(a) gastrin
(b) amylase
(c) trypsin
(d) chemotrypsin
(e) carboxypeptidase

21 The following cause hyperkalaemia

(a) incompatible blood transfusion
(b) blood pH of 7.2
(c) ingestion of 200 mmol of potassium chloride per day by a healthy adult
(d) infusion of 100 mmol of potassium chloride per hour in a healthy adult
(e) Conn's syndrome (primary hyperaldosteronism)

22 Movement of fluid from a capillary into tissue is increased by

(a) a rise in venous pressure
(b) a rise in plasma oncotic pressure
(c) closure of pre-capillary sphincters
(d) a fall in arterial pressure
(e) constriction of arterioles

23 The physiological effects of pregnancy include

(a) increased functional residual volume
(b) a shift of the oxygen dissociation curve to the left
(c) anaemia due to a fall in red cell mass
(d) an increase in plasma fibrinogen concentration
(e) reduced renal threshold for glucose

24 The development of high titres of anti-D antibodies in a Rhesus-negative mother with an Rh-positive fetus

(a) is due to fetal red blood cells entering the maternal circulation
(b) will result in anaemia of the newborn
(c) will result in jaundice of the newborn
(d) is due to antigen alone entering the maternal circulation
(e) always occurs before the third month of gestation

25 Regarding calcium

(a) it is mainly absorbed from the stomach
(b) it is absorbed from the small intestine
(c) calcitonin increases the uptake of calcium into bones
(d) parathyroid hormone increases plasma calcium by activating osteoblasts
(e) hydroxylated vitamin D increases absorption of calcium from the gut

26 The following are true when considering the control of temperature

(a) it involves afferent input from cutaneous cold receptors
(b) the spinal cord is a passive conductor of afferent thermal signals
(c) the central control is in the hippocampus
(d) vasoconstriction occurs at a core temperature of $>37°C$
(e) shivering is activated at a specific temperature

27 Activation of receptors for ANP increases target cell

(a) GTP
(b) IP_3
(c) cAMP
(d) protein kinase A activity
(e) guanylate cyclase activity

28 If the body temperature falls during a long operation

(a) oxygen and carbon dioxide are more soluble in blood
(b) blood viscosity is decreased
(c) there is a shift of the oxygen dissociation curve to the left
(d) the effect of non-depolarising drugs is reduced
(e) alkalosis is a common problem

29 Secretion of corticotrophin

(a) controls glucocorticoid production
(b) controls catecholamine production
(c) is increased by the secretion of a hypothalamic releasing factor
(d) is suppressed by a high level of circulating glucocorticoids
(e) has a circadian variation

30 Gap junctions are responsible for

(a) cellular polarity
(b) connections between cells
(c) transmission of action potentials from one fibre to another in skeletal muscle
(d) rapid transmission of action potentials by Purkinje fibres
(e) transmission of action potentials from one fibre to another in smooth muscle and the gastrointestinal tract

Pharmacology

31 Binding of drugs to plasma proteins

(a) increases their pharmacological activity
(b) depends on pH
(c) allows rapid renal elimination of the drug
(d) can be saturated at high drug concentrations
(e) enhances metabolism of the drug by the liver

32 The following drugs have an oral bioavailability greater than 50%

(a) atenolol
(b) methadone
(c) verapamil
(d) gentamicin
(e) propranolol

33 The blood/gas partition coefficient

(a) is a ratio of solubilities
(b) is a dimensionless measure
(c) is proportional to the time to onset of anaesthesia

(d) determines the MAC
(e) is greater for sevoflurane than for isoflurane

34 The following drugs have membrane-stabilising activity
(a) propranolol
(b) atenolol
(c) esmolol
(d) disopyramide
(e) diltiazem

35 The following drugs are alpha antagonists
(a) phentolamine
(b) clonidine
(c) oxycodone
(d) chlorpromazine
(e) droperidol

36 The following drugs cause dilatation of the pupil when instilled into the conjunctival sac of a normal person
(a) ephedrine
(b) cocaine
(c) timolol
(d) amethocaine
(e) guanethidine

37 The potency of the inhalation anaesthetic agent
(a) is inversely related to MAC
(b) is related to the oil/gas partition coefficient
(c) decreases with increasing molecular weight
(d) sevoflurane is less potent than enflurane
(e) isoflurane is the least potent inhalational anaesthetic agent

38 Sevoflurane
(a) is a fluorinated ether
(b) has a higher blood/gas partition coefficient than isoflurane
(c) causes hepatotoxicity
(d) is non-pungent
(e) is less vulnerable to metabolism than desflurane

39 Ketamine

(a) is presented as a racemic mixture
(b) is a glutamate receptor antagonist
(c) directly causes sympathomimetic effects
(d) is readily metabolised by hydroxylation to form nor-ketamine
(e) increases uterine contractility

40 Methohexitone

(a) is 6 times more potent than thiopentone
(b) causes excitatory movements
(c) in aqueous solution has 6 parts 100 of sodium bicarbonate by weight
(d) has a shorter elimination half-life than thiopentone
(e) is most commonly used for electro-convulsive therapy.

41 The following local anaesthetic agents have a liver biotransformation

(a) lidocaine
(b) procaine
(c) bupivacaine
(d) amethocaine
(e) ropivacaine

42 Cocaine

(a) causes bronchoconstriction
(b) causes vomiting
(c) rarely causes allergic reactions
(d) is excreted largely unchanged in the urine
(e) competes with norepinephrine for reuptake pathways

43 Morphine is metabolised by the following mechanisms

(a) glucuronide formation
(b) *N*-dealkylation
(c) acetylation
(d) hydrolysis of an ester linkage
(e) oxidative deamination

44 Tramadol

(a) is a racemic mixture of two enantiomers
(b) enhances noradrenaline neuronal uptake

(c) has an anti-nociceptive action that is fully blocked by naloxone
(d) has a low incidence of nausea and vomiting
(e) has a greater affinity for mu (μ) receptors than morphine

45 The following drugs reduce the lower oesophageal sphincter tone

(a) atracurium
(b) atropine
(c) morphine
(d) nifedipine
(e) GTN

46 The following drugs are used in the prophylaxis of epilepsy

(a) phenytoin
(b) chlorpromazine
(c) sodium valproate
(d) benzhexol
(e) promethazine

47 Ondansetron

(a) antagonises both peripheral and central $5HT_3$ receptors
(b) undergoes significant hepatic metabolism by hydroxylation
(c) crosses the blood–brain barrier
(d) is associated with cardiac arrhythmias
(e) causes diarrhoea after prolonged usage

48 Edrophonium is employed in clinical practice as

(a) a central respiratory stimulant
(b) a remedy for myotonia congenita
(c) an agent for treating postoperative urinary retention
(d) a diagnostic aid in myasthenia gravis
(e) an antagonist for non-depolarising muscle relaxants

49 Suxamethonium does not cross the feto–placental membrane to a significant degree because

(a) of its elongated molecular configuration
(b) the placenta is rich in cholinesterase
(c) it is bound to plasma proteins

(d) it has low lipid solubility
(e) it is bound to the postsynaptic nicotine receptor

50 Clonidine

(a) is an alpha-2 adrenoreceptor agonist
(b) decreases salivary flow
(c) has an analgesic property
(d) is a dopamine antagonist
(e) increases the MAC of enflurane

51 Compared to sodium nitroprusside, glyceryl trinitate

(a) produces vasodilatation predominantly in the capacitance vessels
(b) has a rapid onset of action
(c) is more potent
(d) produces more cyanide ions
(e) is more effective in the treatment of closed angle glaucoma

52 Verapamil

(a) acts on slow calcium channels
(b) has a high oral bioavailability
(c) vasodilates peripheral vascular smooth muscles
(d) has an extensive hepatic metabolism
(e) has active metabolites

53 Hyoscine compared with atropine

(a) has a shorter duration of action
(b) is a more powerful antisialogogue
(c) has a more marked effect on the eye
(d) causes less confusion in the elderly
(e) is not such a good bronchodilator

54 The following drugs can cause prolongation of the QT interval

(a) sotalol
(b) quinidine
(c) verapamil
(d) flecainide
(e) disopyramide

55 Droperidol

(a) is a piperazone derivative
(b) has alpha adrenergic receptor activity
(c) produces its anti-emetic effect by acting on peripheral (D_2) dopaminergic receptors
(d) causes extrapyramidal side-effects
(e) is predominantly excreted in the urine unchanged

56 The following drugs selectively increase renal blood flow

(a) dopamine
(b) dobutamine
(c) dopexamine
(d) digoxin
(e) mannitol

57 Gastrointestinal pressures are increased by

(a) enflurane
(b) adrenaline
(c) morphine
(d) neostigmine
(e) suxamethonium

58 A solution of 20% human albumin

(a) is isotonic with plasma
(b) contains coagulation factors
(c) its use results in frequent allergic reactions
(d) is prepared by heat treatment at 60°C for 10 h
(e) is not recommended in cardiac failure

59 Low molecular weight heparin

(a) is a mucopolysaccharide
(b) acts as an anticoagulant by binding to factor VIII
(c) is a stronger inhibitor of factor Xa than unfractionated heparin
(d) is mainly eliminated by the kidney
(e) should not be co-administered with warfarin

60 Metronidazole

(a) is well absorbed from the gut
(b) produces a disulfiram-like reaction with alcohol

(c) is excreted mainly unchanged in the urine
(d) it is effective against protozoa
(e) can cause peripheral neuropathy following high doses

Physics, measurement and statistics

61 Applications of the Doppler shift in the measurement of blood flow involve changes in

(a) electrical conductivity of a moving stream of blood
(b) temperature of blood as it moves peripherally
(c) frequency response of the arterial wall
(d) frequency of reflected ultrasound waves
(e) harmonic waves of reflected arterial pulses

62 Viscosity

(a) of a liquid rises as its temperature rises
(b) decreases as the temperature of a gas increases
(c) is dependent on Van der Waal's forces
(d) is dependent on molecular cohesiveness
(e) is measured in pascal/second

63 In the oscilloscope

(a) a hot cathode is used to produce an electron beam, which passes through two deflecting devices
(b) the saw-tooth potential deflects the beam in the *X* direction
(c) for an ECG a 1-mV calibration signal gives 1 cm vertical displacement of the trace
(d) there is a digital record with the simple oscilloscope
(e) there is a phosphorus screen

64 Regarding oxygen failure warning alarms

(a) when activated the auditory alarm shall last 2 s
(b) the energy required to operate the alarm shall be derived solely from the oxygen supply pressure
(c) the alarm shall be activated when the oxygen supply pressure starts to fall
(d) when activated the flow of nitrous oxide shall be shut off
(e) is flow dependent

65 Gases or vapours whose infrared absorption bands overlap those used in the detection of carbon dioxide include

(a) oxygen
(b) water vapour
(c) helium
(d) halothane
(e) nitrous oxide

66 Concerning a vaporiser for use inside a circle system

(a) it must be temperature compensated
(b) it is best situated on the inspiratory limb
(c) its interval volume must be greater than the patient's tidal volume
(d) accurate calibration is not essential
(e) it is generally unsuitable for administration of halothane

67 The following are true of the ideal intravascular pressure measurement device

(a) the resonance frequency is less than 40 Hz
(b) the damping coefficient is 0.6
(c) the manometer tubing is compliant
(d) the manometer tubing is of small diameter
(e) the transducer should have a rigid diaphragm

68 Concerning the chi-squared test

(a) the samples must be drawn randomly from the population
(b) measured variables must be independent
(c) observed frequencies cannot be too small
(d) it includes a calculation for expected values
(e) data must be reported in raw frequencies

69 Regarding electroconvulsive therapy

(a) it uses a current up to 850 mA
(b) it uses a frequency of 10–50 Hz
(c) the pulse duration is about 2.0 s
(d) the potential is about 250 V
(e) the potential depends on the impedance

70 In a process changing exponentially

(a) the time constant is the time taken for 63% of the process to occur
(b) one time constant is the same as two half-lives of the process
(c) after two time constants 87% of the process has occurred
(d) after three time constants all the process has occurred
(e) the rate of change is constant

71 MRI scanners

(a) use two magnetic fields perpendicular to each other
(b) use helium as a coolant
(c) develop a field of 12–14 Tesla
(d) should not be used for patients with non-ferric rings
(e) should be connected to monitoring devices using plastic tubing or fibreoptic cables

72 Oxygen concentrators

(a) contain aluminium silicate
(b) produce at least 92% oxygen
(c) cannot be used in aircraft
(d) can be used to supply hospitals with oxygen
(e) provide a gas with a concentration of argon lower than in air

73 The electromagnetic flow meter

(a) is used to measure blood flow
(b) consists of C-shaped probes and one electrode
(c) uses a steady-state rather than an alternating magnetic field to improve the stability of the measured value
(d) measures an average velocity
(e) is calibrated according to the vessel on which the measurements are to be made

74 Regarding infrared analysis

(a) gases which have two or more different molecules absorb infrared radiation
(b) the Beer–Lambert law applies
(c) the chamber windows absorb infrared radiation

(d) the sample chamber is made small
(e) the response time is about 200 ms

75 Critical pressure
(a) is the pressure at which a gas liquefies at its critical temperature
(b) is the pressure of saturated vapour at critical temperature
(c) for nitrous oxide is about 73 bar
(d) for oxygen is about 50 atm
(e) is directly dependent on the temperature of the gas

76 Regarding humidity
(a) absolute humidity of fully saturated air at 37°C contains 44 mg/l water
(b) the inspired air is saturated by the time it reaches the trachea
(c) humidified gas reduces heat loss by sparing the latent heat of vaporisation
(d) humidity of alveolar gas reduces with altitude
(e) absolute humidity is dependent on the ambient temperature

77 The operation of a standard cylinder pressure gauge is based on the
(a) critical flow rate principle
(b) Bernoulli principle
(c) fixed orifice principle
(d) Hagen–Poiseuille law
(e) Bourdon tube principle

78 The following convert mechanical energy to electrical energy
(a) oscilloscope
(b) photoelectric cell
(c) transducer
(d) transistor
(e) amplifier

79 The saturated vapour pressure
(a) is equal to atmospheric pressure at its boiling point
(b) increases with increased temperature
(c) can be greater than its boiling point

(d) is directly proportional to atmospheric pressure
(e) varies as a function of temperature

80 Regarding biological electrical potentials
(a) the frequency range in the ECG is 0.5–100 Hz
(b) the beta waves of the EEG are in the range of 15–60 Hz
(c) the potentials detected in the EMG range from 100 μV to 100 mV
(d) the EMG gives sharper spikes in place of the complex ECG pattern
(e) the potentials detected in the EEG are about 1000 μV

81 When distribution is positively skewed
(a) the tail on the left is shorter than the tail on the right
(b) the distribution could have more than one mode
(c) most observations are less than the mean
(d) the standard deviation is less than the variance
(e) the median is greater than the mean

82 Refractometers are
(a) non-specific
(b) used for directly measuring the concentration of a variety of different gases
(c) used to identify component gases in a mixture
(d) used to check the performance of vaporisers
(e) unaffected by water vapour

83 Techniques for measuring cardiac output include
(a) measuring oxygen consumption
(b) radioactive xenon
(c) helium inhalation
(d) indocyanine green
(e) thermodilution

84 In a randomised control trial
(a) a power of 60% is normal in medical trials
(b) double blind means the doctor knows which drug the patient has taken
(c) a pilot study is used to determine the number of participants required

(d) a chi-squared test is applied to the distribution of the sexes
(e) small *p* values suggest that the null hypothesis is unlikely to be true

85 Gas chromatography
(a) utilises the principle of selectively retarding the passage of gases through a tube
(b) uses carbon dioxide as a carrier gas
(c) is unsuitable for measuring nitrous oxide concentration
(d) quantifies individual components of a mixture of gases
(e) non-selective detectors respond to all compounds except the carrier gas

86 Pre-mixed 50% nitrous oxide in oxygen (Entonox)
(a) is available in cylinders in a liquid form
(b) separates into its constituents at 0°C
(c) causes bone marrow depression with prolonged use
(d) is contraindicated when there is a closed pneumothorax
(e) is presented in cylinders at 2000 psi (140 bar)

87 Regarding an ideal gas
(a) Boyle's law states that the volume of a gas is inversely proportional to its pressure
(b) the volume of gas at absolute temperature is zero
(c) nitrous oxide is an ideal gas
(d) the volume of a given sample of gas kept at constant pressure varies directly with absolute temperature
(e) it is easy to reach absolute temperature

88 With regard to diathermy
(a) it uses an alternating current of 0.5–1.5 MHz
(b) an alternating sine wave pattern is used in cutting diathermy
(c) a pulsed sine wave pattern is used in coagulation diathermy
(d) about 150–500 W of energy can be delivered using unipolar diathermy
(e) 1 W gives 0.24 cal/s

89 Bispectral analysis
(a) is derived from the heart rate and blood pressure
(b) has a similar response to all anaesthetic agents

(c) predicts the response to surgical stimulation
(d) predicts the prognosis of brain damage after cardiopulmonary bypass
(e) is reduced in normal sleep

90 Regarding surface tension

(a) Laplace's law relates tension to the square root of the radius
(b) it implies that interconnecting bubbles stabilise to equal radii
(c) it equalises the tension in different-sized alveoli
(d) in the wall of a sphere it is directly proportional to the diameter of the sphere
(e) it is measured in newtons per metre

Table for answers for primary paper 2

	(a)	(b)	(c)	(d)	(e)
1					
2					
3					
4					
5					
6					
7					
8					
9					
10					
11					
12					
13					
14					
15					
16					
17					
18					
19					
20					
21					
22					
23					
24					
25					
26					
27					
28					
29					

	(a)	(b)	(c)	(d)	(e)
30					
31					
32					
33					
34					
35					
36					
37					
38					
39					
40					
41					
42					
43					
44					
45					
46					
47					
48					
49					
50					
51					
52					
53					
54					
55					
56					
57					
58					
59					
60					

Paper 2 Questions

	(a)	(b)	(c)	(d)	(e)
61					
62					
63					
64					
65					
66					
67					
68					
69					
70					
71					
72					
73					
74					
75					
76					
77					
78					
79					
80					
81					
82					
83					
84					
85					
86					
87					
88					
89					
90					

Paper 3 Questions

Physiology

1 With respect to blood flow

(a) in the brain autoregulation is mainly controlled by changes in oxygen concentration
(b) in the lung autoregulation is the main determinant of pulmonary vascular resistance
(c) in the kidney autoregulation is primarily to maintain a relatively constant glomerular filtration rate
(d) a constant flow is maintained to an organ over a range of systemic arterial pressures
(e) a rise in blood pressure induces a rise in vascular resistance

2 In a normal 20-kg child the

(a) ratio of weight to surface area is greater than in an adult
(b) resting tidal volume is 7 ml/kg
(c) lung compliance is greater than in an adult
(d) PaO_2 is higher than in an adult
(e) the blood volume is about 1.6 l

3 Venous blood returning from the following organ is likely to have an oxygen content less than mixed-venous oxygen content

(a) heart
(b) liver
(c) brain
(d) kidney
(e) spleen

4 The following nerves are involved in the afferent arc of the baroreceptor reflex

(a) glossopharyngeal
(b) vagus

(c) second cervical
(d) stellate ganglion
(e) long ciliary nerve

5 The features of chronic mountain sickness include
(a) polycythaemia
(b) a decreased ventilatory response to hypoxia
(c) an increased ventilatory response to carbon dioxide
(d) thromboembolism
(e) pulmonary arterial pressure of 40/20 mmHg

6 The carotid body chemoreceptors
(a) have a very high tissue blood flow
(b) are stimulated by a fall in arterial oxygen tension
(c) produce reflex peripheral vasodilatation
(d) are inhibited by a fall in arterial pH
(e) are responsible for increased ventilation in patients with carbon monoxide poisoning

7 The oxygen availability is increased by an increase in
(a) haemoglobin concentration
(b) P_{50}
(c) PO_2
(d) pH
(e) carbon monoxide

8 The alveolar–arterial oxygen tension difference is increased by
(a) nitrous oxide uptake
(b) hepatic failure
(c) a high inspired oxygen concentration
(d) an increase in ventilation/perfusion mismatch
(e) a reduction in functional residual capacity

9 Functional residual capacity
(a) represents about 75% of vital capacity
(b) can be measured by nitrogen washout
(c) is increased in the elderly
(d) is increased in the supine position
(e) is greater than the closing volume

10 The following information is required to calculate the pulmonary shunt fraction (Q_s/Q_t)

(a) F_IO_2
(b) cardiac output
(c) $PaCO_2$
(d) arterial O_2 content
(e) mixed-venous O_2 content

11 A urine specific gravity of 1030 is seen in

(a) diabetes mellitus
(b) diabetes insipidus
(c) physiological oliguria
(d) impaired tubular function
(e) a high-protein diet

12 At 2 atm ambient pressure (about 10 m under water), in a healthy adult, breathing air from a cylinder

(a) the arterial PCO_2 is about twice the normal value
(b) the arterial nitrogen tension is higher than normal
(c) the arterial oxygen tension is about twice the normal value
(d) the alveolar CO_2 concentration is about half the normal value
(e) the tidal volume of the lungs is about half the normal value

13 The sympathetic nervous system

(a) has all un-myelinated preganglionic fibres
(b) synapses are in the lateral horn
(c) transmits pain sensation
(d) has shorter preganglionic fibres than postganglionic fibres
(e) has adrenergic ganglia

14 In smooth muscles

(a) spontaneous pacemaker potentials are generated
(b) contraction is triggered by the binding of calcium to troponin C
(c) there is a variable length-to-tension relationship
(d) calcium influx from extracellular fluid initiates contraction
(e) innervation is either sympathetic or parasympathetic

15 Paraplegic patients with spinal cord transaction at T6 for more than 1 year manifest

(a) hypoventilation
(b) causalagia
(c) a labile blood pressure
(d) mass autonomic reflex
(e) hyperkalaemia after intravenous succinylcholine

16 The end-plate potential

(a) is initiated by the release of acetylcholine
(b) results from a selective increase in sodium permeability
(c) has no refractory period
(d) overshoots zero membrane potential
(e) is blocked by curare

17 The transfer of drugs across the placenta to the fetus is increased by

(a) an increased maternal/fetal concentration gradient
(b) an increased ionisation of the drug at the pH of maternal arterial blood
(c) an increased uterine blood flow
(d) a decreased fetal cardiac output
(e) a fetal metabolic acidosis

18 A painful stimulus to the feet causes

(a) a monosynaptic withdrawal reflex
(b) flexion of the contralateral leg
(c) impulses to be transmitted in the ipsilateral spinothalamic tract
(d) inhibition of ipsilateral extensor muscles
(e) reflex sympathetic stimulation

19 Lactic acid is

(a) formed during anaerobic ATP resynthesis
(b) increased in concentration in the blood during an energy deficit
(c) not formed in red cells
(d) converted to glucose by the Cori cycle
(e) oxidised without conversion back to glucose

20 Platelets

(a) are not involved in primary haemostasis
(b) are eliminated from the circulation by tissue macrophages
(c) are formed in the bone marrow from pro-erythroblasts
(d) have cytoplasm that contains contractile proteins
(e) contain abundant mitochondria

21 Serum osmolarity is

(a) a measure of the number of particles in solution
(b) usually expressed in milliosmols per litre
(c) commonly determined by the temperature at which a solution freezes
(d) proportional to the valency of the particles in solution
(e) dependent on the serum albumin concentration

22 Vasopressin secretion is increased by

(a) decreased pressure in the right ventricle
(b) increased pressure in the aorta
(c) decreased pressure in the right atrium
(d) increased pressure in the right ventricle
(e) increased pressure in the right atrium

23 With regard to the fetal circulation

(a) the ductus venosus drains directly into the inferior vena cava
(b) blood from the superior vena cava goes into the left atrium via the ductus arteriosus
(c) closure of the ductus arteriosus normally takes up to 1 month
(d) it contains blood with a higher P_{50} than in an adult
(e) oxygen saturation in the umbilical vein is 40%

24 Ionised calcium

(a) is measured in a sodium-heparin sample
(b) is affected by pH
(c) is measured in a 'clotted' specimen
(d) falls during a massive blood transfusion
(e) is not affected by changes in serum proteins

25 The cerebral blood flow

(a) is normally 45–50 ml 100 g^{-1} min^{-1}
(b) increases with hypoxaemia
(c) increases with hyperventilation
(d) is independent of temperature
(e) has the autoregulatory curve shifted to the left in chronic hypertension

26 The following contain a sodium concentration over 50 mmol/l

(a) ascitic fluid
(b) oedema fluid
(c) cerebrospinal fluid
(d) intracellular fluid
(e) 0.18% saline in 4% dextrose

27 Thermal sweating

(a) is controlled by a cholinergic sympathetic mechanism
(b) produces a secretion of unvarying composition
(c) can exceed one litre per hour during exercise
(d) is inhibited by adrenaline
(e) is most effective in a hot, humid environment

28 T4 production is

(a) increased by decreased T3 levels
(b) increased by increased iodide absorption from the gut
(c) increased by hypothermia
(d) increased by increased TSH levels
(e) decreased by hypoglycaemia

29 Persistent vomiting for 2 months causes

(a) vitamin B12 deficiency anaemia
(b) a blood urea of 12 mmol/l
(c) hypokalaemia
(d) hypochloraemia
(e) tetany

30 Complement is required for

(a) anaphylaxis
(b) clearance of both endotoxins and bacteraemia

(c) normal C-reactive protein release
(d) membrane attack complex
(e) normal activation of the coagulation cascade

Pharmacology

31 Drugs which block dopamine receptors are likely to

(a) reduce renal perfusion
(b) improve splanchnic blood flow
(c) prevent motion sickness
(d) improve the rigidity seen in Parkinsonism
(e) reduce coronary blood flow

32 With regard to the volatile anaesthetics

(a) solubility is reduced with lowering molecular weight
(b) potency increases with increasing molecular weight
(c) increasing fluorination of the carbon skeleton reduces the boiling point
(d) increasing fluorination of the carbon skeleton decreases SVP
(e) fluoride ions are lighter than chloride ions

33 Halothane hepatotoxicity

(a) exhibits substrate specificity
(b) involves an enzyme induction
(c) is enhanced by hyperthermia
(d) is associated with a rise in hepatic transaminases
(e) is related to the formation of trifluoroacetyl chloride (a reductive metabolite of halothane)

34 Elimination of the following drugs is significantly prolonged in renal failure

(a) digoxin
(b) atracurium
(c) suxamethonium
(d) propofol
(e) indomethacin

Paper 3 Questions

35 Ranitidine compared with cimetidine

(a) is more potent than cimetidine
(b) has fewer anti-androgenic effects
(c) undergoes a greater degree of first-pass metabolism
(d) inhibits cytochrome P450
(e) is used in combination with antibiotics to eradicate *H. pylori*

36 Increasing urinary pH aids the excretion of

(a) amphetamine
(b) phenobarbitone
(c) pethidine
(d) salicylates
(e) tricyclic antidepressants

37 Rapid recovery from a volatile agent is associated with

(a) a high oil to gas partition coefficient
(b) increased minute ventilation
(c) increased cardiac output
(d) a small FRC
(e) second gas effect

38 Isoflurane is

(a) a racemic mixture
(b) inflammable with nitrous oxide
(c) metabolised to trifluroethene
(d) flammable in oxygen
(e) partly metabolised in the liver

39 Propofol

(a) produces its effect by interacting with the GABA receptor complex
(b) has a clearance that exceeds hepatic blood flow
(c) is contraindicated in acute intermittent porphyria
(d) causes significant tachycardia
(e) causes bronchoconstriction

40 Etomidate

(a) has a therapeutic index of approximately 36
(b) has a low incidence of allergy

(c) has an ester linkage
(d) has unpleasant side-effects related to pain on injection in up to 50% of patients
(e) is metabolised by cholinesterase

41 Fetal blood concentrations of lidocaine following maternal administration would be higher than expected
(a) if administered during uterine contraction
(b) in the presence of umbilical cord compression
(c) in the presence of maternal acidosis
(d) in the presence of fetal acidosis
(e) in the presence of increased maternal metabolism

42 Ropivacaine
(a) is a pure *R* (*D*) enantiomer
(b) is less lipid soluble than bupivacaine
(c) has a similar p*K*a and protein binding to bupivacaine
(d) systemic toxicity is not enhanced in pregnancy
(e) blocks C fibres as well as bupivacaine but A fibres less

43 Diamorphine
(a) is a naturally occurring opioid
(b) is more lipid soluble than morphine
(c) has a higher affinity than morphine for opioid receptors
(d) is well absorbed after subcutaneous administration
(e) is converted to mono-acetyl morphine

44 The following inflammatory mediators are involved in the mechanism for the generation of pain
(a) potassium
(b) sodium
(c) prostaglandins
(d) noradrenaline
(e) substance P

45 Tricyclic antidepressants
(a) inhibit the reuptake of noradrenaline
(b) are useful to treat chronic neuropathic pain
(c) have cholinergic effects

(d) do not cause sedation
(e) have drug interactions with adrenaline

46 Anti-emetics include

(a) muscarinic receptor antagonists
(b) H_1 receptor antagonists
(c) $5HT_2$ receptor antagonists
(d) D_1 receptor antagonists
(e) D_2 receptor antagonists

47 Methyldopa

(a) is a phenyl alanine derivative
(b) is a potent alpha 1 agonist
(c) reduces the MAC of volatile anaesthetics
(d) approximately 20% is excreted unchanged in the urine
(e) a positive direct Coombe's test is seen in 50% of patients

48 Repeated doses of suxamethonium in children can cause

(a) hyperthermia
(b) bradycardia
(c) tachyphylaxis
(d) bronchodilatation
(e) phase II block

49 Medetomidine

(a) acts at the alpha 1 receptor
(b) increases MAC
(c) acts principally through peripheral receptors
(d) increases airway secretions
(e) predisposes the patient to preoperative hypertension

50 The following drugs cause bronchospasm in asthmatics

(a) morphine
(b) neostigmine
(c) alfentanil
(d) thiopentone
(e) atracrium

51 Directly acting sympathomimetics include
(a) ephedrine
(b) clonidine
(c) isoprenaline
(d) dopamine
(e) cocaine

52 The following drugs are suitable for the treatment of SVT
(a) adenosine
(b) verapamil
(c) bretylium
(d) lidocaine
(e) amiodarone

53 Pyridostigmine compared with neostigmine
(a) has one-quarter the potency of neostigmine
(b) has a slower onset of action
(c) has a longer duration of action
(d) is less arrhythmogenic
(e) causes bundle branch block

54 Amiodarone
(a) prolongs phase 4 depolarisation
(b) is used in ventricular arrhythmias
(c) causes corneal deposits
(d) has a terminal half-life of about 4 days
(e) potentiates the effects of warfarin

55 Acetazolamide
(a) induces diuresis by inhibiting carbonic anhydrase
(b) decreases potassium excretion
(c) makes the urine alkaline
(d) reduces intraocular pressure
(e) is excreted unchanged by the kidney

56 Left ventricle end-diastolic pressure is decreased following administration of
(a) halothane
(b) isoflurane
(c) thiopentone

(d) fentanyl
(e) ketamine

57 Metoclopramide
(a) is a dopaminergic (D_2) receptor antagonist at the CTZ
(b) blocks 5-HT_3 receptors
(c) crosses the blood–brain barrier
(d) stimulates gastric muscarinic receptors
(e) blocks peripheral dopaminergic (D_2) receptors

58 The following drugs should be given in reduced dosage in patients with renal impairment
(a) erythromycin
(b) metronidazole
(c) midazolam
(d) cephalosporins
(e) paracetamol

59 Sumatriptan
(a) is used as an anti-emetic
(b) is a 5HT receptor antagonist
(c) is used to treat migraine
(d) has been reported to cause cardiac arrhythmias
(e) does not cross the blood–brain barrier

60 The following penicillin compounds are penicillinase resistant
(a) cloxacillin
(b) flucloxacillin
(c) temocillin
(d) benzylpenicillin
(e) methicillin

Physics, measurement and statistics

61 Flow can be measured by
(a) electromagnetic flow meter
(b) Fick principle
(c) pulse oximetry

(d) pulse contour analogue
(e) ballistography

62 Static charges

(a) are generated when two insulators are separated
(b) are dissipated by ionising radiation
(c) are prevented by wetting the surfaces with water
(d) can cause inaccurate rotameter readings
(e) are decreased by conductive anaesthetic breathing systems

63 Measurement of peak expiratory flow rate

(a) reveals a normal diurnal variation of less than 10%
(b) is made approximately using a vitalograph
(c) with a Wright's peak flow meter uses the principle of a constant orifice with variable pressure drop
(d) can be achieved using a 'rapid' capnograph
(e) produces a reading which is normally between 450 and 600 litres per minute in the adult

64 The following are gases at room temperature

(a) nitrogen
(b) xenon
(c) Entonox
(d) air
(e) carbon dioxide

65 At sea level the boiling point of sevoflurane is 23.5°C. This means that at this temperature

(a) sevoflurane becomes flammable
(b) the partial pressure of sevoflurane above the liquid in a closed space is 33% of atmospheric pressure
(c) sevoflurane vapour cannot be liquefied whatever the pressure used at this temperature
(d) the vapour pressure of sevoflurane equals atmospheric pressure
(e) the latent heat of vaporisation of sevoflurane is zero

66 If a pressure gauge reads 50% this can give a guide to the amount of substance remaining in the cylinder of

(a) nitrous oxide
(b) carbon dioxide
(c) air
(d) oxygen
(e) helium

67 The air in an operating theatre

(a) has a dew point of 37°C
(b) is tested for pollution with anaesthetic gases by means of an infrared analyser
(c) is used in the calibration of an oxygen analyser
(d) has a higher PO_2 when the temperature is raised
(e) contains more oxygen per millilitre than does arterial blood from a normal adult breathing air

68 In a collection of statistical values, measures of scatter within the sample are given by

(a) $P = 0.05$
(b) the mean
(c) standard deviation
(d) centiles
(e) standard error of the mean

69 The likely causes of a severely damped radial blood pressure trace include

(a) malfunctioning of the continuous flushing system
(b) a bubble in the connecting tubing
(c) more than one stopcock included in the connecting tubing
(d) the use of a 20-gauge arterial cannula
(e) the length of the connecting tubing exceeding 120 cm

70 The TEC5 vaporiser

(a) is non-spill at an angle of 180°
(b) has a greater wick area than that in the TEC4
(c) delivers enflurane at a constant concentration over 15 min when the dial is set at 4%

(d) has the same capacity as a TEC 4
(e) has the thermostat in the vaporising chamber

71 Sources of error in pulse oximetry include

(a) HbF
(b) HbS
(c) jaundice
(d) acute severe hypoxia
(e) severe anaemia

72 Regarding saturated vapour pressure (SVP)

(a) a liquid boils when SVP equals atmospheric pressure
(b) SVP is only dependent on ambient temperature
(c) at high altitude water will boil at a lower temperature than at sea level
(d) SVP is proportional to atmospheric pressure
(e) SVP of a liquid is lowered if a gas is dissolved in it

73 Temperature compensation within a vaporiser

(a) relies on the high specific heat of the constituent metals
(b) often works by the incorporation of a bimetallic strip
(c) is managed by alteration of the splitting ratio
(d) can be avoided by adding liquid anaesthetic directly to the gas stream
(e) is unnecessary with volatile agents of high liquid density

74 The following gases absorb infrared light

(a) oxygen
(b) nitrogen
(c) carbon monoxide
(d) water vapour
(e) helium

75 A solution of pH 7.4

(a) contains a concentration of $10^{-7.4}$ moles of hydrogen ions per litre
(b) contains approximately 40×10^{-8} moles of hydrogen ions per litre
(c) is a chemically neutral solution

(d) will maintain the pH irrespective of changes in temperature
(e) contains one gram equivalent weight of hydrogen ions per 22.4 litres

76 Flow of fluid through a tube is more likely to be turbulent if
(a) heliox is breathed rather than air
(b) there is a sudden increase in the flow through the tube
(c) the viscosity of the fluid increases
(d) the density of the fluid increases
(e) the velocity of the fluid increases

77 Devices for indirect non-invasive automated mean arterial pressure measurement (DINAMAP)
(a) under-read at low pressures
(b) over-read at high pressures
(c) over-read if the cuff size is too narrow
(d) over-read if the cuff contains too much air
(e) read mean blood pressure at the onset of rapidly decreasing oscillation

78 The mass spectrometer
(a) is agent specific
(b) analyses mixtures of substances according to their molecular weights
(c) allows the differentiation of different volatile anaesthetic agents
(d) should not return the sample gas to the breathing circuit
(e) responds partially to water vapour

79 Carbon dioxide in a blood sample can be measured by
(a) capnography
(b) flame ionisation
(c) mass spectrometry
(d) Clark's electrode
(e) Severinghaus electrode

80 With regard to pressure
(a) the gauge pressure equals the measured pressure plus the atmospheric pressure
(b) mercury barometers have a vacuum

(c) mercury manometers are closed at the top to air to prevent dust contamination
(d) if the diameter of the plunger is reduced by half then the pressure generated is reduced by a factor of four
(e) the pressure of the oxygen cylinder is approximately 138 bar

81 The Principles involved in intraoperative oxygen analysis include

(a) the volumetric method
(b) Graham's law
(c) oxygen extraction
(d) paramagnetism
(e) absorption of oxidative energy

82 With regard to radiation

(a) an alpha particle is a combination of two protons and two electrons
(b) an alpha particle has a low energy but penetrates matter poorly
(c) beta particles are electrons or positrons with variable energy and velocity
(d) the SI unit of radioactivity is the becquerel
(e) the process of one element changing into another is known as an isotope

83 Radiofrequency current burns result from the earth electrode

(a) area being too small
(b) not being in full contact with the patient
(c) being insulated from the skin by clothing
(d) and the electrocautery unit being improperly earthed
(e) drying out

84 The amount of gas dissolved in a liquid

(a) is proportional to the pressure of gas above the liquid
(b) is proportional to the molecular weight of the gas
(c) equals its solubility coefficient
(d) increases as the temperature rises
(e) has the same partial pressure as the gas above the liquid at equilibrium

Paper 3 Questions

85 The risk of operating room staff receiving an electrical shock from contact with theatre equipment is reduced by

(a) conductive shoes
(b) conductive flooring
(c) bipolar diathermy
(d) electrically isolated monitoring equipment
(e) a relative humidity of more than 50%

86 Measures for reducing the risk of accidental diathermy burns include

(a) using small needle electrodes for monitoring
(b) placing the earth electrode as close to the operative site as possible
(c) running all leads to the patient together in a parallel bundle
(d) not earthing monitoring electrodes
(e) using bipolar diathermy forceps

87 The reaction of carbon dioxide with soda lime includes the

(a) release of heat
(b) binding of water
(c) formation of calcium carbonate
(d) formation of sodium carbonate
(e) liberation of phosgene

88 Paramagnetic oxygen analysers

(a) consist of nitrogen-filled dumbbells
(b) utilise the principle of null deflection
(c) are sensitive to expired nitrogen
(d) consume oxygen during analysis
(e) can measure gas dissolved in a liquid

89 The following can be compressed into a liquid at room temperature

(a) nitrous oxide
(b) carbon dioxide
(c) Entonox
(d) air
(e) xenon

90 Transducers used in physiological monitoring include

(a) pH meter
(b) ear oximeter
(c) ECG electrode
(d) strain gauge
(e) fuel cell

Table for answers for primary paper 3

	(a)	(b)	(c)	(d)	(e)
1					
2					
3					
4					
5					
6					
7					
8					
9					
10					
11					
12					
13					
14					
15					
16					
17					
18					
19					
20					
21					
22					
23					
24					
25					
26					
27					
28					
29					

	(a)	(b)	(c)	(d)	(e)
30					
31					
32					
33					
34					
35					
36					
37					
38					
39					
40					
41					
42					
43					
44					
45					
46					
47					
48					
49					
50					
51					
52					
53					
54					
55					
56					
57					
58					
59					
60					

Paper 3 Questions

	(a)	(b)	(c)	(d)	(e)
61					
62					
63					
64					
65					
66					
67					
68					
69					
70					
71					
72					
73					
74					
75					
76					
77					
78					
79					
80					
81					
82					
83					
84					
85					
86					
87					
88					
89					
90					

Paper 4 Questions

Physiology

1 The cardiovascular response to cooling to 31°C in a healthy 20-year-old is likely to include

(a) asystole
(b) bradycardia
(c) ventricular fibrillation
(d) prolongation of the PR interval
(e) prolongation of the QT interval

2 The pulse pressure increases with an increase in

(a) PaO_2
(b) LVEDV
(c) stroke volume
(d) blood viscosity
(e) systematic vascular resistance

3 The arterial pulse pressure wave

(a) is normally transmitted as far as the venules
(b) travels faster than the flow of blood
(c) amplitude increases with exercise
(d) has a larger amplitude in the peripheral arteries
(e) central amplitude increases with advancing age

4 An increase in inotropy

(a) increases heart rate
(b) increases dp/dt
(c) increases end-diastolic volume
(d) decreases contraction time
(e) increases ejection fraction

5 The oxygen dissociation curve is shifted to the right

(a) if fetal haemoglobin is replaced by adult haemoglobin
(b) by a raise in temperature
(c) by an increase in 2,3-DPG in the erythrocytes
(d) by a fall in pH
(e) by the passage of blood through the lungs

6 A $PaCO_2$ of 8 kPa

(a) causes vasodilatation
(b) increases cardiac output
(c) increases cerebral blood flow
(d) causes sympathetic stimulation
(e) causes alkalosis

7 When calculating the dead space using the Bohr equation

(a) there must be a steady state
(b) the assumption is of two fractions in each tidal volume
(c) the result is equivalent to a volume of each breath that takes no part in gas exchange
(d) arterial and end-tidal samples taken to estimate the CO_2 are equivalent
(e) the result is usually expressed at s.t.p.

8 An area in the lung with increased ventilation/perfusion ratio

(a) represents dead space
(b) represents shunt
(c) is responsible for a decrease in the PaO_2 with no change in $PaCO_2$
(d) may be compensated for by an increased FiO_2
(e) may be compensated for by an increased minute ventilation

9 Lung compliance

(a) depends on lung volume
(b) decreases with age
(c) the pressure/volume curve is approximately linear at normal tidal volume

(d) has the units of cmH_2O/l
(e) when measured dynamically is more during exhalation than inhalation

10 Physiological dead space
(a) is equal to the sum of the anatomical and the alveolar dead spaces
(b) is increased with use of PEEP
(c) increases with increased lung volumes
(d) can be calculated from $PaCO_2$ and PaO_2
(e) the ratio of V_d/V_t is approximately 0.3

11 Glomerular filtration rate is reduced by
(a) increased extracellular fluid volume
(b) increased secretion of antidiuretic hormone
(c) obstruction of the urethra
(d) hypovolaemia
(e) a high plasma concentration of angiotensin II

12 Antidiuretic hormone (ADH)
(a) acts on the peritubular capillary side of the collecting duct
(b) is synthesised in the paraventricular nucleus of the hypothalamus as a precursor molecule
(c) has a plasma half-life of about 2 min
(d) travels to the anterior pituitary via the hypothalamic–hypophyseal tract
(e) acts on vasopressin VIb receptors to release ACTH

13 In a healthy, alert adult, with the eyes closed, the dominant EEG rhythm observed over the occipital lobes is
(a) alpha (8–13 kHz)
(b) delta (0.5–4 Hz)
(c) beta (18–30 Hz)
(d) theta (4–7 Hz)
(e) fast irregular low voltage activity

14 Excitability of nerves
(a) is increased by a decrease in extracellular calcium ion concentration
(b) is dependent on the resting membrane potential

(c) is reduced by an influx of chloride ions
(d) is increased by reducing the extracellular sodium ion concentration
(e) is increased by increasing the extracellular potassium ion concentration

15 Fasting for longer than 24 h is associated with
(a) increased hepatic glycogenolysis
(b) increased hepatic gluconeogenesis
(c) increased protein catabolism
(d) increased muscle gluconeogenesis
(e) ketoacidosis

16 Cerebrospinal fluid (CSF)
(a) has the same PaO_2 as arterial blood
(b) has fewer proteins than venous blood
(c) has the same pH as arterial blood
(d) has the same sodium ion concentration as venous blood
(e) has the same chloride ion concentration as venous blood

17 The parasympathetic nervous system
(a) includes the third cranial nerve
(b) includes the seventh cranial nerve
(c) when stimulated causes slowing of the heart
(d) when stimulated causes relaxation of the sphincter of Oddi
(e) has nerve fibres in the second sacral nerve

18 Stimulation of postganglionic thoracolumbar autonomic nerve fibres produces
(a) bronchodilatation
(b) an increase in myocardial rhythmicity
(c) an increase in myocardial contractility
(d) cutaneous vasoconstriction
(e) secretion by sweat glands

19 Fetal haemoglobin
(a) has no alpha chains
(b) represents 8% of haemoglobin in the normal adult
(c) represents 90% of haemoglobin at birth

(d) has the same molecular weight as myoglobin
(e) the saturation of HbF in the descending aorta is more than in the aortic arch

20 Corticotrophin
(a) has a diurnal variation
(b) is under the control of hypothalamic releasing factor
(c) regulates glucocorticoid secretion
(d) regulates catecholamine release
(e) release is decreased with prolonged steroid therapy

21 Slow, high voltages on an electroencephalogram are associated with
(a) deep anaesthesia
(b) $PaCO_2$ of 6.5
(c) cerebral hypoxia
(d) hypertension
(e) hypothermia

22 The following respiratory changes occur during pregnancy
(a) functional residual capacity is reduced by about 45% at term
(b) dead space increases by 25% during pregnancy
(c) closing capacity remains unchanged
(d) residual volume decreases by 15%
(e) expiratory reserve volume increases by about 25%

23 Withdrawal reflex to pain involves
(a) ipsilateral inhibition of extensors
(b) contralateral flexion of the limb
(c) reflex sympathetic stimulation
(d) transmission via ipsilateral spinothalamic tract
(e) a monosynaptic reflex

24 During pregnancy
(a) total peripheral vascular resistance decreases
(b) haemoglobin concentration decreases
(c) plasma cholinesterase concentration increases
(d) blood glucose concentration increases
(e) functional residual capacity increases

Paper 4 Questions

25 The following factors decrease gastric emptying

(a) acidity in the duodenum
(b) high-protein meal
(c) alcohol ingestion
(d) vagal stimulation
(e) ingestion of ferrous gluconate

26 The passage of ions across a cell membrane

(a) takes place through permanently open channels
(b) requires the expenditure of energy
(c) can occur through ligand-gated channels
(d) can occur through voltage-gated channels
(e) involves thyroxine release

27 The following variables are employed in the Bohr equation

(a) mean expired CO_2 concentration
(b) tidal volume
(c) inspired PCO_2
(d) cardiac output
(e) P_cCO_2 (partial pressure of capillary CO_2)

28 The action potential of skeletal muscle

(a) spreads inwards to all parts of the muscle via the T tubules
(b) has a prolonged plateau phase
(c) causes the immediate uptake of Ca^{2+} into the lateral sacs of the sarcoplasmic reticulum
(d) is longer than the action potential of cardiac muscle
(e) returns to a resting value of about -85 mV in the interior of a resting muscle fibre

29 Interruption of the cervical sympathetic chain results in

(a) dilation of the pupil; on the affected side
(b) loss of taste sensation over the anterior two-thirds of the tongue
(c) partial ptosis on the same side
(d) dryness of the mouth
(e) absence of thermal sweating on the same side of the face

30 Muscarinic receptors are

(a) sensitive to acetylcholine and are found in smooth muscle and glands
(b) not found in the brain
(c) serpentine in nature
(d) blocked by atropine
(e) coupled to adenyl cyclase via G protein

Pharmacology

31 A drug that acts rapidly on the central nervous system and has a high plasma clearance will

(a) have a long terminal half-life
(b) be readily soluble in aqueous solution at pH 7.0
(c) produce a bolus effect
(d) have a large distribution volume
(e) be rapidly excreted unchanged by the kidney

32 Metabolic acidosis can result from the administration of

(a) paracetamol
(b) frusemide
(c) sodium nitroprusside
(d) ammonium chloride
(e) diazepam

33 Clearance of a drug

(a) is reduced when the drug is strongly protein bound
(b) is increased in liver failure
(c) represents the volume of blood from which the drug is completely eliminated in unit time
(d) is not dependent on renal function
(e) cannot exceed glomerular filtration rate

34 Alkalisation of urine can increase the excretion of the following drugs

(a) pethidine
(b) amphetamine
(c) salicylates

(d) amphetamine
(e) ecstasy

35 The speed of uptake of an anaesthetic agent from the lung
(a) is temperature dependent
(b) is proportional to the minimum alveolar concentration
(c) is proportional to the blood/gas solubility
(d) is proportional to the cardiac output
(e) is proportional to the minute ventilation

36 The following drugs relax uterine muscle
(a) terbutaline
(b) isoflurane
(c) prostaglandin F2α
(d) ranitidine
(e) alcohol

37 Isoflurane compared with enflurane
(a) has a higher oil/gas solubility coefficient
(b) has a higher blood/gas solubility coefficient
(c) is more respiratory depressant at equipotent doses
(d) produces more fluoride ions on metabolism
(e) has a lower boiling point

38 Sevoflurane
(a) has an analgesic effect at sub-anaesthetic concentrations
(b) has a boiling point of 56°C
(c) forms more compound A the higher the temperature within the carbon dioxide absorber
(d) 3%–5% is metabolised in the liver by cytochrome P450
(e) causes bradycardia

39 Regarding barbiturates
(a) the potency is increased by increasing the number of carbon atoms in the side chains at position 5
(b) substitution of a sulfur atom for an oxygen atom at position 2 increases the duration of action

(c) substitution of a methyl group at position 1 increases the incidence of excitatory phenomena
(d) the presence of a sulfur atom at position 6 enhances the lipid solubility
(e) the presence of a phenyl group at position 5 produces a compound with convulsive properties

40 Propofol
(a) causes significant myocardial depression
(b) is partly metabolised to phenol
(c) is used in status epilepticus
(d) is partly excreted unchanged in the urine
(e) has a clearance that exceeds hepatic blood flow

41 The dose of bupivacaine required for spinal anaesthesia is reduced in the pregnant patient at term because of decreased
(a) CSF volume
(b) spinal cord blood flow
(c) metabolism of bupivacaine
(d) CSF pressure
(e) turnover of CSF

42 Local anaesthetic drugs
(a) increase the threshold potential
(b) increase the resting membrane potential
(c) block potassium channels
(d) cause a marked depression of the rate of depolarisation
(e) inhibit propagation of the action potential

43 Alfentanil compared to fentanyl
(a) is more lipid soluble
(b) is more potent
(c) is more protein bound
(d) has a smaller volume of distribution
(e) has a more rapid elimination

44 The following are cyclo-oxygenase-2-selective inhibitors
(a) etodolac
(b) parecoxib

(c) rofecoxib
(d) etoricoxib
(e) meloxicam

45 Prochlorperazine

(a) acts mainly on thalamic nuclei
(b) is a potent ventilatory depressant
(c) is highly lipid soluble
(d) is metabolised in the liver
(e) is a trigger of the neuroleptic malignant syndrome

46 Dopexamine

(a) does not increase renal blood flow through direct vasodilatation
(b) exerts its predominant effect by stimulating beta-1 adrenoreceptors
(c) has significant alpha-adrenergic activity
(d) is a weak beta-2 adrenoreceptor agonist
(e) does not stimulate dopamine receptors

47 Remifentanil

(a) is a synthetic anilidopiperidine derivative
(b) does not cause histamine release
(c) acts at all opioid receptors
(d) is metabolised by tissue esterases
(e) undergoes extensive first pass metabolism in the lung

48 The following drugs are bactericidal

(a) penicillin
(b) chlorhexidine
(c) sulphonamides
(d) neomycin
(e) erythromycin

49 In agonist–antagonist interactions

(a) the steepness of the log dose–response curve indicates the duration of action
(b) competitive antagonism shifts the log dose–response curve to the right in a parallel manner

(c) competitive antagonism shifts the log dose–response curve to the left in a non-parallel manner
(d) non-competitive antagonism shifts the log dose–response curve to the left in a non-parallel manner
(e) non-competitive antagonism can be overcome by increasing the concentration of the agonist

50 Dopamine
(a) increases splanchnic oxygen requirement
(b) decreases intracellular calcium concentration
(c) has vasoconstrictor effects with increasing dose
(d) stimulates alpha and beta adrenergic receptors
(e) crosses the blood–brain barrier

51 Nifedipine
(a) causes tremor
(b) causes tachycardia
(c) reduces blood glucose concentrations
(d) dilates skeletal muscle arterioles
(e) has active metabolites

52 Clonidine
(a) inhibits the alpha-2 presynaptic receptors to stimulate release of noradrenaline
(b) acts on imidazole receptors
(c) decreases salivary secretion
(d) slows the pulse
(e) reduces adrenaline-induced dysrrhythmias due to halothane

53 Bumetanide
(a) inhibits the sodium, potassium chloride co-transport in the descending loop of Henle
(b) is secreted into the tubular lumen
(c) increases oxygen consumption in the nephrons
(d) can reduce ventricular preload
(e) causes metabolic acidosis

54 Hyoscine
(a) has a sedative effect
(b) causes extrapyramidal side-effects

(c) causes tachycardia
(d) causes mydriasis
(e) has an antiemetic action

55 Thiazide diuretics

(a) are chemically related to sulphonamides
(b) act on the proximal convoluted tubules
(c) increase lipid levels
(d) decrease urate levels
(e) enhance the effects of non-depolarising neuromuscular blockers

56 The renal clearance of a drug involves

(a) filtration at the glomerulus
(b) active secretion at the proximal tubules
(c) passive diffusion at the distal tubules
(d) breakdown of protein binding
(e) enzyme inhibition

57 The rate of transfer of a molecule across the placenta is

(a) proportional to the size of the molecule
(b) directly related to the lipid solubility of the molecule
(c) related to the blood flow to the placenta
(d) dependent on the duration of pregnancy
(e) dependent on the amount of the fetal haemoglobin

58 Treatment with lithium

(a) induces hyperkalaemia
(b) causes an exaggerated reaction to sedation drugs
(c) causes leucopenia
(d) is associated with hypothyroidism
(e) antagonises the action of suxamethonium

59 The anticoagulant effect of warfarin is

(a) reversed by protamine sulphate
(b) apparent within 2 h of the first dose
(c) increased by tolbutamide
(d) increased by prolonged barbiturate
(e) increased by prolonged NSAID administration

60 Concerning oral hypoglycaemic agents

(a) sulphonylureas increase insulin secretion
(b) tolbutamide has a longer half-life than chlorpropamide
(c) relatively contraindicated in diabetic nephropathy
(d) biguanides increase hepatic and renal gluconeogenesis
(e) biguanides cause hypoglycaemia

Physics, measurement and statistics

61 The working principles of capnography depend on

(a) infrared absorption
(b) acoustic photometry
(c) the Haldane principle
(d) katharometry
(e) Raman spectrometry

62 The standard deviation of a normally distributed population

(a) is the square root of the variance
(b) is small in a distribution curve with a tall peak
(c) defines the limits above and below the mean containing two-thirds of the population
(d) is greater than the standard error of the mean
(e) defines the range of the population

63 The fuel cell

(a) acts as an oxygen-dependent battery
(b) is unaffected by temperature
(c) current flow depends on the uptake of oxygen at the anode
(d) gives a high reading if oxygen pressure increases
(e) has a typical response time of 30 to 40 seconds

64 Concerning the Ayre's T piece or its Jackson Rees modification

(a) a fresh gas flow of 2–3 times greater than the spontaneous minute ventilation is required to ensure normocapnia
(b) it is more efficient for controlled ventilation than spontaneous ventilation

Paper 4 Questions

(c) in a normocapnic ventilated patient, doubling the length of the tubing from the T piece does not affect the PaO_2
(d) it is classified as a Mapleson F system if an open bag is attached to the expiratory limb
(e) the expiratory limb must have a 32 mm internal diameter to avoid excessive resistance

65 A *P* value of less than 0.05 indicates that

(a) the null hypothesis should be rejected
(b) that the difference between two sample means is statistically significant
(c) there is less than 1 chance in 100 that the differences between two sample means could have occurred by chance
(d) the results are not clinically significant
(e) the distribution of the measured variable is normal

66 The following are found on anaesthetic gas cylinders the

(a) weight of the empty cylinder
(b) chemical formula of the contents
(c) date of pressure testing
(d) test pressure
(e) name of the owner

67 Non-ionising radiation includes

(a) infrared radiation
(b) X-rays
(c) ultraviolet
(d) gamma rays
(e) visible light

68 The following work on a variable-orifice, constant-pressure principle

(a) mass spectrometry
(b) pneumotacograph
(c) Bourdon gauge
(d) rotameter
(e) Wright's respirometer

69 Regarding gauge pressure

(a) when the cylinder is empty the gauge records 0 bar
(b) the absolute pressure in the empty cylinder is about 1 bar
(c) a full oxygen cylinder has an absolute pressure of 137 bar
(d) absolute pressure equals atmospheric pressure minus gauge pressure
(e) arterial blood pressure readings are absolute pressures

70 In a Venturi-type oxygen therapy mask

(a) the delivered flow should exceed 20 litres per minute
(b) oxygen concentration remains the same if the oxygen flow rate is reduced
(c) plugging the holes in the side of the mask will increase the delivered oxygen concentration
(d) rebreathing does not occur
(e) increasing the diameter of the orifice increases the concentration of the oxygen delivered

71 Regarding vacuum-insulated evaporators (VIE)

(a) they create a pressure of 1055 kPa if no oxygen is used
(b) they display the amount of the oxygen present as a weight
(c) they convert one volume of liquid oxygen at 15°C and atmospheric pressure to over 800 times the volume of gas
(d) oxygen is stored below its critical temperature
(e) they utilise the latent heat of evaporation

72 Considering direct intra-arterial blood pressure measurement

(a) in an under-damped transducer system ($D < 0.7$) significant overshoot and subsequent oscillation occur
(b) in an optimally damped system ($D = 0.7$) overshoot is limited to 6%–7% of the initial pressure change and no oscillation will occur
(c) in a critically damped system ($D = 1.0$) the change in pressure is measured accurately with no overshoot
(d) in an overdamped system ($D > 1.0$) the response is progressively slower
(e) flushing the system can assess optimal damping

73 The Bourdon gauge

(a) is based on a bellows or a capsule which expands or contracts according to the pressure across it
(b) has the advantage over a manometer in that it has no liquid to spill
(c) is calibrated for each gas used on the anaesthetic machine
(d) is colour coded
(e) scale should extend to a pressure at least 50% greater than the filling pressure of the cylinder

74 The concentration of volatile anaesthetic agent can be measured using

(a) a refractometer
(b) ultraviolet radiation
(c) absorption of infrared radiation
(d) the changes in elasticity of silicone rubber
(e) a paramagnetic analyser

75 With regard to temperature measurement

(a) the mercury thermometer has a high coefficient of expansion
(b) the alcohol thermometer is suitable for high temperatures as mercury boils at 78°C
(c) the fixed point on the Kelvin scale is the freezing point of water at one atmosphere pressure
(d) mercury thermometers are too inaccurate for use in intensive care
(e) a Bourdon gauge can be used to measure temperature

76 The hazards of microshock can be reduced by the use of

(a) battery-powered appliances
(b) isolated power supply
(c) equipment with a maximum leakage current of $<100\,\mu A$
(d) 5% dextrose-filled intracardiac catheters
(e) COELCB

77 High-frequency jet ventilators

(a) are time cycled
(b) deliver positive end-expiratory pressure (PEEP) if the respiratory rate is greater than 100 per minute

(c) employ a Venturi injector and solenoid valves to deliver gases to the trachea
(d) provide a fixed fraction of inspired oxygen (FiO_2)
(e) generate a range of frequency from 20 to 500 cycles per second

78 Confidence intervals

(a) are normally defined by the *P* value
(b) are wider if the sample size is small
(c) are wider if the variance of the population is small
(d) the 95% confidence intervals for a value are calculated as ±1.96 SEM from that value
(e) a 95% confidence interval has a 95% chance of containing a population mean

79 Core temperature may be reliably measured in the

(a) external auditory canal
(b) axilla
(c) lower third of the oesophagus
(d) nasopharynx
(e) rectum

80 The likelihood of the onset of the turbulent flow is predicted by

(a) the density of the fluid in kg/m^3
(b) the viscosity of the fluid in pascals
(c) the velocity of the flow
(d) the diameter of the tube
(e) the square root of the driving pressure

81 With regard to heat

(a) specific heat is the heat energy required to raise the temperature of 1 kg of a given object by 1°C
(b) heat capacity is the amount of heat energy required to change the structure of a substance without a change in temperature
(c) frost on a nitrous oxide cylinder can be explained by latent heat of vaporisation

(d) the specific heat capacity of a gas is less than that of liquids
(e) the units of heat capacity are joules/K

82 The Magill breathing system

(a) is an example of a semi-closed Mapleson A breathing system
(b) has a reservoir bag and APL valve at the patient end of the system
(c) is very efficient for spontaneous ventilation because alveolar gas is reused with the next breath
(d) is inefficient for IPPV
(e) can be used in paediatrics

83 The systolic blood pressure may be overestimated when

(a) using too narrow a cuff
(b) the patient's arm is very fat
(c) the cuff is deflated in less than 30 s
(d) measuring the pressure in a paralysed limb
(e) the arm muscles are held tight

84 A thermistor

(a) has a high heat capacity
(b) uses a platinum wire resistor
(c) resistance falls exponentially with temperature
(d) accuracy is improved by incorporation in a Wheatstone bridge
(e) can be used to measure flow

85 With regard to humidity

(a) in hair hygrometers the hair becomes shorter and wider with increased humidity
(b) Regnault's hygrometer contains mercury
(c) high humidity reduces the risk of electrocution
(d) relative humidity equals actual vapour pressure $\times$ SVP at that temperature
(e) if the temperature of a gas increases the relative humidity falls

86 Concerning damping

(a) it increases the natural frequency of the system
(b) the optimal damping is given a value of 0.7
(c) critical damping is given the value of 1
(d) there is minimal phase shift when $D = 1$
(e) it is proportional to the cube of the tubing diameter

87 In a normally distributed sample of 25 patients, with a mean Hb of 10 and standard deviation of 2

(a) the SEM is 0.4
(b) the maximum Hb value is 14
(c) the range is 6–14
(d) the lowest Hb value is 8
(e) the variance is 2

88 Transcutaneous electrical nerve stimulation

(a) uses a frequency of 0–100 Hz
(b) uses a voltage from 0–100 V
(c) excites C afferent nerve fibres
(d) is contraindicated in patients with a pacemaker
(e) is effective in thalamic pain

89 Pulse oximeters

(a) can cause burns to the skin under the probe
(b) are inaccurate in the presence of HbF
(c) are inaccurate in the presence of methaemoglobin
(d) are inaccurate in patients with pigmented skin
(e) have a slower response time than transcutaneous oxygen electrodes

90 The following gases interfere with CO_2 measurement by capnography

(a) N_2O
(b) water vapour
(c) halothane
(d) oxygen
(e) nitrogen

Table for answers for primary paper 4

	(a)	(b)	(c)	(d)	(e)
1					
2					
3					
4					
5					
6					
7					
8					
9					
10					
11					
12					
13					
14					
15					
16					
17					
18					
19					
20					
21					
22					
23					
24					
25					
26					
27					
28					
29					

	(a)	(b)	(c)	(d)	(e)
30					
31					
32					
33					
34					
35					
36					
37					
38					
39					
40					
41					
42					
43					
44					
45					
46					
47					
48					
49					
50					
51					
52					
53					
54					
55					
56					
57					
58					
59					
60					

	(a)	(b)	(c)	(d)	(e)
61					
62					
63					
64					
65					
66					
67					
68					
69					
70					
71					
72					
73					
74					
75					
76					
77					
78					
79					
80					
81					
82					
83					
84					
85					
86					
87					
88					
89					
90					

Paper 5 Questions

Physiology

1 Myocardial contractility is increased by

(a) atropine
(b) isoprenaline
(c) a raised end-diastolic pressure
(d) an increased heart rate from 70 to 140 beats per minute
(e) a reduced arterial pH from 7.4 to 7.3

2 Changing from supine to the standing position is associated with

(a) an increased pulmonary blood volume
(b) an increased heart rate
(c) a decreased venous pressure in the lower limb
(d) increased baroreceptor neuronal firing
(e) an increased stoke volume

3 Pulmonary vascular resistance is increased by

(a) serotonin
(b) hypocarbia
(c) hypoxia
(d) decreased pH
(e) adrenaline

4 Sinus arrhythmia

(a) is very marked in the elderly
(b) is most marked during breath-holding
(c) is more marked during exercise
(d) is associated with variation of the PR interval
(e) is associated with variation of the RR interval

5 After placement of a pulmonary artery floatation catheter, the following can be measured directly or derived

(a) left ventricular stroke work index
(b) pulmonary venous admixture or shunt fraction ($Q_S/(Q_T)$
(c) left ventricular end-diastolic volume
(d) aortic valve pressure gradient
(e) oxygen consumption VO_2 (ml/min)

6 At the start of a forced expiration against a closed glottis there is

(a) an increased intra-thoracic pressure
(b) an increased systolic blood pressure
(c) an increased heart rate
(d) a raised right ventricular output
(e) a decrease in left ventricular output

7 The rate of gastric emptying is delayed by

(a) the presence of fat in the duodenum
(b) the acidity of the duodenum content
(c) the presence of hypertonic duodenal contents
(d) large gastric food volume
(e) anticholinergic drugs

8 Closing capacity

(a) is normally lower than FRC and higher than residual volume
(b) decreases in supine position
(c) decreases with age
(d) can be measured by body plethysmography
(e) equals FRC in infants

9 Surfactant

(a) is a mucopolysaccharide
(b) allows alveoli of different diameter to have the same surface tension
(c) production decreases with prolonged pulmonary artery occlusion
(d) increases compliance
(e) concentration per unit area is directly proportional to the surface tension

10 Prolonged respiratory alkalosis

(a) increases the ionised calcium in the blood
(b) increases bicarbonate concentration in the urine
(c) decreases the pH inside the red blood cells
(d) shifts the oxygen dissociation curve to the left
(e) causes hypokalaemia

11 Total body water

(a) is increased during pregnancy
(b) can be measured using deuterium oxide
(c) is half to two-thirds of the body weight in young adults
(d) is a smaller proportion of body weight in men than in women
(e) is a lower proportion of body weight in neonates than in young children

12 Regarding glucose handling by the kidney

(a) glucose is reabsorbed in the proximal tubule against a concentration gradient along with sodium
(b) insulin promotes the renal excretion of glucose
(c) the tubular maximum for glucose reabsorption is about 12 mmol/l
(d) glucose reabsorption occurs passively along its concentration gradient
(e) glucose reabsorption in the kidney is similar to glucose reabsorption in the intestine

13 A diver at 30 m breathing air

(a) would expend more work breathing at this depth than at sea level
(b) has a venous PO_2 of about 5.3 kPa
(c) would not get nitrogen narcosis
(d) would experience a pressure of about 3 times that at sea level
(e) would develop bubbles of nitrogen in the CNS at this depth

14 It is possible to induce the appearance of an abnormal EEG by

(a) forced hyperventilation to induce an alkalosis
(b) having the patient close their eyes

(c) turning the patient from the prone to the supine position
(d) altering the plasma vasopressin concentrations
(e) asking the patient to perform arithmetical calculations

15 Somatic nerves

(a) synapse in the ventral horn
(b) have a conduction velocity of more than 5 m/s
(c) exhibit saltatory conduction if they are unmyelinated
(d) have no ganglia
(e) have acetylcholine as a neurotransmitter

16 In normal individuals with a normal $PaCO_2$, cerebral blood flow

(a) autoregulates between cerebral perfusion pressures of 50 and 100 mmHg
(b) is reduced when breathing 100% oxygen
(c) increases with hypothermia
(d) is normally 45 ml/mg per min
(e) increases following administration of 0.5 g/kg mannitol

17 In the kidney

(a) over 99% of the filtered load of bicarbonate is recovered in the kidney
(b) urine has a maximum concentration of 1400 mosmol/l
(c) ammonium ion is secreted into the tubule instead of hydrogen ion on the Na/H^+ transporter
(d) urinary phosphate buffering mainly takes place in the distal convoluted tubules
(e) urine osmolality of 700 equals a specific gravity of 1040

18 Afferent muscle spindle activity is increased by

(a) active muscle contraction
(b) passive muscle shortening
(c) painful stimuli
(d) reticulo-spinal tract activity
(e) vestibulo-spinal tract activity

19 Prothrombin level is reduced in

(a) hepatic immaturity
(b) vitamin K deficiency
(c) obstructive jaundice
(d) hypothermia
(e) anaemia

20 Transferrin

(a) aids the uptake of iron from the gut
(b) carries the iron to the liver
(c) carries the iron to the stores
(d) carries the iron to the muscles
(e) is metabolised after it gives up the iron

21 The following are the causes of low urine output after major surgery

(a) the supine position
(b) hypotension
(c) catecholamine release
(d) ADH release
(e) hypoglycaemia

22 The following are parasympathetic ganglia

(a) ciliary
(b) sphenopalatine
(c) superior cervical
(d) otic
(e) stellate

23 Measurement of the ECF compartment involves

(a) radiolabelled albumin
(b) Evan's blue
(c) radiolabelled sulphate
(d) H_2O deuterium
(e) inulin

24 The physiology of the neonate is characterised by

(a) obligatory nose breathing
(b) increase in alveolar ventilation predominantly achieved by an increase in tidal volume

(c) a relatively fixed stroke volume
(d) low levels of vitamin-K-dependent clotting factors at birth
(e) a normal maintenance fluid requirement of 80 ml/kg per day in a neonate

25 Gastric secretions are increased by
(a) vagal stimulation
(b) gastric secretion
(c) secretin
(d) sympathetic stimulation
(e) acidic stomach contents

26 The Na^+/K^+ pump
(a) is confined to nerve and muscle tissues
(b) is associated with the removal of two Na^+ ions and entry of three K^+ ions into the cell
(c) requires Mg^{2+} for pump activity
(d) is the cause of high extracellular Na^+ compared with K^+
(e) keeps the osmotic balance within the cell

27 Maternal hyperventilation produces a decrease in
(a) maternal arterial pH
(b) fetal cerebral blood flow
(c) maternal cerebral blood flow
(d) maternal uterine artery flow
(e) fetal arterial PO_2

28 Parathyroid hormone secretion increases in response to
(a) a decrease in extracellular calcium concentration
(b) an increase in extracellular magnesium concentration
(c) an increase in vitamin D
(d) propranolol
(e) prednisolone

29 The following will increase the secretion of thyroxine (T_4)
(a) a decrease in circulating tri-iodothyronine (T_3)
(b) increased secretion of calcitonin
(c) somatostatin
(d) a cold environment
(e) an increase in iodide absorbed from the gastrointestinal tract

30 Aldosterone

(a) is released from the posterior pituitary
(b) is released from the adrenal cortex
(c) decreases renal sodium secretion
(d) increases potassium secretion
(e) is excreted in response to angiotensin

Pharmacology

31 Total clearance is

(a) the rate of drug elimination (mg/min) per unit of blood or plasma concentration
(b) inversely proportional to the volume of distribution
(c) directly proportional to the reciprocal of rate constant
(d) equal to the individual hepatic and renal clearance
(e) not dependent on renal function

32 Sodium nitroprusside

(a) decreases cerebral perfusion pressure
(b) decreases PO_2
(c) decreases pulmonary pressure
(d) decreases heart rate
(e) causes methaemoglobulinaemia

33 The following drugs act by enzyme inhibition

(a) allopurinol
(b) ibuprofen
(c) enalapril
(d) lansoprazole
(e) enoximone

34 The bronchial tone is increased by

(a) morphine
(b) ketamine
(c) PGE_2
(d) $PGF_{2\alpha}$
(e) indomethacin

35 Some of the effects of acetylcholine can be reversed by

(a) amitriptyline
(b) metoclopramide
(c) clonidine
(d) trimetaphan
(e) morphine

36 In uncomplicated isoflurane anaesthesia

(a) the stoke volume is decreased
(b) the intracranial pressure is decreased
(c) the skeletal blood flow is increased
(d) splanchnic blood flow is decreased
(e) skeletal muscle tone increases

37 The volume of distribution of a drug

(a) can be calculated from a graph which plots plasma concentration against time after giving an intravenous bolus dose
(b) is greater with more lipid-soluble drugs
(c) depends on p*K*a
(d) changes with age
(e) is altered by changes in protein binding

38 Inorganic fluoride is a normal metabolite of

(a) halothane
(b) desflurane
(c) enflurane
(d) isoflurane
(e) cyclopropane

39 Desflurane

(a) has a boiling point of 33.5°C
(b) has a MAC of 6.0% in oxygen
(c) at 37°C has a blood/gas partition coefficient of 1.4
(d) reacts with soda lime
(e) molecules contain six fluoride atoms

40 Factors that influence the activity of local anaesthetics

(a) molecular weight does not affect pharmacological activity
(b) the higher the lipid solubility the lower the penetration of the nerve membrane
(c) ionisation is affected by the p*K*a
(d) acidosis decreases the proportion of ionised drug
(e) protein binding affects the duration of action

41 A eutectic mixture of local anaesthetic (EMLA)

(a) can be formed by any local anaesthetic drug
(b) contains 5.0% lidocaine and 5.0% prilocaine when formulated as EMLA cream
(c) results in an alteration in the melting point of anaesthetic bases
(d) can be formed from the carbonated salts of local anaesthetics
(e) contains adrenaline

42 Pethidine

(a) is a naturally occurring opiate
(b) is insoluble in water
(c) has no active metabolites
(d) decreases ventilatory response to hypoxia
(e) shifts the ventilatory carbon dioxide response curve to the right

43 The following drugs can be reversed by naloxone

(a) buprenorphine
(b) codeine
(c) dextropropoxyphene
(d) morphine
(e) paracetamol

44 The following drugs are metabolised by esterases

(a) aspirin
(b) atracurium
(c) esmolol
(d) procaine
(e) edrophonium

45 Atracurium

(a) is a monoquaternary benzyl-isoquinolinium
(b) metabolism is slowed by hypothermia
(c) a decrease in pH will increase its shelf-life
(d) is inactivated by a high pH
(e) is compatible with 0.9% saline

46 The following drugs are known to cause cholestatic jaundice

(a) erythromycin
(b) sulphonylureas
(c) NSAIDs
(d) tricyclic antidepressants
(e) rifampicin

47 Salbutamol

(a) increases pulmonary vascular resistance
(b) inhibits uterine contraction
(c) decreases serum potassium levels
(d) causes hypoglycaemia
(e) decreases blood pressure

48 Potentiation of neuromuscular blockade by neomycin is

(a) antagonised by neostigmine
(b) antagonised by giving calcium
(c) commoner with non-depolarising agents than with depolarising agents
(d) enhanced by enflurane
(e) augmented if trimethoprim is also given

49 The following drugs exert their action by competing with neurotransmitter

(a) atropine
(b) propranolol
(c) morphine
(d) tramadol
(e) atracurium

50 Concerning isomerism

(a) structured isomers have identical molecular formulae but different chemical structures
(b) mivacurium contains a mixture of three optical isomers
(c) atracurium contains ten different stereoisomers
(d) hyoscine and ropivacaine are single enantiomers
(e) equal mixtures of two enantiomers have no optical activity

51 Adenylate cyclase

(a) is indirectly coupled to beta receptors
(b) is inhibited by aminophylline
(c) is a *trans* membrane-bound enzyme
(d) catalyses the conversation of ATP to cAMP
(e) crosses the membrane 7 times

52 Hepatic blood flow is decreased by

(a) propranolol
(b) vasopressin
(c) somatostatin
(d) halothane
(e) cimetidine

53 Aprotinin

(a) is a serine protease inhibitor
(b) inhibits platelet aggregation
(c) is a thrombotic agent
(d) causes release of histamine
(e) converts inactive plasminogen into active plasmin

54 Insulin

(a) acts by interacting with enzyme-linked receptors located on the cell surface
(b) promotes glycogen synthesis in the liver
(c) facilitates protein metabolism
(d) inhibits lipogenesis
(e) stimulates fatty acid release from adipose tissue

55 Non-steroidal anti-inflammatory drugs have the following side effects

(a) reduce platelet aggregation
(b) cause pancreatitis
(c) precipitate congestive heart failure
(d) cause constipation
(e) cause angioneurotic oedema

56 Heparin

(a) is a mucopolysaccharide
(b) inhibits the release of a lipoprotein lipase from tissues
(c) crosses the placenta
(d) binds to histidine residues in the mast cell
(e) causes thrombocytopenia

57 Omeprazole

(a) is a reversible inhibitor of the proton pump of the parietal cells
(b) is a pro-drug
(c) biochemical availability increases with repeated administration
(d) has a short-life
(e) inhibits hepatic oxidative drug metabolism

58 The following drugs are best given via a central line

(a) adenosine
(b) amiodarone
(c) digoxin
(d) phenytoin
(e) dopexamine

59 The intra-ocular pressure is increased by

(a) methohexitone
(b) suxamethonium
(c) ecothiopate
(d) atracurium
(e) acetazolomide

60 Benzylpenicillin

(a) acts by decreasing DNA synthesis
(b) acts by decreasing RNA synthesis

(c) acts by decreasing bacterial cell wall synthesis
(d) is effective in mycoplasma infection
(e) can cause hypersensitivity in some individuals

Physics, measurement and statistics

61 Concerning the Mapleson E breathing system (Ayres T piece)

(a) during spontaneous ventilation the fresh gas flow should be 2.5–3.0 times the patient's minute volume
(b) the volume of the corrugated tube must exceed the patient's tidal volume
(c) Jackson-Rees modified the system by adding a closed bag to the end of the corrugated tube
(d) it should be used in children of 20 kg or less
(e) during ventilation by hand there should be no positive expiratory pressure

62 The risk of fire in the operating room may be reduced by

(a) connecting trolleys through a high resistance to the floor
(b) avoiding battery-operated equipment whenever possible
(c) the use of an isolated transformer
(d) the use of footwear with a resistance of 10 000 Ω
(e) placing electrical sockets higher than 1.5 m above the floor

63 An earth fault detector indicates

(a) faulty drainage of static electrical charges from equipment to the conductive floor
(b) the presence of equipment with a broken earth connection
(c) an excessive load on the isolation transformer
(d) an excessive electrical leakage from mains to earth
(e) too low a conductance in the theatre floor

64 A thermistor

(a) demonstrates the Seebeck effect
(b) shows a linear relationship between resistance and temperature
(c) has a resistance that changes with time

(d) exhibits hysteresis
(e) may have a positive or negative temperature coefficient

65 During controlled ventilation the following may cause hypercarbia

(a) Bain circuit tubing longer than 3 m
(b) decreased apparatus dead space
(c) low fresh gas flow in a circle system
(d) lack of a unidirectional valve in a circle system
(e) increasing the expiratory time on a Penlon Nuffield 200 ventilator

66 The following are correct pin index configurations

(a) oxygen 2 and 6
(b) nitrous oxide 3 and 5
(c) Entonox 3 and 6
(d) carbon dioxide 1 and 6
(e) helium 2 and 5

67 Blood filters

(a) have a pore size of 100 μm
(b) may be screen or depth types
(c) remove micro aggregates
(d) become less efficient with each unit passed
(e) may damage red cells

68 Light emitting from a laser source

(a) consists of two parallel wavelengths when the source is carbon dioxide
(b) is in the region of the visible spectrum when the source is carbon dioxide
(c) has a wavelength of about 500 nm when the source is argon
(d) may be transmitted around corners using fibreoptics
(e) may penetrate mucous membranes up to a depth of 1 cm when the source is carbon dioxide

69 In cardioversion

(a) it is the voltage that is important
(b) only 10%–30% of the energy applied to the chest wall will pass through the myocardium

(c) direct current capacitor discharge is the preferred technique
(d) if alternating current is used it must be synchronised with the R wave
(e) the maximum energy applied should not exceed 100 J

70 Concerning ultrasound

(a) it has a frequency of 30 kHz
(b) low frequencies are audible to the human ear
(c) it is the Doppler shift of signals that allows visualisation of structures
(d) it is efficiently transmitted through air
(e) it has shorter wavelengths than sound

71 When recording an electrical signal

(a) isolating equipment from an earth eliminates mains interference
(b) electrical filters reduce the signal-to-noise ratio
(c) the frequency response of a suitable recorder should be linear to about the 10th harmonic of the fundamental
(d) matching of equipment impedances is important
(e) zero stability may depend on temperature

72 In a step-down transformer

(a) the voltage across the secondary coil is greater than the voltage across the primary coil
(b) there are fewer turns on the secondary coil than the primary
(c) the output power is greater than the input power
(d) the current in the secondary coil is greater than the current in the primary coil
(e) there is an earthed circuit

73 Concerning biological potentials

(a) the normal signal amplitude of the electrocardiogram is of the order of 1 mV
(b) the frequency components of the ECG signal are between 0.5 and 80 Hz
(c) the normal signal amplitude of the EEG is of the order of microvolts

(d) electrical activity from muscle does not interfere with the electrocardiogram
(e) the electroencephalogram does not interfere with the ECG

74 The following apply to gauge sizes
(a) a catheter of 28 FG will have a circumference of 28 mm
(b) a needle of 21 SWG is smaller than one of 23 SWG
(c) a short cannula of 14 SWG external diameter will allow a maximum flow of 1 l in about 5 min
(d) an endotracheal tube size 7 mm will have an external diameter of 8 mm
(e) the standard BS tapers are 15, 22 and 32 mm

75 The following reduce intra-operative heat loss
(a) a condenser–humidifier in the breathing circuit
(b) low-flow anaesthesia
(c) laminar flow in an orthopaedic theatre
(d) use of a bowel bag during laparotomy
(e) use of a volatile surgical preparation sterilising agent

76 With regards to computers
(a) random access memory (RAM) is known as volatile memory
(b) read only memory (ROM) retains its contents when the power supply is removed
(c) they use the binary system for processing data
(d) a digit in the binary system of counting can have only two values
(e) a digit in the decimal system can have ten values

77 Regarding cylinders
(a) they are made of molybdenum steel
(b) the colour of the plastic disc around the neck of the cylinder denotes the year of manufacture
(c) they are tested every 3 years
(d) they are designed to operate to a 60%–70% higher pressure than the usual filling pressure
(e) the large ball-nosed cylinders have different thread connections for flammable and non-flammable gases

78 Concerning magnetic resonance imaging (MRI)

(a) the MRI uses a field strength of 6 Tesla
(b) the magnetic field causes alignment of tissue atoms
(c) the radiofrequency pulses cause deflection of the atoms with absorption of energy
(d) monitors used in the MRI are manufactured from desensitised ferrous materials
(e) it uses a super conductor magnet cooled by liquid helium and nitrogen

79 Amplifiers

(a) are transducers
(b) need protection during defibrillation
(c) amplify the signal and the random noise to the same degree
(d) are not affected by interference
(e) measure the difference between the currents from two sources

80 With regard to fluid dynamics

(a) the flow is double the mean flow in the centre and half the mean flow at the edge of the tube
(b) the flow drops by a unit of 16 if the diameter is reduced by half
(c) the flow drops by a unit of 4 if the length is reduced by half
(d) the resistance is inversely proportional to flow
(e) the flow is proportional to pressure in turbulent flow

81 Regarding the confidence interval

(a) 95% of the confidence interval has a 95% chance of containing the population mean
(b) the population mean has a 95% chance of lying within the 95% confidence interval
(c) if the *P* is less than 0.01 the result is significant at the 1% level
(d) it is standard practice to use the 99% confidence interval
(e) the confidence interval will be large if the size sample is small

82 When analysing categorical variables the following statistical methods may be used

(a) paired *t* test
(b) chi-squared test
(c) simple linear regression
(d) Spearman's rank test
(e) Kendall's rank correlation coefficient

83 Errors in measuring cardiac output by thermal dilution may occur

(a) if the injection is erratic
(b) if the injectate is at room temperature
(c) if the injection is repeated at different phases of the ventilation cycle
(d) in the presence of tricuspid incompetence
(e) in the presence of atrial fibrillation

84 Regarding heat

(a) the specific heat capacity is the heat energy required to raise the temperature of a unit mass of a substance by 1 K
(b) the latent heat capacity of a substance is the amount of heat energy required to change its structure without a change in temperature
(c) the copper heat sink in a vaporiser has a low specific heat capacity
(d) the specific heat capacity of gases is less than that of liquids
(e) the unit of specific heat capacity is joules/K

85 Accidental burns associated with the use of electrocautery result from

(a) too high a current density
(b) a faulty indifferent patient electrode
(c) faulty earthing of the operating table
(d) a leakage current induced by capacitative coupling
(e) simultaneous use of an ECG monitor

86 Humidity can be measured by

(a) the detection of the dew point
(b) gas chromatography
(c) mass spectrometry

(d) weighing
(e) changes in the length of biological tissues

87 In a time-cycled ventilator providing a constant pressure during the inspiratory phase

(a) a driving gas of 400 kPa (4 bar) is required
(b) the tidal volume is unaffected by leaks around the tracheal tube
(c) an exponential inspiratory flow waveform is produced
(d) the tidal volume is unaffected by changes in lung volume
(e) the peak inspiratory pressure is an indication of airway pressure

88 The application of the Doppler effect in clinical practice involves the measurement of a change in the

(a) frequency of reflected ultrasound waves
(b) electrical conductivity of a moving stream of blood
(c) frequency response of the arterial wall
(d) temperature of the blood as it moves to the periphery
(e) harmonic waves of reflected arterial pulses

89 In a Venturi-type oxygen therapy mask

(a) the delivered flow into the mask should exceed 20 l/min
(b) oxygen concentration remains the same if the oxygen flow rate is reduced
(c) plugging the holes in the side of the mask will increase the concentration of the delivered oxygen
(d) rebreathing does not occur
(e) increasing the diameter of the orifice of the Venturi increases the concentration of delivered oxygen

90 A paramagnetic analyser

(a) measures the concentration of a diamagnetic gas
(b) measures gas dissolved in a liquid
(c) utilises the principle of null deflection
(d) is used to measure the concentration of oxygen in a mixture of gases
(e) does not need calibration

Table for answers for primary paper 5

	(a)	(b)	(c)	(d)	(e)
1					
2					
3					
4					
5					
6					
7					
8					
9					
10					
11					
12					
13					
14					
15					
16					
17					
18					
19					
20					
21					
22					
23					
24					
25					
26					
27					
28					
29					

	(a)	(b)	(c)	(d)	(e)
30					
31					
32					
33					
34					
35					
36					
37					
38					
39					
40					
41					
42					
43					
44					
45					
46					
47					
48					
49					
50					
51					
52					
53					
54					
55					
56					
57					
58					
59					
60					

	(a)	(b)	(c)	(d)	(e)
61					
62					
63					
64					
65					
66					
67					
68					
69					
70					
71					
72					
73					
74					
75					
76					
77					
78					
79					
80					
81					
82					
83					
84					
85					
86					
87					
88					
89					
90					

Paper 6 Questions

Physiology

1 If a fit healthy adult is hyperventilated to twice his minute ventilation

(a) the $PaCO_2$ will be halved
(b) the PaO_2 will double
(c) cerebral vasoconstriction will be induced
(d) cardiac output will fall
(e) the mean arterial blood pressure will fall

2 Injury to the cervical sympathetic chain causes

(a) miosis
(b) enophthalmos
(c) nasal congestion
(d) conjunctival congestion
(e) anhidrosis

3 The following are synthesised in the hypothalamus

(a) prolactin
(b) growth hormone
(c) vasopressin
(d) thyroid-stimulating hormone
(e) corticotrophin-releasing hormone

4 With regard to calcium absorption

(a) it is passive
(b) it is increased by parathyroid hormone
(c) calcium is so effectively absorbed that there is hardly any calcium in the stool
(d) it is increased by calcitonin
(e) it is reduced by the fat-soluble vitamin D

5 Minute ventilation in a healthy adult male is reduced by

(a) bilateral transection of the vagus nerve
(b) unilateral damage to the phrenic nerve
(c) bilateral damage to the recurrent laryngeal nerve
(d) transection at C2
(e) unilateral damage to the vagus nerve

6 Regarding cerebrospinal fluid

(a) it is an ultrafiltrate of plasma
(b) it is actively secreted
(c) it is mostly stored in the lateral ventricle
(d) it is absorbed via the venous plexus of the spinal cord
(e) the specific gravity is reduced during pregnancy

7 The *D* (A–a) O_2 difference is increased by

(a) increased left atrial pressure
(b) increased plasma oncotic pressure
(c) abdominal distension
(d) air trapping
(e) a high inspired oxygen tension

8 In the Fetal circulation the

(a) blood can flow from the inferior vena cava to the aorta without passing through the left atrium or left ventricle
(b) ductus arteriosus carries blood with a higher oxygenation saturation than the ductus venosus
(c) blood in the descending aorta is better oxygenated than blood in the arch of aorta
(d) closure of the ductus arteriosus is due to increased pulmonary artery pressure at birth
(e) closure of the foramen ovale is due to a reversal of pressure

9 Glomerular filtration rate is reduced by

(a) hypovolaemia
(b) increased ADH production
(c) increased angiotensin II production
(d) obstruction of distal urethra
(e) renin

10 Cardiac output can be accurately assessed from

(a) the arterio-venous oxygen differences
(b) the oxygen extraction ratio
(c) the oxygen delivery
(d) tissue oxygenation
(e) indocyanine green dye injection

11 Basal metabolic rate

(a) is proportional to oxygen consumption
(b) is increased by dobutamine
(c) is the same obtained by measuring oxygen consumption as by measuring heat production by calorimetric methods
(d) of a 70-kg man is 100 W or $58 Wm^2$
(e) is twice as much, per kg, in the newborn compared to an adult

12 With regard to fat metabolism

(a) fat is mainly present in the diet as triglycerides
(b) fat is absorbed by the lymphatics
(c) fat has a respiratory quotient of 1.0
(d) fat needs acetyl CoA for its metabolism
(e) insulin increases fat synthesis from glucose in the liver

13 Functional residual capacity

(a) can be estimated by subtracting the inspiratory capacity from the total lung capacity
(b) can be measured by use of the Bohr equation
(c) is increased in obesity
(d) is increased with pregnancy
(e) is reduced with exercise

14 Increased afferent input discharge by the baroreceptors

(a) increases vagal stimulation
(b) causes peripheral vasoconstriction
(c) increases heart rate
(d) increases sympathetic stimulation
(e) increases renin secretion

15 Changing from the erect to the supine position

(a) increases systolic blood pressure
(b) decreases baroreceptor discharge

(c) increases venous leg pressure
(d) increases pulmonary blood volume
(e) is associated with no change in heart rate

16 During the expulsive phase of a cough the

(a) airway diameter decreases
(b) diaphragm contracts
(c) venous return decreases
(d) cerebral perfusion pressure increases
(e) intrapulmonary pressure exceeds 50 mmHg

17 The pulse pressure is increased by

(a) anaemia
(b) hypercarbia
(c) an increase in end-diastolic volume
(d) a decrease in vessel compliance
(e) measuring at the periphery of the vascular tree

18 Pain transmission can be interrupted by

(a) ablation of the median lemniscus
(b) ablation of the contralateral cortex
(c) transection of the dorsal root ganglia
(d) contralateral cordotomy
(e) injection of encephalin into the hippocampus

19 Insulin

(a) increases fat storage
(b) stimulates the release of glucagon
(c) decreases potassium ion movement out of the cells
(d) reduces protein synthesis
(e) increases gluconeogenesis

20 The carbon dioxide ventilatory response curve is shifted to the right during

(a) normal sleep
(b) hypoxia
(c) isoflurane anaesthesia
(d) pain
(e) pregnancy

21 The liver parenchymal cells are involved in

(a) the synthesis of clotting factors
(b) glycogen storage
(c) drug metabolism
(d) bile synthesis
(e) phagocytosis

22 Stimulation of gamma motor neurone fibres causes

(a) uterine contraction
(b) skeletal muscle hypertonia
(c) hyperactive tendon reflexes
(d) vasodilatation
(e) smooth muscle relaxation

23 Total body water (TBW)

(a) can be measured using deuterium
(b) minus plasma volume gives a measure of red cell volume
(c) is proportionally greater in infants than in neonates as a fraction of body weight
(d) is increased in pregnancy
(e) is proportionally greater in infants than adults as a fraction of body weight

24 The effects of intrapulmonary shunt may be distinguished from those of $\dot{V}/\dot{Q}$ mismatch by

(a) carbon monoxide transfer
(b) the helium steady-state test
(c) calculation of the arteriovenous PO_2 difference
(d) giving 100% inspired oxygen
(e) calculation of the A–a PCO_2 difference

25 Gastric emptying time is increased by

(a) acid in the duodenum
(b) fat in the oesophagus
(c) an increase in blood secretin concentration
(d) an increase in the size of a meal
(e) sympathetic stimulation

26 Concerning hepatic blood flow

(a) portal venous pressure is less than 20 mmHg
(b) 50% is from the hepatic artery
(c) total flow is 1.5 1/min
(d) the liver derives most of its oxygen needs from the portal supply
(e) the oxygen saturation of portal blood is 95%

27 Concerning compliance

(a) lung compliance is less than total compliance
(b) dynamic compliance is less in a paralysed patient
(c) in IPPV tidal volume depends only on compliance
(d) compliance is directly proportional to $\dot{V}/\dot{Q}$ ratio
(e) compliance in a 5-year-old is double that of a 20-year-old

28 Hypoxaemia stimulates respiration by an action on

(a) the carotid sinus
(b) central pH
(c) central respiratory neurones
(d) the carotid and aortic bodies
(e) central chemoreceptors in the hypothalamus

29 The velocity of nerve impulse propagation

(a) increases with pressure on the nerve
(b) increases with metabolic acidosis
(c) increases with myelination of the nerve
(d) increases proportionally with the diameter of the nerve
(e) is greater in motor than in sensory nerves

30 In the control of body temperature

(a) shivering is a spinal reflex
(b) energy from brown fat is released via beta-adrenergic receptors
(c) brain amines play an important role
(d) PGEI may cause pyrexia
(e) control is independent of higher centres

Pharmacology

31. With regard to half-life

(a) half-life depends only on clearance
(b) half-life is inversely related to the elimination constant
(c) at a steady-state the plasma concentration is affected by the rate of clearance
(d) the amount of drug distributed to the extracellular fluid is unlikely to affect the half-life
(e) the half-life of a drug is shorter than its time constant

32 The following drugs are highly alkaline in solution

(a) Ringer's lactate
(b) suxamethonium
(c) propofol
(d) thiopentone
(e) lidocaine

33 Heparin

(a) is derived from amino acids
(b) levels cannot normally be detected in plasma
(c) is metabolised in the reticuloendothelial system
(d) readily crosses the placenta
(e) affects platelet aggregation

34 Buprenorphine

(a) is less potent than morphine
(b) does not cause respiratory depression
(c) is a partial agonist
(d) effects are only partially reversed by naloxone
(e) duration of action is 4 h

35 Flumazenil

(a) has an effect on NMDA receptors
(b) has an inverse agonist activity
(c) has a half-life of 2 h
(d) has an active metabolite
(e) causes convulsions

36 Atracurium

(a) metabolism is reduced by hypothermia
(b) is metabolised by ester hydrolysis
(c) produces laudanosine as a metabolite
(d) when given in very high doses acts quicker than suxamethonium
(e) as the *cis* isomer has the molecules on the same side of the double bond to give less histamine release

37 The following drugs cause histamine release

(a) etomidate
(b) atracurium
(c) hyoscine
(d) morphine
(e) amitriptyline

38 The following drugs cause bradycardia

(a) atracurium
(b) nifedipine
(c) neostigmine
(d) verapamil
(e) desflurane

39 The following drugs can readily cross the placenta

(a) atropine
(b) suxamethonium
(c) warfarin
(d) aspirin
(e) pancuronium

40 The following drugs increase urinary potassium excretion

(a) spironolactone
(b) acetazolamide
(c) ethacrynic acid
(d) thiazides
(e) frusemide

41 The following drugs exert their effects by affecting the calcium concentration in excitable tissues

(a) isoflurane
(b) nifedipine
(c) atropine
(d) caffeine
(e) flecainide

42 Monoamine oxidase inhibitors

(a) are enzyme inhibitors
(b) should be ideally stopped 2 weeks before surgery
(c) and pethidine interact to cause a hypertensive crisis
(d) and morphine are safe
(e) increase body stores of noradrenaline

43 The following drugs cause methaemoglobinaemia

(a) paracetamol
(b) acetazolamide
(c) sodium nitroprusside
(d) prilocaine
(e) sulphonamide antibiotics

44 Phase I depolarizing block

(a) shows tetanic fade
(b) shows post-tetanic facilitation
(c) can be prolonged by pretreatment with small doses of non-depolarising drugs
(d) can be reversed by anticholinesterases
(e) is prolonged with hypermagnesaemia

45 Regarding antimicrobial therapy

(a) erythromycin causes more ototoxicity than gentamicin
(b) dose reduction is needed for cefotaxime in renal failure
(c) flucloxacillin is penicillinase resistant
(d) rifampicin potentiates the action of warfarin
(e) trimethoprim potentiates the action of sulphonamides

46 The following drugs induce the cytochrome P450 enzyme system

(a) carbamazepine
(b) phenytoin
(c) imipramine
(d) benzodiazepines
(e) propranolol

47 Methaemoglobinaemia

(a) can be caused by the higher oxides of nitrogen
(b) is clinically detectable at 10g/l
(c) is caused by prilocaine
(d) is caused by paracetamol
(e) can be treated by intravenous methylene blue

48 The flowing substances transfer freely across the placenta

(a) neostigmine
(b) thyroxine
(c) insulin
(d) warfarin
(e) glucose

49 In a patient suffering from digoxin toxicity

(a) the ECG characteristically shows widespread ST segment depression
(b) intravenous calcium gluconate may temporarily reverse the toxic effects on the myocardium
(c) propranolol is helpful in the treatment of digoxin-induced heart block
(d) intravenous potassium can be therapeutic
(e) intravenous lidocaine is indicated for ventricular arrhythmias

50 Clopidogrel

(a) acts by direct stimulation of adenosine diphosphate (ADP)
(b) action last up to 5 days, after stopping treatment, and before the bleeding time returns to normal
(c) causes diarrhoea

(d) crosses placenta–blood barrier
(e) is excreted in milk

51 Cocaine

(a) competes with noradrenaline binding sites
(b) may produce vomiting
(c) depresses respiration
(d) hypersensitivity is rare
(e) is largely excreted unchanged in urine

52 Enoximone

(a) is an imidazoline derivative
(b) is a non-selective phosphodiesterase inhibitor (PDE111)
(c) increases the calcium concentration by mechanisms other than increasing cAMP
(d) causes vasoconstriction of small arterioles
(e) is metabolised in the liver

53 Pupillary dilatation is caused by

(a) cocaine
(b) ganglion blockers
(c) alpha-1 agonists
(d) anticholinesterases
(e) codeine

54 Theophylline may cause

(a) an increase in cardiac output
(b) an increase in GFR
(c) an increase in alveolar dead space
(d) feelings of anxiety
(e) life-threatening ventricular arrhythmias

55 Alfentanil

(a) has a smaller volume of distribution than fentanyl
(b) has a higher lipid solubility than fentanyl
(c) is metabolised by the same hepatic enzyme as midazolam
(d) anticholinesterase drugs will prolong its duration of action
(e) is less protein bound than fentanyl

56 Concerning benzodiazepines

(a) they act on both $GABA_A$ and $GABA_B$ receptors
(b) they decrease serum chloride levels
(c) diazepam has a duration of action of more than 20 h
(d) there is a wide range in their potency
(e) they displace warfarin from protein-binding sites

57 The following may be administered via the oral mucosa/ mucous membranes

(a) heparin
(b) amethocaine
(c) nifedipine
(d) GTN
(e) lidocaine

58 Compared with bupivacaine, ropivacaine

(a) is a pure *S* (L) enantiomer
(b) has a similar p*K*a
(c) has a similar protein binding
(d) has an equivalent duration of sensory block
(e) has a faster clearance

59 Local anaesthetic agents exert their action on the following receptor channels

(a) K^+ channels
(b) ligand-gated channels
(c) ion channels
(d) Na^+ channels
(e) voltage-gated channels

60 Phosphodiesterase (PDE) inhibitors

(a) prevent breakdown of cAMP to 5′AMP
(b) reduce afterload
(c) cause vasodilatation
(d) increase myocardial contractility
(e) significantly increase survival in ischaemic heart disease

Physics, measurement and statistics

61 Gas chromatography works on

(a) a Venturi principle
(b) an electron capture technique
(c) an acoustic technique
(d) a thermal-dilution technique
(e) a selective retardation technique

62 Regarding electrical safety

(a) a current passing from the right to the left hand at 100 mA and 240 V is safe
(b) a current passing from the right to the left hand at 100 mA and 2 V is safe
(c) an operating theatre floor has a very low resistance to reduce the risk of static electricity build up
(d) class I devices have two connecting wires (neutral and live)
(e) a relative humidity over 50% reduces the risk of static charge building up

63 A gauge pressure is a reliable measure of the pressure in the following cylinders

(a) N_2O
(b) CO_2
(c) oxygen
(d) helium
(e) air

64 The pneumotachograph

(a) directly measures a change across a resistance
(b) must have a resistance of sufficient diameter to ensure laminar gas flow
(c) is not suitable for accurate breath-by-breath monitoring
(d) accuracy is affected by a change in temperature
(e) accuracy is unaffected by alterations in gas composition

65 Intraoperative heat loss due to convection may be minimised by

(a) increasing the ambient theatre temperature
(b) using HME filters

(c) using a reflective space blanket
(d) the use of a heated mattress
(e) the avoidance of evaporation of spirit-based skin preparations

66 Likely causes of severely damped radial artery blood pressure trace include

(a) malfunctioning of the continuous flushing system
(b) a bubble in the connecting tubing
(c) more than one stopcock included in the connecting tubing
(d) the use of a 20-gauge arterial cannula
(e) the length of the connecting tubing exceeding 120 cm

67 The following can be measured utilising the Doppler principle

(a) arterial vascular compliance
(b) depth of structures in the tissues
(c) the presence of a ventricular septal defect
(d) left ventricular wall function
(e) gestational age of a fetus

68 Bispectral analysis (BiS)

(a) is measured in hertz
(b) is used as a measure of depth of anaesthesia
(c) values are affected by a natural sleep
(d) values are decreased by opioids used preoperatively
(e) is a reliable monitor to predict recall under anaesthesia

69 Critical pressure

(a) is the pressure at which a gas liquefies at its critical temperature
(b) is 5100 kPa
(c) is the same for all gases
(d) is the pressure of the saturated vapour at the critical temperature
(e) is the pressure above which a liquid cannot be boiled

70 Transducers

(a) convert one form of energy to another
(b) can be used in the measurement of temperature

(c) convert the arterial pressure signal so that it can be displayed on an oscilloscope
(d) include a photocell as an example
(e) measure changes in electrical current

71 If the results from a study are 0, 1, 1, 1, 2, 4, 5, 10

(a) the standard deviation would be a good measure of spread in this sample
(b) the median is 1.5
(c) the sample is normally distributed
(d) there is a negative skew
(e) the 95% confidence limits will be at 1.96 standard deviations

72 With regard to positively skewed data

(a) the median will be greater than the mode
(b) a *P* value of less than 0.05 is more significant than a *P* value of less than 0.01
(c) the Student's *t* test will give a reliable test of the null hypothesis
(d) the distribution of the data would be well described using percentiles
(e) SEM is the variance divided by the square root of the numbers in the sample

73 Expiratory flow rate measurement

(a) in a normal adult is 500l/min
(b) by a peak expiratory flow meter operates on a variable-orifice principle
(c) displacement of the vane is proportional to the gas flow
(d) by the Wright peak flow meter under-reads when compared to the Wright respirometer
(e) can be achieved using a rapid capnograph

74 Henry's law describing the solubility of gases in blood applies to

(a) N_2O
(b) nitrogen

(c) helium
(d) CO_2
(e) halothane

75 In an electrocardiogram movement of the trace reading from the baseline can be caused by
(a) drift
(b) mains interference
(c) gain
(d) the use of filters
(e) common mode rejection

76 An infrared analyser
(a) can be used for any gas
(b) is not affected by water vapour
(c) is not affected by infrared absorption by glass
(d) can cause collision broadening
(e) sample chamber is made small

77 Resistance to flow in a tracheal tube is determined by
(a) curvature
(b) length
(c) being made of silicone
(d) expiratory flow rate
(e) the viscosity of the gases

78 The properties of a gas that influence the resistance during laminar flow include
(a) viscosity
(b) density
(c) critical temperature
(d) diffusion rate
(e) molecular weight

79 The assessment of neuromuscular blockade
(a) uses a unipolar stimulus with a wavelength of 0.3 ms
(b) uses a painful stimulus of 20–60 mA
(c) uses a train of four at 4 Hz

(d) with a double-burst stimulation lasting 3 s is more sensitive to fade than the train of four
(e) by a sustained head lift for 5 s indicates less than 20% blockade

80 Magnetic resonance imaging
(a) uses magnets with air cores
(b) has a field strength of 40 tesla
(c) can be safely used in the presence of aluminium cylinders
(d) uses phosphorus to study metabolic processes
(e) uses hydrogen which has a strong response to a magnetic field

81 With regard to the Venturi principal
(a) potential energy is associated with flow
(b) kinetic energy is associated with pressure
(c) at the constriction there is gain in the kinetic energy at the expense of potential energy
(d) beyond the constriction the kinetic energy decreases and the pressure increases
(e) an increase of kinetic energy can only occur if there is a fall in potential energy

82 Alveolar vapour pressure of anaesthetic inhalational agents is dependent on
(a) barometric pressure
(b) ambient temperature
(c) body temperature
(d) respiratory rate
(e) minute volume

83 With regard to derived SI units
(a) one joule is the work done when a force of one newton moves one square metre
(b) one newton is the force required to accelerate a mass of one kilogram by one metre per second
(c) one watt is the power of one joule per second

(d) pressure of one pascal equals one newton per metre
(e) one kelvin is 1/273.16 of the thermodynamic temperature of the triple point of water

84 Interference in the ECG monitor can be reduced by
(a) the use of amplifiers
(b) the use of gel
(c) checking the electrodes
(d) earthing
(e) the use of low-pass filters

85 With regard to electrical safety the risk of electrocution is reduced by the use of
(a) transformers
(b) isolating capacitor in the diathermy circuit
(c) battery-powered equipment
(d) circuit breakers and fuses within electrical equipment
(e) frequencies in megahertz when using surgical diathermy

86 The Bain circuit
(a) is a partial rebreathing circuit
(b) has one metre length
(c) can be used in children
(d) requires a fresh gas flow of 2–3 times the minute ventilation during mechanical ventilation to prevent rebreathing
(e) increases its dead space if the inner tube disconnects from the patient's end

87 A pressure reducing valve
(a) has a diaphragm made of metallic or rubber material
(b) offers protection to the patient
(c) is incorporated in an oxygen cylinder
(d) maintains constant pressure within the anaesthetic machine
(e) prevents equipment damage

88 Regarding Entonox
(a) the cylinder requires a one-stage reducing valve
(b) the cylinder must be stored vertically
(c) the cylinder contents are 50:50 NO_2 and O_2 by weight

(d) the gas mixture has a pseudocritical temperature of 5.5°C
(e) the full cylinder has a gauge pressure of 140 bar at room temperature

89 The following are correct concerning the colligative properties of a solution when more solute is added to the solvent

(a) a lower vapour pressure
(b) a lower pH
(c) an increased osmotic pressure
(d) a reduced boiling point
(e) an increase in density

90 Regarding medical ultrasound

(a) ultrasound is a form of pressure wave
(b) the frequency of ultrasound is between 20 Hz and 20, 000 Hz
(c) the speed of ultrasound is 1540 m/s
(d) the Doppler shift is a change in wavelength when either the source of the ultrasound or the detector is moving
(e) a piezoelectric material vibrates rapidly to create ultrasound

Table for answers for primary paper 6

	(a)	(b)	(c)	(d)	(e)
1					
2					
3					
4					
5					
6					
7					
8					
9					
10					
11					
12					
13					
14					
15					
16					
17					
18					
19					
20					
21					
22					
23					
24					
25					
26					
27					
28					
29					

	(a)	(b)	(c)	(d)	(e)
30					
31					
32					
33					
34					
35					
36					
37					
38					
39					
40					
41					
42					
43					
44					
45					
46					
47					
48					
49					
50					
51					
52					
53					
54					
55					
56					
57					
58					
59					
60					

Paper 6 Questions

	(a)	(b)	(c)	(d)	(e)
61					
62					
63					
64					
65					
66					
67					
68					
69					
70					
71					
72					
73					
74					
75					
76					
77					
78					
79					
80					
81					
82					
83					
84					
85					
86					
87					
88					
89					
90					

Paper 1 Answers

1 (**a**) false (**b**) true (**c**) true (**d**) false (**e**) false

Pulse pressure reflects the intermittent ejection of blood into the aorta by the heart. The difference between systolic and diastolic blood pressure is the pulse pressure.

The principle factors that alter pulse pressure in the arteries are as follows:

- *Left ventricular stroke volume*: the larger the stroke volume the greater is the volume of blood that must be accommodated in the arterial vessels with each contraction, resulting in an increased pulse pressure
- *Velocity of blood flow*: pulse pressure increases when the flow of blood from arteries to veins is accelerated, i.e.:
  - patent ductus arteriosus (reflection of rapid run off of blood into the pulmonary circulation or left ventricle)
  - aortic regurgitation (reflection of rapid run off of blood into the left ventricle)
  - pulse pressure increases when systemic vascular resistance decreases
  - an increase in heart rate while the cardiac output remains constant causes the stroke volume and pulse pressure to decrease
- *Compliance of arterial tree*: pulse pressure is inversely proportional to compliance (distensibility) of the arterial system; for example, with aging the distensibility of the arterial walls often decreases and pulse pressure increases

2 (**a**) false (**b**) true (**c**) true (**d**) true (**e**) true

The main determinants of myocardial oxygen consumption are:

- ventricular wall tension
- heart rate
- velocity of myocardial shortening

Cardiac cells have a greater mitochondrial content than skeletal muscle probably because they are required to contract repetitively over a life time and are incapable of developing a significant oxygen debt – so they need a ready source of energy. To further enhance its metabolic capability, the myocardium has a rich capillary supply.

The important factors affecting myocardial oxygen consumption are supply and demand balance:

Supply

- Heart rate
  - diastolic time
- Coronary perfusion pressure
  - aortic diastolic pressure
  - ventricular end-diastolic pressure (EDP)
- Arterial O_2 content
  - arterial oxygen tension
  - haemoglobin concentration
- Coronary vessel diameter

Demand

- Basal requirements
- Heart rate
- Wall tension
  - preload (ventricular radius)
  - afterload
- Contractility

The heart rate and, to a lesser extent, ventricular EDP are important determinants of both supply and demand. The changes in the stroke volume are the least expensive metabolically for the work of the heart.

3 **(a)** false **(b)** false **(c)** true **(d)** true **(e)** false

Fetal haemoglobin (Hb F)

- The blood of the human fetus normally contains Hb F, which consists of two alpha chains and two gamma chains (i.e. there are no beta chains). Consequently the P_{50} (the partial pressure of oxygen (oxygen tension) at which haemoglobin is 50% saturated with oxygen) is lower than that of adult haemoglobin because Hb F is less sensitive to the effects of 2,3-DPG
- Forms 80% of circulating haemoglobin at birth, replaced by haemoglobin A normally within 3–5 months. May persist in the haemoglobinopathies

- The curve has a sigmoid shape very similar to the normal dissociation curve for adult haemoglobin but slightly left-shifted

4 **(a)** true **(b)** true **(c)** false **(d)** false **(e)** false

In the normal ECG:

- standard speed 25 mm/s
- one small square represents 0.04 s
- one large square represents 0.2 s
- two large squares vertically = 1 mV
- P–R interval = 0.12–0.21 s
  = 3–5 small squares
- P wave max height = 2.5 mm
- mean frontal QRS axis $\rightarrow -30°$ to $+110°$ and maximum duration 0.1 s
- normal QRS complex = 0.08–0.15 s
- maximum QT interval < 0.42 s

Not all Q waves are indicators of myocardial infarction. There is a Q wave in lead aVR.

Small 'septal' Q waves are normally seen in the left chest leads (V4 to V6) and in one or more of leads I, aVL, II, III, and aVF.

Normally septal Q waves are characteristically narrow and of low amplitude (less than 0.04 s). However, Q waves in leads V1 and V2 may be the only evidence of anterior septal myocardial infarction.

Between V1 and V6 as you move across the chest (in the direction of the electrically predominant left ventricle) the R wave tends to become relatively large and the S wave relatively small. This increase in height of the R wave, which usually reaches a maximum around lead V4 or V5, is called normal R wave progression.

The normal T wave in lead aVR is always negative, while in lead II it is always positive in left-sided chest leads, such as V4 to V5, which normally show a positive T wave.

The duration of the QRS complex is constant, no matter which lead is used for the recording.

5 (**a**) true (**b**) false (**c**) true (**d**) true (**e**) true

Resistance in the pulmonary circulation is distributed more evenly than in the systemic circulation with approximately 50% residing in the arteries and arterioles, 30% in the capillaries and 20% in the veins.

PVR is affected by:

(a) Passive factors
- *Lung expansion*: at lung volumes below functional residual capacity (FRC), the radial forces acting on the extraalveolar vessels and holding them open are reduced, thus increasing PVR. However, at high lung volumes, the increased airway pressures associated with hyperexpansion may compress the vessels also increasing PVR. PVR is lowest at lung volumes around FRC
- *Intravascular pressures*: PVR falls when either pulmonary artery pressure or pulmonary venous pressure increases, because of recruitment of previously closed vessels or the distension of individual capillary segments
- *Cardiac output*: as pulmonary blood flow increases, vessel diameter increases, thus reducing PVR

(b) Active factors, via changes in muscle tone
- Systemic hypoxia increases vessel resistance by inducing muscle constriction
- Hypercapnia and acidosis increase PVR
- Humoral control, vasoconstrictors:
  - thromboxane A_2
  - prostaglandin F
  - histamine
  - serotonin
  - angiotensin
- Humoral control, vasodilators:
  - acetylcholine
  - prostaglandin E
  - prostacyclin
  - bradykinin
- Neural control:
  - sympathetic nervous system supplies vasoconstrictor (α-adrenergic receptor) and vasodilator (β-adrenergic receptor) fibres of the pulmonary vessels
  - parasympathetic nervous system supplies cholinergic vasodilator fibres

- Local control, PVR may be increased by:
  - pulmonary embolism
  - atelectasis
  - pleural effusion

6 (**a**) true (**b**) true (**c**) false (**d**) false (**e**) true

Baroreceptors are stretch receptors.

(a) They are located in carotid sinuses at the bifurcation of the internal and external carotid arteries

(b) They are also located in the aortic arch

(c) A few are located in the wall of almost every large artery of the thoracic and neck region

Stimulus

Since they are mechanoreceptors, any mechanical deformation of the barosensitive areas can cause a burst of action potentials to be generated and provoke a baroreceptor reflex response. They are mainly stimulated by an increase in intraluminal pressure, which stretches the arterial wall and causes the receptor to fire.

Afferent

Afferent information is conveyed to the brain via myelinated and unmyelinated fibres in the sinus nerve (a branch of the glossopharyngeal nerve) from the carotid sinus and via the vagus nerve from the aortic arch.

CNS

The primary relay is found in the nucleus tractus solitarius in the medulla.

Efferent pathways

Efferent pathways are carried by the autonomic nervous system:

- vagus nerve (parasympathetic) to the heart, primarily the sinoatrial (SA) node and atrioventricular (AV) nodes, influencing heart rate
- sympathetic nerves to the heart, affecting both heart rate and the force of ventricular contraction
- sympathetic nerves to the vasculature
- adrenal medulla releases adrenaline to affect both heart rate and the vasculature

Effect

Simulation of the baroreceptors will initiate mechanisms tending to decrease arterial pressure to normal (inhibit tonic discharge).

- Receptors within the aortic arch have a higher threshold pressure and are less sensitive than the carotid sinus receptors
- The receptors in the carotid sinus show adaptation, and therefore are more responsive to constantly changing pressures than sustained ones
- An increase in the mean arterial pressure produces stretch of the baroreceptor nerve endings and an increase in the number of nerve impulses transmitted to the depressor portion of the vasomotor centre. This leads to a relative decrease in the sympathetic nervous system outflow

7 **(a)** false **(b)** false **(c)** true **(d)** true **(e)** true

Lung compliance is defined as the volume change caused by unit pressure change $= \frac{\text{Volume}}{\text{Pressure}}$.

It reflects the *elastic recoil of the lung.*

Lung compliance is the change in lung volume caused by a unit change of transmural pressure. This is the pressure difference between the alveolar pressure measured at the mouth with no flow, i.e. breath held, and the intrapleural pressure measured by a balloon in the oesophagus, across the lung wall.

$$C_{\text{lung}} = \frac{\text{Change in lung volume}}{\text{Change in transmural pressure}} \quad \text{ml/cmH}_2\text{O}.$$

Normal lung compliance in a conscious erect man is 1.5–2.0 l/kPa (150–200 ml/cmH_2O).

Factors reducing lung compliance:

- small lung volume
- increased pulmonary blood volume
- increased extravascular lung water
- inflammation, acute respiratory distress syndrome (ARDS), pneumonia
- fibrosis, emphysema
- extremes of age, e.g. neonatal compliance = 20 ml/cmH_2O
- many studies have failed to demonstrate any change in compliance when allowing for changes in lung volumes

Surfactant improves lung compliance especially at low lung volumes. Chest wall compliance is a change in chest volume caused by a unit change in transthoracic pressure. Transthoracic pressure equals alveolar pressure minus intrapleural pressure. (Difficult to measure due to the effect of muscle contraction.)

$$C_{chest} = \frac{\text{Change in chest volume}}{\text{Change in transthoracic pressure}}$$

Normal chest wall compliance is 2 l/kPa or 200 ml/cmH_2O.

Total compliance is the change in lung volume that occurs with a unit change in the alveolar/ambient pressure.

Total compliance (lung and chest together) is 0.85 l/kPa (85 ml/cmH_2O).

Total compliance is expressed as

$$\frac{1}{C_{total}} = \frac{1}{C_{chest}} + \frac{1}{C_{lung}}.$$

Compliance is inversely proportional to elastance. With age elastance decreases so compliance increases.

8 **(a)** false **(b)** false **(c)** true **(d)** true **(e)** false

Initiation of a breath starts in the inspiratory neurones of the respiratory centre in the floor of the fourth ventricle. The diaphragm is the main muscle of respiration and contraction of the inverted J-shaped fibres causes it to descend with a consequent decrease in intrapleural pressure.

The increasing subatmospheric intrapleural pressures expand the lung and dilate the intrathoracic airways. Air is drawn through the nose where it is warmed and humidified.

Both intrapleural and alveolar pressure fall by 2 cmH_2O as inspiration starts.

9 **(a)** true **(b)** true **(c)** true **(d)** true **(e)** true

Factors affecting alveolar dead space include:

(a) Age
- Alveolar dead space increases with increasing age

(b) Pulmonary arterial (PA) pressure
- A decrease in PA pressure (e.g. hypotension) decreases perfusion to the upper parts of the lung, which increases zone 1 and increases alveolar dead space

(c) Posture
- Alveolar dead space increases in the upright and lateral position, due to exaggeration of hydrostatic differences – increased in zone 1

(d) Intermittent positive-pressure ventilation (IPPV)
- Increases alveolar dead space due to exaggeration of hydrostatic failure of perfusion
- Also decreases total pulmonary blood flow

(e) Tidal volume
- As tidal volume increases, so alveolar dead space increases, but their ratio remains constant

(f) Oxygen
- Hypoxaemic vasoconstriction decrease dead space, whereas hyperoxaemic vasodilatation increases it

(g) Anaesthetic gases
- Increase alveolar dead space (but it is not known why)

(h) Lung disease
- ARDS increases microembolic and vasodilatation of non-vascular air spaces
- IPPV and the lateral posture increase gross ventilation/perfusion mismatch

10 (**a**) false (**b**) false (**c**) false (**d**) true (**e**) false

Functional residual capacity is the volume of air (about 3 l in an adult) that is present in the lungs at the end of normal expiration, i.e. when the elastic recoil of the lung is balanced with the elastic recoil of the chest and the diaphragm.

It is the sum of two volumes:
- residual volume
- expiratory reserve volume

Functional residual capacity is the resting volume of the lung where gases are exchanged.

Factors which increase FRC include:
- height (FRC is directly proportional to height)
- position (upright)
- continuous positive airways pressure (CPAP)
- positive end-expiratory pressure (PEEP)

Factors which decrease FRC include:

- sex (10% less in females)
- obesity
- supine position
- rest
- age: There is a slight increase with age of 16 ml/year. (Lumb, A. B. *Nunn's Respiratory Physiology*, 6th edn. Amsterdam: Elsevier, 2005)

The FRC is measured by:

- body plethysmography
- nitrogen washout method
- helium dilution

Body plethysmography

- The subject is enclosed in an air-tight chamber
- At the end of normal expiration a shutter occludes the mouth piece
- The subject attempts to expand his or her lungs, by a series of panting breaths while the mouth and nose are closed
- The resultant pressure changes within the chamber can be related to the lung volume by the application of Boyle's Law

Nitrogen washout method

- The subject breathes 100% O_2 from the end of a maximum expiration
- The expired gas is collected and analysed for N_2
- Nitrogen expired comes from the FRC at a concentration of 79%
- The FRC can be derived from the washout concentration

Helium dilution

- Based on a closed-circuit equilibration method
- At the end of expiration the subject is connected to the system with:
    - a known volume of inert gas helium
    - a known concentration of inert gas helium
- The subject then breathes until a new steady-state is reached and a new lower concentration of helium (diluted by the FRC) is recorded
- During the procedure CO_2 is absorbed by soda lime and the O_2 consumed is replaced

- The FRC is calculated from the equation:

$He[^1] \times$ circuit volume $= He[^2] \times$ (circuit volume + FRC), where $He[^1]$ is the initial concentration of inhaled helium and $He[^2]$ is the helium concentration in the respirometer.

Relevance to anaesthesia of the FRC

- FRC is a respiratory gas buffer zone
- After adequate preoxygenation it is the O_2 store in the FRC which will be utilised during any subsequent period of apnoea (O_2 replaces N_2) during:
  - rapid sequence induction
  - difficult intubation
  - laryngospasm
  - upper airway obstruction
  - induction of anaesthesia

Breathing 100% oxygen for 10 maximum volume breaths will replace the FRC nitrogen and give a reserve of 2000 ml oxygen. Breathing 100% O_2 for a further 3–5 min will replace some of the small amount of nitrogen dissolved in the body tissues. Clinically it is important that 100% O_2 is breathed.

Patients with smaller O_2 stores desaturate more rapidly, e.g.:

- small FRC
- infants
- pregnancy
- obese
- low Hb concentration

Causes of a reduced FRC

The FRC is reduced after induction of anaesthesia by around 15%–20% regardless of the mode of ventilation.

Causes

- Nitrogen in the alveoli is replaced by more soluble gases
- Elevation of the diaphragm – due to loss of end-expiratory muscle tone
- Inward movement of the chest wall (reduced thoracic cross-sectional area)
- Blood moved from thorax and pooled in abdomen

11 (**a**) false (**b**) false (**c**) false (**d**) false (**e**) true

The loop of Henle (LOH) employs a sodium countercurrent mechanism to provide hypertonic conditions – approximately 1200 mmol/l, mainly sodium chloride and urea, in the deep medulla of the kidney. This permits the production of concentrated urine if required.

The active component of the LOH is the ascending limb. Here chloride, and hence sodium, is pumped out of the tubule into the interstitium.

The ascending limb of the LOH is impermeable to water. The descending limb of the LOH is permeable to sodium chloride and water.

The net effect is for sodium chloride to leave the ascending limb and to enter the descending limb, having first passed through the renal medullary interstitium. Some water is also lost from the descending limb.

As the tubular fluid passes through the ascending limb it becomes increasingly dilute as the sodium chloride is removed. As a result the fluid entering the distal convoluted tubule is hypotonic (150 mmol/l).

12 (**a**) false (**b**) true (**c**) false (**d**) true (**e**) true

In the awake, healthy individual assuming the lateral position, gravity favours greater blood flow to the dependent lung while spontaneous ventilation also favours greater gas flow to that lung, so that normal *ventilation|perfusion* ($\dot{V}/\dot{Q}$) matching is maintained.

Ventilation is greater to the dependent lung because:

- contraction of the dependent diaphragm is more efficient as a result of its higher position in the chest (from the weight of abdominal contents)
- the dependent lung is on a more favourable part of the compliance curve

(a) Anaesthetised, spontaneously breathing patient in lateral position
Anaesthesia decreases FRC. The upper lung moves down to a more favourable part of the compliance curve while the lower lung moves to a position that is less favourable. This results in greater ventilation to the upper lung whereas the perfusion remains greater to the dependent lung, resulting in a mismatched ($\dot{V}/\dot{Q}$).

(b) Anaesthetised, mechanically ventilated patient in lateral position
In a mechanically ventilated patient, an even greater proportion of tidal volume goes to the upper lung because the mechanical advantage of the dependant diaphragm is lost.
Muscle paralysis allows the abdominal contents to rise up further against the dependent diaphragm and impede ventilation of the lower lung because ventilation is mechanical; the path chosen by the airflow is that of least resistance.

(c) Anaesthetised, mechanically ventilated patient with an open chest
When the chest wall is open the restriction of lung expansion caused by the chest wall is lost (its compliance increases). This effect favours even greater ventilation of the upper lung. Perfusion remains unaltered. The potential for severe $\dot{V}/\dot{Q}$ mismatch is at its greatest.

13 (**a**) false (**b**) true (**c**) false (**d**) false (**e**) false

The technique for measuring the pressure/volume (*P*/*V*) curve was first used clinically in 1949 and is the only clinical method for directly assessing the elastic properties of the pulmonary parenchyma. The *P*/*V* curve is obtained by having the patient swallow, into the stomach, a balloon-tipped catheter that is connected to a pressure transducer. The catheter is then withdrawn until a negative deflection in the pressure tracing is observed during inspiration, indicating that the catheter tip is in the thorax. Then the catheter is withdrawn 10 cm further, in order to centre the tip in the thorax; this is also where the maximal pressure swings are found. The patient is then asked to inhale to total lung capacity (TLC) and to expire slowly, while the exhaled volume is measured. While the patient is expiring, the test operator manually closes a shutter for approximately 0.5 s, thereby allowing for the measurement of static pressure at several different volumes. Using the obtained static pressure and volume measurements, a *P*/*V* curve is plotted. Because of the skill required in measuring and interpreting a *P*/*V* curve, it is not a commonly used test.

From the *P*/*V* curve, one can calculate several indices, which are used to characterise the elastic recoil of the lung. These indices are:

- the compliance (the slope of the *P*/*V* curve)
- the coefficient of retraction
- the shape factor (*k*)

The *P*/*V* curve is not linear, because as the lung becomes more distended the compliance falls and elastance rises. The non-linear shape of the *P*/*V* curve means that the value of the calculated compliance will vary depending on where on the curve the slope is calculated. The most common practice is to calculate the slope of the line between functional residual capacity and 0.5 l, but there are many other approaches.

The coefficient of retraction is calculated by dividing the maximal pressure generated by the TLC. A high coefficient of retraction is indicative of a stiff lung.

14 **(a)** true **(b)** false **(c)** false **(d)** false **(e)** false

Cerebrospinal fluid (CSF) is a clear aqueous solution that, compared with plasma, contains:

(a) a higher concentration of
- Na^+
- Cl^-
- magnesium

(b) a lower concentrations of
- glucose
- protein
- K^+
- Ca^{2+}
- HCO_3^-
- PO_4^-

- The rate of CSF formation is 0.35–0.40 ml/min or 500–600 ml/day
- The turnover time of total CSF volume is 4–5 h
- Total CSF volume 40 ml
- CSF is formed in the choroid plexus in the two lateral ventricles and then passes through the paired interventricular foramina of Monro into the third ventricle. CSF then flows caudally through the aqueduct of Sylvius and fourth ventricle and into the subarachnoid space by one of

Table 1.14 CSF and plasma composition

	CSF	Plasma
Specific gravity	1.007	1.025
Osmolarity (mosmol/l)	289	289
pH	7.31	7.41
PCO_2 (kPa)	6.6	5.4
Na^+(mmol/l)	141	140
Cl^- (mmol/l)	124	101
Mg^{2+} (mmol/l)	1.2	0.85
Bicarbonate (mmol/l)	23	28
K^+ (mmol/l)	2.9	4.6
Glucose (mmol/l)	2–4	4
Protein (g/l)	0.2–0.4	60–80

three exits. Two are the lateral foramina of Luschka and the third is the midline foramen of Magendie, from which CSF flows into the subarachnoid space around the brain and spinal cord. A small proportion of CSF may also leave the fourth ventricle through the central canal of the spinal cord

- 85%–90% of CSF is absorbed at intracranial sites through arachnoid villi and granulations bordering the superior sagittal sinus and venous lacunae
- 10%–15% of CSF is reabsorbed at spinal sites
- Normal CSF pressure is less than 15 mmHg
- CSF pressure values in the lumbar region are:
  - lateral (60–100 mm CSF)
  - sitting (200–250 mm CSF)

15 (**a**) false (**b**) true (**c**) false (**d**) true (**e**) false

The proximal tubule is considered the bulk reabsorber as it is responsible for:

- reducing the volume of glomerular filtrate by 80%
- reabsorbing 70% of Na^+ and Cl^-
- reabsorbing 90% of Ca^{2+}, HCO_3, Mg^{2+}
- reabsorbing 100% of glucose, phosphate and amino acids during their passage through the proximal tubule

- The fluid entering the proximal tubule from Bowman's capsule has a composition similar to that of plasma except for the absence of protein
- As the reabsorptive process is iso-osmotic, the osmolality remains identical at the beginning and at the end of the proximal tubule (290 mosmol/kg)

16 (**a**) true (**b**) true (**c**) false (**d**) true (**e**) true

When a muscle is stretched, primary sensory fibres (group Ia afferent neurones) of the muscle spindle respond to both the velocity and the degree of stretch, and send this information to the spinal cord. Likewise, secondary sensory fibres (group II afferent neurones) detect and send information about the degree of stretch (but not the velocity thereof) to the CNS.

Afferent and efferent

This information is transmitted monosynaptically to an alpha efferent motor fibre; it activates extrafusal fibres of the muscle to contract, thereby reducing stretch, and polysynaptically through an interneurone to another alpha motoneurone, which inhibits contraction in opposing muscles.

Neurotransmitters

- At the central synapse is glutamate
- The stretch reflex is a monosynaptic reflex

17 **(a)** true **(b)** false **(c)** false **(d)** false **(e)** false

Normal daily excretion is affected by a number of factors.

(a) The metabolic response to trauma results in the following changes:
- urine volume is reduced and its Na content is reduced
- urine K and nitrogen (N_2) content are raised
- plasma Na and albumin are decreased
- plasma antidiuretic hormone (ADH), aldosterone, cortisol, catecholamines, insulin, glucose, free fatty acids (FFA) and amino acids (AA) are increased

(b) Intraoperative factors
(c) Fluid administration
(d) Renal impairment

Table 1.17 Principle urine constituents

	Normal	Effect of operation
Water (ml)	1500 (1000–2500)	500
Na^+ (mmol/l)	70–160	5–20
K^+ (mmol/l)	40–120	90–180
Urea (g)	16–350	20–60

18 **(a)** true **(b)** true **(c)** false **(d)** false **(e)** true

Starvation is a complete absence of dietary food intake which can result in death after 60 days, in contrast to the state of malnutrition, when a calorie intake may be present. Biochemical adaptations to starvation aim to supply glucose to tissue that needs it. A patient needs 180 g glucose/day.

Changes in starvation

(a) Glycogenolysis
- First few hours
- Breakdown of glycogen to glucose

- Takes place in the liver
- After 24 h hepatic glycogen is exhausted

(b) Gluconeogenesis

- Glucose can be formed from glycerol formed in the liver by lipolysis
- Occurs as glycogen sources become depleted
- Protein loss: amino acids from the muscles
    - pyruvate
    - alanine
- Glucose can be formed from oxaloacetate

(c) Ketogenesis

- After about 3 days
- Adipose tissue fat
- FFA and ketones are the major energy sources
- Later most of the body tissues, including the ketone bodies, are used as a fuel source
- Glucose requirements fall
- Increased ketone bodies with mild acidosis
- Increased fatty acids, which inhibit gluconeogenesis
- Thus body adapts to preserve proteins and use fats
- Once the fat stores are depleted, protein is then mobilised to provide energy (death occurs afterwards)
- Free fatty acid (FFA) used directly or indirectly as a source of energy

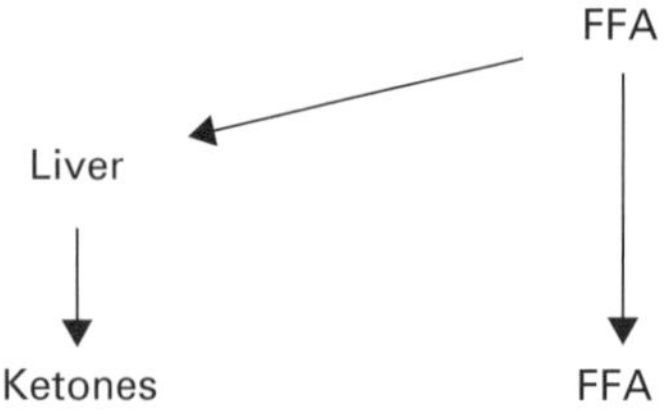

19 (**a**) true (**b**) false (**c**) true (**d**) false (**e**) false

In utero, the placenta acts as the fetal lung, and oxygenated blood (saturated by about 80%) from the placenta passes through a single umbilical vein to the fetus. This blood flows predominantly through the ductus venosus and into the inferior vena cava, thus by-passing the liver. Most of the oxygenated blood entering the right atrium from the inferior vena cava preferentially passes through the foramen ovale into the left atrium, thus by-passing the lungs. Passage of this oxygenated blood directly to the left atrium allows perfusion of the fetal brain with maximal available concentrations of oxygen.

Blood entering the right atrium from the superior vena cava is mainly oxygenated blood from the fetal head regions. This blood enters the right ventricle for delivery into the pulmonary artery and then to the descending thoracic aorta via the ductus arteriosus.

As a result, this deoxygenated blood is delivered distal to the blood vessels that supply the fetal brain.

Blood is returned to the placenta by two umbilical arteries for oxygenation.

The pressure gradient across the foramen ovale causes the flag-like valve to occlude the opening.

Flow through the ductus arteriosus decreases after birth due to constriction of the muscular wall of this vessel upon exposure to higher concentrations of oxygen.

Table 1.19 Fetal circulation: oxygen saturation (SPO_2 %) and oxygen tension (PO_2 *K*Pa)

	Saturation (SPO_2 %)	O_2 tension (kPa)
Umbilical vein	80	5.3
Inferior vena cava	67	4.4
Superior vena cava	30	2.5
Right atrium and ventricle	52	3.2
Left atrium and ventricle	62	4.0
Ductus arteriosus	52	3.2
Descending aorta	58	3.5

20 (**a**) true (**b**) false (**c**) true (**d**) false (**e**) true

The EEG measures brainwaves of different frequencies within the brain. Electrodes are placed on specific sites on the scalp to detect and record the electrical impulses within the brain.

A **frequency** is the number of times a wave repeats itself within a second. It can be compared to the frequencies that you tune into on your radio. If any of these frequencies are deficient, excessive, or difficult to access, our mental performance can suffer.

Amplitude represents the *power* of electrical impulses generated by brain.

Volume or intensity of brain wave activity is measured in microvolts.

The raw EEG is usually described in terms of frequency bands:

- gamma greater than 30 Hz
- beta 13–30 Hz
- alpha 8–12 Hz
- theta 4–8 Hz
- delta less than 4 Hz or 0.1–3 Hz

The lowest frequencies are ***delta.*** These are less than 4 Hz and occur in deep sleep, in some abnormal processes, and also during experiences of 'empathy state'. Delta waves are involved with our ability to integrate and let go. They reflect the unconscious mind. It is the dominant rhythm in infants up to 1 year of age and it is present in stages 3 and 4 of sleep.

Peak performers decrease delta waves when high focus and peak performance are required.

Lack of oxygen initially produces frontal alpha rhythm. Delta waves appear as consciousness is lost.

Moderate hypercarbia produces an arousal pattern in the EEG.

21 (**a**) true (**b**) true (**c**) true (**d**) false (**e**) true

Erythropoietin is a haemopoietic glycoprotein growth factor derived from a single gene on chromosome seven, which is expressed in cells of the renal cortex. Some 10% is produced by the liver by unknown cells; this amount is not enough for normal functioning. Its key action is to control erythropoiesis. Normally erythropoietin is produced as a result of hypoxia detected by an oxygen sensor; it then acts back on an effector receptor. There is normally a rise in levels in anaemia. Erythropoietin secretion is stimulated by:

- hypoxia
- cobalt salts
- androgens
- alkalosis
- catecholamines
- adenosine

Erythropoietin secretion is inhibited by:

- increased red cell volume
- theophylline

22 (a) true (b) false (c) true (d) false (e) true

Chemoreceptor trigger zone (CTZ) receptors receive inputs from:

- cholinergic (muscarinic) receptors
- $5HT_3$ receptors
- histamine receptors (H_1)
- dopaminergic (D_2) receptors

It is located in the area postrema on the floor of the fourth ventricle (outside the blood–brain barrier).

The main pathways by which the emetic reflex can be induced appear to be:

- abdominal vagal afferents
- area postrema
- ventricular system

23 (a) false (b) false (c) false (d) false (e) true

Vomiting reflex

- Vomiting starts with salivation and the sensation of nausea
- Reverse peristalsis empties material from the upper part of the small intestine into the stomach
- The glottis closes, preventing aspiration of vomitus into the trachea
- The breath is held in mid inspiration
- The muscles of the abdominal wall contract, and because the chest is held in a fixed position the contraction increases intra-abdominal pressure
- The lower oesophageal sphincter and the oesophagus relax and the gastric contents are ejected
- The vomiting centre in the formation of the medulla at the level of the olivary nuclei controls these activities

24 (a) true (b) true (c) true (d) false (e) true

Aldosterone is a 21-carbon steroid derived from the precursor cholesterol. It is the main endogenous mineralocorticoid hormone. It is produced from corticosterone by the zona glomerulosa of the adrenal cortex mainly in response to angiotensin II.

Aldosterone probably causes activation of a specific Na^+/K^+ active pump in the distal renal tubule. This leads to reabsorption of sodium and water from the urine in exchange for potassium and hydrogen ions. Sodium retention causes a secondary retention of water.

Aldosterone causes a reduction in the sodium and an increase in the potassium concentration of both sweat and saliva. This effect is not seen in cystic fibrosis.

Regulation of aldosterone release is by:

- angiotensin II via the renin–angiotensin system
- potassium, via a direct action on the zona glomerulosa
  - low levels of serum potassium appear to have an inhibitory effect on aldosterone secretion
  - high levels of serum potassium increase aldosterone secretion
- ACTH has a minimal effect except at very high concentrations when it stimulates secretion
- hyponatraemia increases aldosterone secretion via a direct effect on the zona glomerulosa

Aldosterone may be competitively inhibited by drugs such as spironolactone.

25 (**a**) false (**b**) true (**c**) false (**d**) false (**e**) true

The respiratory quotient (RQ) is the ratio of CO_2 production to O_2 consumption per unit time in steady state.

Respiratory exchange ratio (R) is the ratio at any time not in the steady state.

R is affected by

- Severe exercise (increased due to CO_2 blown off and increased CO_2 produced from lactic acid)
- Hyperventilation (increased due to CO_2 being blown off)
- Post exercise (decreased as O_2 dept paid)
- Metabolic acidosis (increased due to respiratory compensation)
- Metabolic alkalosis (decreased due to respiratory compensation)
- Average values
  - CHO 1
  - fat 0.7
  - protein 0.8

26 (**a**) false (**b**) false (**c**) true (**d**) true (**e**) false

Compensatory reactions activated by haemorrhage include:

- vasoconstriction
- tachycardia
- increased thoracic pumping
- increased skeletal muscle pumping
- increased movement of interstitial fluid into capillaries
- increased secretion of epinephrine and norepinephrine
- increased secretion of vasopressin
- increased secretion of glucocorticoid
- increased secretion of renin and aldosterone
- increased secretion of erythropoietin
- increased plasma protein synthesis
- increased filtration fraction

The glomerular filtration rate is depressed, but renal plasma flow is decreased to a greater extent.

27 (**a**) true (**b**) false (**c**) true (**d**) true (**e**) true

Hydrogen ions are actively secreted into renal tubules by epithelial cells lining proximal renal tubules, distal renal tubules and collecting ducts. At the same time sodium ions are reabsorbed and replaced by secreted hydrogen ions. Bicarbonate ions, formed in renal tubular epithelial cells, move into the peritubular capillaries to combine with sodium ions. As a result, the amount of sodium bicarbonate in the plasma is increased during the secretion of H^+ in renal tubules.

Hydrogen ions must combine with buffers in the lumen of renal tubules to prevent tubular fluid pH from decreasing below the pH that allows continued secretion of H^+ ions by the renal tubular epithelial cells.

Ammonia combines with H^+ to form ammonium.

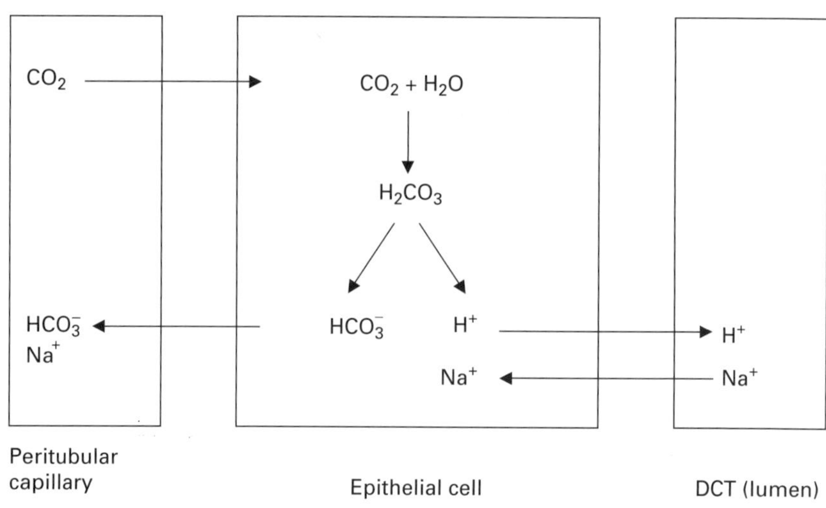

28 (**a**) true (**b**) true (**c**) false (**d**) true (**e**) false

Both at rest and at any given level of exercise, trained athletes have a larger stroke volume and lower heart rate than untrained individuals and tend to have larger hearts.

Training increases the maximal oxygen consumption.

The changes that occur in skeletal muscles with training include:

- increased numbers of mitochondria
- increased numbers of enzymes
- increased numbers of capillaries
- a smaller increase in lactate production
- a smaller increase in blood flow to muscles

29 (**a**) false (**b**) false (**c**) true (**d**) true (**e**) false

Plasma proteins are mostly in the form of anions and are responsible for about 15% of the buffering capacity of the blood. They are involved in the transportation of thyroid, adrenocortical and gonadal hormones. The osmotic pressure of plasma proteins plays an important role in the exchange of fluid across capillaries (however, plasma proteins only provide approximately 25 mmHg of the osmotic pressure – a small proportion).

Plasma proteins consist of

(a) Albumins
  - 60%–80% of plasma proteins
  - Most important in maintenance of osmotic balance
  - Produced by liver

(b) Globulins
  - Alpha and beta
  - Some are important for transport of materials through the blood (e.g. thyroid hormone and iron)
  - Some are clotting factors
  - Produced by liver
  - Gamma globulins are immunoglobulins (antibodies) produced by lymphocytes

(c) Fibrinogen produced by liver
  - Important in clotting

The plasma proteins have different electrical charges, which permits electrophoretic separation.

The concentration of plasma protein is maintained in starvation.

Plasminogen is a single-chain glycoprotein consisting of 791 amino acid residues. It is the inactive precursor of plasmin, which is found in body fluids and blood plasma.

30 **(a)** false **(b)** false **(c)** false **(d)** true **(e)** true

Normally gastric emptying results from peristaltic waves of contraction passing through the cardia, antrum, pylorus and duodenum.

The waves occur up to 3 times per minute after a meal. Liquids leave faster than solids.

Carbohydrates leave faster than protein, which leave faster than fats.

Gastric emptying is increased by:

- gastric distension
- drugs: metoclopramide, domperidone, cisapride, erythromycin

Gastric emptying is slowed by:

- lying down, anxiety, fear and pain
- mechanical obstruction and duodenal distension
- labour

- drugs
- opioids, anticholinergics, alcohol

31 (**a**) false (**b**) false (**c**) true (**d**) true (**e**) true

Receptors

A receptor is a part of a cell that interacts in a selective manner with an extracellular compound to start a biochemical change.

There are a number of ways of trying to classify receptors.

By site of action:
- surface membrane with a hydrophobic transmembrane region
- intracellular effect mediated by a second messenger
- intracellular effect on a protein system, e.g. hormones

Surface or transmembrane receptors can be divided into three sub-groups:
- voltage-sensitive ion channels, e.g. sodium, potassium, calcium and chloride
- ligand-gated ion channels, e.g. nicotinic, GABA, NMDA
- transmembrane receptors, e.g. adrenoreceptors, muscarinic cholinergic, opioid, serotonin, dopamine

Receptor function or activation

(a) Surface
  - Ion channels. Ion pumps are one type of excitable membrane protein, e.g. sodium-potassium ATPase pump
  - Ligand gated ion channels. The channel has 4 or 5 subunits

  The drug activates excitable cell membrane proteins which modulate the ion channels and the permeability of electrically excitable membranes, e.g. GABAA, nicotinic and acetylcholine receptors are enzyme and amino-acid-linked receptor ion channels. These receptors are involved in rapid synaptic transmission between cells.

(b) Coupled to an intermediary, e.g. G protein or guanine nucleotide proteins. Most hormones and neurotransmitters are water-soluble signalling molecules that interact with G protein.

  This is an intermediary called a second messenger or the sequence of events is called the second messenger. The binding of the drug or hormone to such an intracellular receptor sets off a series of biochemical events, which couple the receptor binding to the clinical effect. Many membrane receptors are coupled to their primary second messenger through intermediate membrane proteins called guanine nucleotide regulatory proteins (G proteins). This G protein, when stimulated, will increase cAMP activity, e.g. by glucagon, beta-adrenergic agonists. Inhibiting G protein will decrease cAMP activity, e.g. alpha-2 adrenergic agonists, muscarinic agonists.

The phosphatidylinositol system is another second messenger.

(c) Tyrosine kinase linked, e.g. the insulin receptor, which is made up of two alpha and two beta subunits. Receptor binding activates kinase activity. This receptor is effective in minutes or hours.
(d) Intracellular effect on protein synthesis, e.g. steroid and thyroid hormones.

Membrane receptors have hydrophobic transmembrane regions.

Ion channels have changed transmembrane regions.

Ligand-gated ion channels have both hydrophobic and charged transmembrane regions.

32 **(a)** false **(b)** false **(c)** true **(d)** true **(e)** true

Drugs which undergo extensive metabolism include:

(a) Analgesics
- Paracetamol
- Aspirin
- Morphine
- Pethidine

(b) Cardiovascular drugs
- GTN
- Lidocaine
- Verapamil
- Nifedipine
- Propranolol
- Metoprolol
- Isoprenaline

(c) Drugs acting on CNS
- Chlorpromazine
- Levodopa

(d) Respiratory drugs
  - Salbutamol
  - Terbutaline

(e) Oral contraceptives

33 (**a**) false (**b**) false (**c**) false (**d**) false (**e**) false

Acidic drugs (e.g. aspirin) are unionised in the highly acidic medium of the stomach, and therefore are absorbed more rapidly than the basic drugs.

In practice even acidic drugs are predominantly absorbed from the small bowel, as its surface area for absorption is so much greater as a result of mucosal villi.

Of the basic drugs, those that are weak bases (e.g. propranolol), though ionised in the stomach, are relatively unionised in the duodenum and are therefore absorbed.

Morphine is highly ionised in the acidic environment of the stomach and so is poorly absorbed.

34 (**a**) false (**b**) false (**c**) false (**d**) true (**e**) true

The rate of transfer across the blood–brain barrier is dependent on:
- lipid solubility
- degree of ionisation
- protein binding
- molecular weight

35 (**a**) false (**b**) true (**c**) true (**d**) true (**e**) false

- Midazolam is water soluble but when subjected to a pH of 7.4 in the body the midazolam ring closes and becomes lipid soluble so it can cross the blood–brain barrier
- Diazepam does not show this phenomenon
- Local anaesthetics are weak bases and hence their structure is pH dependent
- Atracurium undergoes irreversible Hofmann degradation at certain pH values

36 (**a**) true (**b**) false (**c**) false (**d**) false (**e**) true

Drugs which induce metabolising enzymes in the liver include:
- carbamazepine
- phenobarbitone

- phenytoin
- rifampicin
- chronic ethanol
- griseofulvin

37 (**a**) false (**b**) false (**c**) true (**d**) false (**e**) false

All inhalation agents adversely affect the cardiovascular system to some extent. Several mechanisms are involved:

- direct depression of the vasomotor centre
- depression of baroreceptor reflexes
- depression of cardiac contractility
- dilatation of peripheral vessels causing a fall in systemic vascular resistance
- autonomic effects
- sensitisation of myocardium to catecholamines

The combined effect is a dose-related fall in mean arterial pressure. Sevoflurane has the best cardiovascular profile and halothane the worst. Desflurane is associated with a sympathetically medicated sinus tachycardia when the concentration is increased rapidly above 1 MAC, where MAC is the minimal alveolar concentration, i.e. the concentration that prevents movement in response to skin incision in 50% of subjects studied.

38 (**a**) false (**b**) false (**c**) false (**d**) true (**e**) false

The following factors influence the uptake of anaesthetic agents from inhaled gas to the blood:

(a) Inhaled concentration
- The higher the tension or inhaled partial pressure the higher the levels achieved in the blood

(b) Alveolar ventilation
- Increasing alveolar minute volume speeds up the approximation of alveolar to inspired levels

(c) Blood/gas partition coefficient
- This is the ratio of the amount of anaesthetic in blood to that in gas when the two phases are of equal volume and pressure and in equilibrium at 37 ° C.
- It is the partial pressure of the agent in the blood and hence the brain that gives rise to anaesthesia. Therefore, agents with a low

blood/gas coefficient exert a high partial pressure and therefore a more rapid onset/offset of action.

(d) Small FRC

(e) Second gas effect

- Administration of a rapidly absorbed gas given in a high concentration (typically N_2O, blood/gas partition coefficient of 0.47) together with a volatile agent of lower solubility produces an increasing alveolar concentration of the second agent thus promoting its absorption

(f) Cardiac output

- A low cardiac output favours a more rapid equilibration and so onset of anaesthesia will also be more rapid

39 (**a**) false (**b**) true (**c**) false (**d**) true (**e**) true

Dystonic reactions are adverse extrapyramidal effects that often occur shortly after the initiation of neuroleptic drug therapy. These reactions may occur with a wide variety of medications such as neuroleptics (antipsychotics) and antiemetics. Antidepressants are the most common causes of drug-induced dystonic reactions. Acute dystonic reactions have been described with every antipsychotic. Alcohol and cocaine use increases the risk of developing such reactions.

40 (**a**) true (**b**) true (**c**) true (**d**) false (**e**) false

Etomidate is a carboxylated imidazole so unstable it is formulated in a mixture of water and 35% propylene glycol.

Etomidate has two isomers:

(a) dextro: (hypnotic effect)

(b) laevo:

Pharmacokinetics

molecular weight	342
pH	8.1
p*Ka*	4.2
protein binding	75%
volume of distribution	3 l/kg
clearance	10–20 $ml.kg^{-1}.\ min^{-1}$

Elimination

Non-specific hepatic esterases and possibly plasma cholinesterase hydrolyse etomidate to ethyl alcohol and its carboxylic acid metabolite.

It may inhibit plasma cholinesterase; 87% excreted in urine, 3% unchanged.

Side-effects

- Pain on injection in up to 25% of patients
- Postoperative nausea and vomiting (2%–15%)
- Excitatory movements
- Inhibits steroidogenesis which lasts 3–6 h after a single dose by inhibition of the enzyme 11β-hydroxylase and 17α-hydroxylase

41 (**a**) false (**b**) false (**c**) false (**d**) false (**e**) false

Prilocaine is closely related to lidocaine. It has the following characteristics:

- the same p*K*a (7.9)
- the same speed of onset
- a similar duration of action
- less lipid soluble
- less toxic because of
  - high tissue fixation
  - rapid metabolism

It is metabolised in the liver, lung, kidney to o-toluidine and then hydroxyl-toluidine.

O-Toluidine is responsible for methaemoglobinaemia.

42 (**a**) false (**b**) false (**c**) false (**d**) false (**e**) true

- Lidocaine is primarily classified as a local anaesthetic agent but is also a class Ib anti-arrhythmic
- It has a relatively rapid onset of action and intermediate duration
- It is metabolised in the liver by microsomal oxidases and amidase; *N*-dealkylation followed by hydrolysis produces ethylglycine

- Kinetics
  - p*Ka*: 7.9
  - plasma protein bound: 70%
  - elimination half-life: 100 min

43 (**a**) false (**b**) false (**c**) true (**d**) true (**e**) true

Table 1.43 Mechanisms of opioid actions

Receptor	Drugs	Natural ligand	Action	Clinical effects
Mu	Morphine Pethidine Fentanyl	Endorphin	Increase K^+ conductance	Analgesia dependence, Respiratory depression, GIT effects
M_I				Supraspinal and peripheral analgesia
M_2				Spinal analgesia, dependence, respiratory depression, GIT effects
M_3		M6G Ligand		
Kappa	Pentazocine Nalbuphine Keto-cyclazocine	Dynorphin	Reduce Ca^{2+} conductance	Analgesia Dysphoria Diuresis Psychomimetic
Delta		Enkephalin	Increase Ca^{2+} conductance	Spinal & supra spinal

Opioid receptors

Opioid receptors exist throughout the:

- CNS with particularly high concentrations in:
  - periaqueductal grey area
  - substantia gelatinosa of the spinal cord
- gastrointestional tract

The more recent classification scheme for opioid receptors = op classification.

There are three distinct opioid receptors identified by their prototype agonists:

- OP3 μ (Mu)
- OP2 κ (kappa)
- OP1 δ (delta)

All three receptors have now been successfully cloned and their amino acid sequences defined.

A fourth variant σ (sigma) was originally classified as an opioid receptor.

Buprenorphine is a partial mu receptor agonist.

Nalbuphine is a:

- partial agonist at kappa receptors
- antagonist at mu receptors

44 (**a**) false (**b**) false (**c**) false (**d**) true (**e**) false

Naloxone is a pure opioid antagonist and will reverse opioid effects at mu, kappa and delta receptors.

Its affinity is highest for mu receptors.

Side-effects:

- increased BP
- pulmonary oedema
- cardiac arrhythmia

NB It has a duration of action of 30–40 min which is shorter than morphine. Oral bioavailability is only 2%.

45 (**a**) false (**b**) false (**c**) false (**d**) false (**e**) true

The following drugs are $5HT_3$ antagonists:

- dolasetron
- granisetron
- ondansetron
- tropisetron

46 (**a**) true (**b**) false (**c**) true (**d**) false (**e**) false

Table 1.46 Characteristics of flumazenil

Action	Competitive benzodiazepine receptor antagonist High affinity and specificity for this receptor Its agonist properties are very weak, and of no importance Reverses the respiratory depression
Pharmacokinetics	Rapidly distributed, with peak effect within 5 min of iv injection Metabolised in liver Action duration <1 h so repeat doses or infusion may be needed
Cautions	Rapid injection in high-risk or anxious patients, or after major surgery Elderly Head injuries (may raise intracranial pressure) Liver impairment Overdoses
Contraindications	Epileptics on prolonged therapy with benzodiazepines
Side-effects	Nausea and vomiting, flushing, agitation, anxiety, fear Pulse and BP increase, convulsions (especially in epileptics)
Dose	300–600 μg (first 200 μg over 15 s and then 100 μg every min) Maximum 1 mg (2 mg in intensive care) Infusion: 100–400 μg/h

47 (**a**) true (**b**) false (**c**) true (**d**) false (**e**) true

Midazolam is an imidazole benzodiazepine.

Differences from diazepam:

- has an imidazole ring
- soluble in water
- no active metabolites

- short duration of action
- high extraction ratio

Midazolam is water soluble in the ampoule but when introduced into the blood with a pH of 7.4 the midazolam ring closes and the molecule becomes lipid soluble.

48 (**a**) false (**b**) true (**c**) true (**d**) true (**e**) false

Neostigmine is a quaternary ammonium, alkyl carbamic acid ester. Produces reversible inhibition of acetylcholinesterase by acylation of the esteratic site – forming a carbamate–ester complex at the esteratic site of the enzyme. The carbamylated acetyl esterase cannot hydrolyse acetylcholine until the carbamate enzyme bond dissociates.

Kinetics

- Poorly lipid soluble
- Does not penetrate the blood brain barrier or the gastro-intestinal tract
- Volume of distribution 0.26l/kg
- Clearance 8ml/kg/min
- t1/2 40min

Effects

- CNS
  - miosis
  - blurred vision
- Cardiovascular system
  - decreased heart rate
  - decreased cardiac output
- Respiratory system
  - decreased anatomical dead space
  - bronchoconstriction

Others

- increased peristalsis (gastrointestinal, ureteric)
- increased lacrimation, sweating
- increased gastric tone

49 **(a)** true **(b)** true **(c)** true **(d)** true **(e)** true

Potentiation of neuromuscular block

Drugs

(a) Volatile anaesthetic agents
- Dose dependent
- Enflurane > isoflurane > desflurane > sevoflurane > halothane
- Mechanism
  - CNS depression
  - decreased skeletal muscle tone

(b) Aminoglycoside antibiotics
- Especially streptomycin and neomycin

(c) Local anaesthetics
- Mechanism
  - decreased prejunctional (acetylcholine) release
  - stabilise postsynaptic membrane
  - direct depolarisation of skeletal muscles

(d) Anti-arrhythmic drugs
- Lidocaine
- Quinidine

(e) Diuretics
- Frusemide

(f) Others
- Magnesium
- Lithium
- Phenytoin
- Steroids
- Cyclosporines
- Ganglionic blocker

Hypothermia

(a) Slows the enzymatic activity in the liver
(b) Decreases clearance

Electrolyte disturbances

(a) Hypokalaemia
(b) Hyperkalaemia
(c) Hypocalcaemia

Acid–base disturbances
(a) Acidosis
(b) Hypocapnia

50 (**a**) true (**b**) false (**c**) true (**d**) false (**e**) true

Class Ia anti-arrhythmic drugs have local anaesthetic properties that exhibit membrane-stabilising activity and affect conduction, refractory period and action potential.

Class Ia drugs have three subdivisions based on their effect on action potential duration:
- slow d*v*/d*t* of phase zero
- decrease conduction velocity
- prolong repolarisation
- prolong PR, QRS, Q-T
- increase action potential duration

51 (**a**) false (**b**) false (**c**) true (**d**) false (**e**) true

Drugs that slow emptying of the stomach and so increase the time for gastric emptying include:
- opioids (systemic and via epidural)
- anticholinergics
- tricyclic antidepressants
- aluminium and magnesium hydroxides
- sympathomimetic drugs
- alcohol
- antihistamines

Drugs that increase the rate of gastric emptying include:
- metoclopramide
- pancuronium
- suxamethonium

52 (**a**) true (**b**) true (**c**) true (**d**) false (**e**) false

Examples of ACE inhibitors include:
- captopril
- enalapril (a pro-drug hydrolysed into enalaprilat)
- lisinopril

- perindopril
- ramipril

Action

- ACE inhibitors block the action of the carboxypeptidase (ACE) in the lungs which converts the inactive angiotensin I (AngI) into the active angiotensin II (AngII)
- Inactivate bradykinin and other kinins

Effects

The effects of ACE inhibitors include a reduction in:

- Na^+ and H_2O retention
- vasomotor tone
- preload
- afterload
- myocardial work

Side-effects

Major:

- angio-oedema
- agranulocytosis
- thrombocytopenia

Minor:

- loss of taste
- rash
- pruritus
- fever
- aphthous ulcer

53 **(a)** true **(b)** true **(c)** true **(d)** false **(e)** true

The effects of intravenous/intramuscular adrenaline vary according to dose.

(a) CVS (at low doses beta effects predominate)
  - Increased cardiac output, which means that venous return must increase and so pulmonary blood flow increases
  - Increased myocardial oxygen consumption
  - Coronary artery dilatation
  - Decreased threshold for arrhythmias

- Decreased diastolic blood pressure
- Decreased systemic vascular resistance (SVR)

At high doses alpha effects predominate

- Increased SVR

(b) Respiratory
- Increased minute volume
- Bronchodilation
- Increased pulmonary vascular resistance

(c) CNS
- When adrenaline is given the minimum alveolar concentration of an anaesthetic rises
- Increased peripheral pain threshold

(d) Renal
- Decreased renal blood flow
- Increased bladder sphincter tone

(e) Metabolic
- Decreased basal metabolic rate
- Increased glucose level

54 (**a**) true (**b**) true (**c**) false (**d**) true (**e**) true

Adenosine is a nucleoside comprising adenine (6-amino purine) and D-ribofuranose (pentose sugar).

Action

It has a specific action on the sinoatrial and atrioventricular (AV) node mediated by adenosine A1 receptors. Opening of K^+ channels, causing hyperpolarisation, and G_i-linked proteins cause a reduction in cAMP. This results in a negative chronotropic effect within the AV node.

Kinetics

Half-life is 8–10 s

Effects

(a) CVS
- Inhibits AV nodal conduction
- Decreases contractility
- Vasodilatation
- Palpitation
- Flushing
- Hypotension
- Severe bradycardia

(b) CNS
- Headache, dizziness
- Blurred vision

(c) Respiratory system
- Dyspnoea
- Bronchospasm

(d) Gastrointestinal system
- Nausea

Contraindications

- Second and third degree heart block
- Sick sinus syndrome
- Asthma

55 (**a**) true (**b**) false (**c**) false (**d**) false (**e**) true

Mannitol is an osmotic diuretic derived from dahlia tubers.

Action

(a) In the tubule lumen, it exerts an osmotic effect, reducing the effective Na concentration thus reducing the reabsorptive gradient for Na^+.

(b) It increases the flux of Na^+ from the interstitial fluid back into the tubular fluid.

(c) It expands extracellular and intravascular fluid volume:
- decreases blood viscosity
- increases medullary blood flow

- impairs medullary concentration gradient
- decreases concentration ability
- increases urine flow

Effects

- Freely filtered at the glomerulus but not reabsorbed at the tubules
- Available as 10% or 20%
- Onset 30 min

Problems

- It does not work if the nephrons are blocked by a disease (e.g. rhabdomyolysis)
- Fluid overload and oedema
- Toxic effects on distal convoluted tubules and the collecting duct

56 (**a**) true (**b**) true (**c**) true (**d**) false (**e**) false

Doxapram acts via the carotid sinus chemoreceptors (and also centrally causing stimulation of the respiratory centre). Its clinical effects last only 5–10 min. Has a high therapeutic index.

57 (**a**) true (**b**) false (**c**) true (**d**) false (**e**) true

Omeprazole is a substituted piperidinyl benzamide.

Action

It is a pro-drug being converted within the parietal cell to sulphonamide, the active form which blocks the proton pump (K^+ /H^+ ATPase) in the membrane of the parietal cell.

Kinetics

Bioavailability	35%
Protein binding	95%
Half-life	24 h
p*Ka*	3.97

Side-effects

CNS	headache, dizziness
CVS	no effect

RS	no effect
Others	rash, pruritus
	eosinophilia
	gynaecomastia
	liver dysfunction
	inhibition of hepatic microsomal P450

58 (**a**) false (**b**) true (**c**) true (**d**) true (**e**) true

Context-sensitive half-time is defined as the time taken for the plasma concentration to decline by half, after termination of an infusion designed to maintain a constant plasma concentration. (Context refers to infusion duration.)

Context-sensitive half-time, in contrast to elimination half-time, considers the combined effects on drug pharmacokinetics of:

- distribution
- metabolism
- infusion duration

Thus, it depends on:

- lipid solubility
- clearance

Context-sensitive half-time increases in parallel with duration of continuous intravenous administration.

In contrast to most agents, remifentanil has a relatively constant context-sensitive half-time.

59 (**a**) true (**b**) true (**c**) false (**d**) true (**e**) true

The side-effects of heparin include

(a) Haemorrhage due to relative overdose

(b) Thrombocytopenia
  - Mild
    - after initial administration
    - due to an anaphylactoid reaction
  - Severe
    - occurs later
    - associated with heparin resistance, serious thrombotic events and high mortality
    - due to hypersensitivity of reaction.

(c) CVS
   - Decreased BP following rapid, large-dose IV
(d) Osteoporosis
(e) Alopecia

60 (**a**) true (**b**) true (**c**) true (**d**) false (**e**) true

Glibenclamide is an antidiabetic sulphonyl/urea derivative.

Uses

- Non-insulin-dependent diabetes mellitus (NIDDM)

Action

- Works at the pancreas
- Displaces insulin from B cells
- Induces B cell hyperplasia
- Reduces glucagon secretion
- Reduces hepatic insulinase activity
- Reduces peripheral resistance to insulin by increasing number and sensitivity of insulin receptors
- Decreases absorption of glucose from the intestine

Kinetics

- Oral bioavailability > 80%
- Highly protein bound (90%–98%)
- Principally bound to albumin

61 (**a**) false (**b**) false (**c**) true (**d**) true (**e**) true

Laminar flow rate is determined by the Hagen–Poiseuille equation.

$$\text{Flow rate } \alpha \ \frac{\Delta P \pi r^4}{8 \eta l}$$

Where ΔP is the pressure gradient along the tube, r is the radius of the tube, l is the length of the tube and η (eta) is the viscosity of the fluid.

62 (**a**) true (**b**) true (**c**) false (**d**) false (**e**) true

The critical temperature is the temperature above which a gas cannot be liquefied by pressure alone.

$$N_2O = 36.5\ ^\circ C$$
$$O_2 = -119\ ^\circ C$$

At or below the critical temperature liquefaction under pressure is possible.

Critical pressure is the pressure at which a gas liquefies at its critical temperature.

$$N_2O = 73 \text{ bar } (7300 \text{ kPa}) \text{ at } 36.5\,^\circ C, \text{ but } O_2 = 51 \text{ bar } (5100 \text{ kPa}) \text{ at } -118\,^\circ C.$$

A gas is a substance in the gaseous phase above its critical temperature.

A vapour is a substance in the gaseous phase below its critical temperature.

Pseudo-critical temperature

For a mixture of gases at a specific pressure, this is defined as the specific temperature at which the individual gases may separate from the gaseous phase.

$$N_2O\ 50\% : O_2\ 50\% = -5.5\,^\circ C \text{ for cylinders (most likely at 117 bar or 11700 kPa)}$$

$$N_2O\ 50\% : O_2\ 50\% = -30^\circ C \text{ for piped gas}$$

63 (**a**) true (**b**) false (**c**) true (**d**) false (**e**) false

A capacitor consists of a pair of conductors (e.g. metal plates) separated by an insulator called a dielectric. Conductors lose and gain electrons easily and therefore allow current to flow. Insulators do not lose their electrons and so do not allow a current to flow.

The function of the capacitor is to store a large amount of energy in the form of electrical charge, then to release it over a short period of time.

The maximum working voltage is the voltage which, when exceeded, causes the dielectric to break down and conduct, often with catastrophic results.

The unit of electrical charge is the coulomb (C), where 1 C is the quantity of electricity transported in 1 s by a current of 1 amp (A). It is equivalent to 6.24×10^{18} electrons.

Capacitance is the ability to store charge.

A capacitance has 1 farad (F) of capacitance if a potential difference of 1 V is present across its plates, when a charge of 1 C is held by them.

$$\text{Capacitance} = \frac{A}{D\,E_0},$$

where A is the area which the plates overlap, D the distance between the plates and E_0 the dielectric constant.

A capacitor prevents a DC current from flowing and allows an AC current to flow.

64 (**a**) true (**b**) false (**c**) false (**d**) false (**e**) false

The latent heat of vaporisation is the amount of heat required to convert 1 kg of a liquid to the gaseous phase at the same temperature.

The latent heat of crystallisation is the amount of heat required to convert 1 kg of a solid into the liquid phase without a change in temperature.

65 (**a**) false (**b**) true (**c**) false (**d**) true (**e**) false

Classification of electrical medical devices

There are number of ways of classifying electrical equipment

(a) Classification by class. This refers to the degree of protection from electrical shock to the operator by insulation and fuses
- Classes I, II, III

(b) Classification by type. This refers to the degree of protection given to the patient from micro shock
- Type B, BF, CF
- Type B and BF can be class I, II or III
- Type CF can be class I or II

(c) Classification by suitability for use in a flammable atmosphere
- AP and APG

(d) Classification based on protection from ingress of water
- IPX classification

Class I, II, III classification

- *Class 1.* Earthed metal outer casing. These devices have a metal case which is insulated and earthed in such a way that exposed metal parts cannot become live. There are fuses on the live and neutral supply in the equipment and a fuse on the live mains supply

- *Class 2.* These devices are double insulated. They are not earthed and only have live and neutral leads with one fuse on the live
- *Class 3.* These devices use a safety extra low-voltage (SELV) power supply. SELV means >24 V (AC) or >40 V (DC). **There is still a risk of micro shock**

All diagnostic, therapeutic, life-support or patient-handling equipment is also classified and labelled as type B, BF or CF. This classification is based on the amount of permissible leakage current. A leakage current is any current which returns by a pathway other than the neutral wire. All electrically operated equipment has some leakage current. This current is not the result of a fault but is a natural consequence of electrical wiring and components. Leakage currents have two major parts: capacitative and resistive.

Type B, BF and CF classification

- Type B: Symbol – matchstick man. Can be class I, II or III, battery or mains powered. The leakage current is low but the device is not safe for connection to the heart. The maximum permissible leakage current is below the threshold for skin sensation (100 μA) and therefore unlikely to cause any pain or injury. These devices have no conductor connection to the patient and include blood pressure monitors, thermometers, manometers, gas analysis, and ventilator alarms

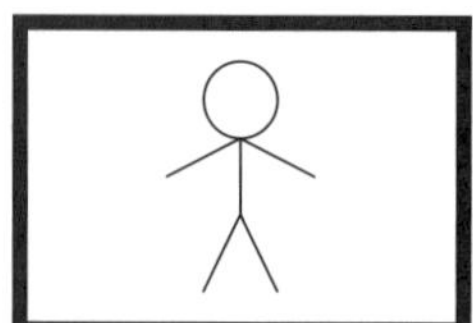

- Type BF symbol – matchstick man in a box. Any part in contact with the patient is isolated from the rest of the device ensuring a very low leakage current so wires can have surface contact with the patient. Safer than Type B but may still cause micro shock to the heart

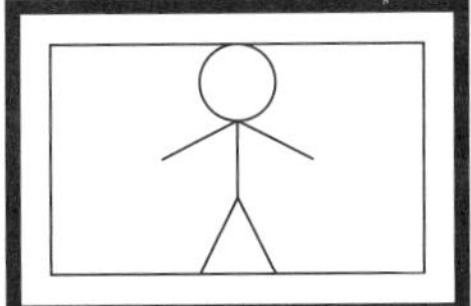

- BF stands for devices fitted with type F isolated circuits (F = floating circuit). The maximum permissible leakage current (100 μA) is similar to that for type B, with the addition of a maximum 5 mA patient leakage when the applied part is raised to mains voltage. These devices are ECG, EEG and EMG monitors and pulse oximeters
- Type CF symbol – heart in a box, can be Class I or II. There is an internal power source, which is separate from, but may be charged from the mains. This allows direct heart contact

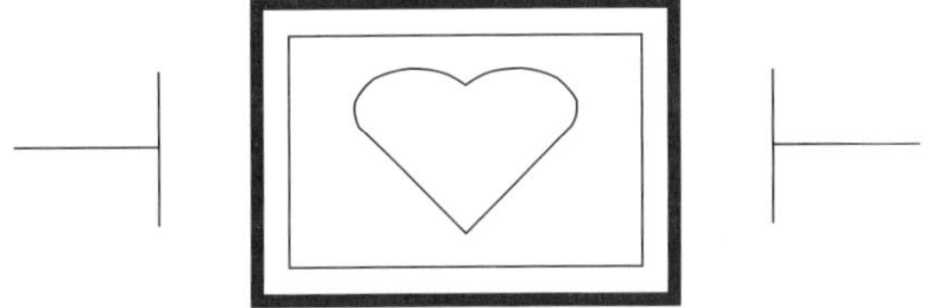

These devices have the most stringent protection against shock hazard, specifically intended for applications where an intra-cardiac connection is likely. The maximum permissible patient leakage current is set at 1/10 (<10 μA) of that for type BF devices. These devices are likely to be connected to cardiac catheters such as syringe drivers, ECG monitors, pacemakers and pressure transducers.

The symbols ⊣ ⊢ are placed either side of the symbol for BF and CF equipment to indicate that the device is safe to use with a defibrillator. The defibrillator current will not short back through the device.

Paper 1 Answers

66 (**a**) true (**b**) false (**c**) false (**d**) false (**e**) true

SI units

- Système International d'Unités (or International System of Units)
- Introduced by a general conference on weights and measures in 1960
- Based on the metric system
- There are base units and derived units

Table 1.66a Base units

Unit	Unit of	Definition
Metre	Length	The distance occupied by 1 650 763.73 wavelengths of light from gaseous krypton It was originally a bar of platinum-iridium against which the metre was calibrated. This ceased to be used after concerns about its loss of a consistent length over time
Second	Time	The definition relates to the frequency of radiation emitted by caesium-133. It is also roughly $\frac{1}{24 \times 60 \times 60}$ of the time taken for the earth to complete one revolution
Kilogram	Mass	There is a standard cylinder of platinum-iridium against which the kilogram is calibrated It is about 37 mm in each dimension and is kept near Paris
Ampere	Electrical current	The current in two straight parallel wires 1 m apart in a vacuum which will produce a force of 2 × 107 newtons/meter on each of the wires
Kelvin	Temperature	0 K – 273.16 °C. The exact definition is 1 K = 1/273.16 of the thermodynamic scale temperature of the triple point of water The triple point of water is the temperature at which water in solid, liquid and gaseous states are in equilibrium
Candela	Luminous intensity	This is the light intensity of a body at the freezing point of platinum
Mole	Substance	The quality of substance containing Avogadro's number of particles (6.022×10^{23}). The number of particles as atoms in 12 g of carbon-12

Table 1.66b Derived units

Unit	Unit of	Definition
Newton	Force	Force = mass × acceleration 1 N is the force required to accelerate a mass of 1 kg by 1 m/s^2
Pascal	Pressure	Pressure is force/area 1 Pa is 1 N/m^2
Joule	Energy work	Potential energy is the energy possessed by a body by virtue of its position Kinetic energy is the energy of the body due to its motion 1 Joule is the work done (energy used) when a force of 1 newton moves 1 metre.
Watt	Power	Power is the rate of doing work. This is work/time 1 W = 1 J/s
Hertz	Frequency	1 H = 1 cycle/s

67 **(a)** true **(b)** false **(c)** true **(d)** true **(e)** false

The term 'diathermy' is terminologically incorrect. Diathermy literally means heat (going) through. However, when diathermy is used it is the electrical current that goes through the body, while the heat that it produces is confined to the intended site of action. Therefore, the correct term should be 'electrosurgery'.

Definition

Diathermy relies on the heating effect of an electrical current.
Current density refers to the current per unit cross-sectional area (watts/unit area). With a large conductive area there is very low current density and the heat generated is rapidly conducted away. At a contact point of an active electrode the current density is very high and the heat is generated over a very small area, thereby creating a surgical effect.

Types of diathermy

- Monopolar
- Bipolar

They are optimised for cutting or coagulation of the tissues.

Types of current

The current can be

- DC
- High-frequency AC

If the household electricity, which is of a frequency of 50 cycles per second (Hz), passes through the body the electrical energy causes excitation of body tissue. In the case of the heart this can lead to ventricular fibrillation (VF) or sustained cardiac contraction (tetanus). For this to happen the organ must be energised with at least a threshold quantity of electrical energy. Electrical charge is measured in coulombs (c) or ampere × seconds.

In the case of a diathermy current, its frequency is of the order of 0.4–3.0 (Mhz) and therefore whatever the current (amperes) it does not flow in one direction for a sufficient length of time to reach the threshold quantum of electrical energy to stimulate the heart.

The sensitivity markedly decreases as the frequency is increased beyond 10 kHz.

Energy delivered

The rate of heat produced depends on:

- current I (measured in amperes)
- resistance R (measured in ohms)

$$\text{Power } (W) = I^2R$$

For a definition of a watt in terms of heat equivalent:

$$1 \text{ W} = 0.24 \text{ cal/s}$$

Note

- Monopolar diathermy generates 50–500 W
- Bipolar diathermy generates 40 W

Monopolar diathermy

Genenosrates electrical energy at 200 kHz to 6 MHz. The energy is applied between two electrodes: neutral and active

(a) The neutral electrode has a large conductive surface area producing a low current density with no measurable heating effect.

(b) The active electrode has a very small contact area producing a very high current density. Therefore, the heating effect beneath the active electrode is considerable.

Bipolar diathermy

The output is applied between the points of a special pair of forceps producing a high local current density with no current passing through the rest of the body.

Dangers and precautions

(a) Electrical burns due to poor contact between the neutral plate and the patient. This can be prevented by an audible warning if the plate is not plugged in or the lead is broken.

(b) Inadvertent depression of the foot switch can be prevented by:
- keeping the forceps in a protective quiver
- installation of a buzzer which is activated when the switch is depressed

(c) If the electrical circuit is completed via the operating table or other points through which the patient may be earthed.

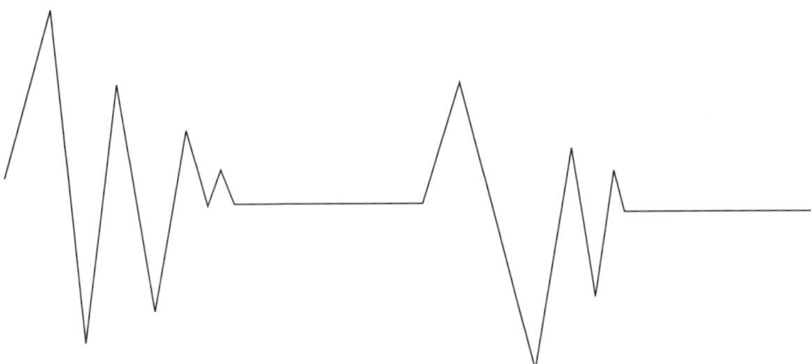

Risks are reduced by the use of

(a) Isolating capacitors in diathermy equipment. This is because capacitors have a high impedance to low-frequency (50 Hz) current, but a low impedance to high-frequency (1 Mhz) current, so damaging effects of all stray mains current are minimised.

(b) Isolating transformer. The design of the circuit prevents the flow of current to earth by any alternative earth-linked path from a fault in the generator; should the circuit be broken, the diathermy is deactivated.

Paper 1 Answers

68 (**a**) true (**b**) false (**c**) true (**d**) true (**e**) false

- The mean is the average of the population
- Arithmetical mean = (sum of observation)/number of observation
- Geometric mean is calculated using:
  - the logarithm of the values measured
  - the arithmetic mean of logarithms
  - the antilog of the calculated arithmetic mean

$$G_Y = (Y_1 \times Y_2; \text{times } Y_3 \ldots Y_N)^{1/N}, \text{ or } \log G = (\Sigma \log Y)N,$$

where Y_1, Y_2, Y_3, ... Y_N, the individual measurements, are multiplied together and the *N*th root taken; or, the arithmetic mean of their logarithms is calculated and the antilog of this is taken.

- Mode is the most commonly observed value in a series of values; it is the maximum point in the frequency distribution
- Median is that measurement that lies exactly halfway between each end of a range of values ranked in order; it is not sensitive to extreme values in arteries
- Standard deviation is a measure of the spread of the observations about the mean:

$$\text{SD} = \sqrt{\text{Variance}}$$

69 (**a**) false (**b**) false (**c**) false (**d**) true (**e**) true

- This type of gauge is a mechanical device that uses the pressure being measured to operate a mechanism coupled to a point
- It can be used to measure high and low pressures
- Usually employed when measuring pressure greater than 1 bar (100 k Pa)

Advantages

- Simple technology
- Mechanically robust
- Convenient to use
- Operate in any position
- Does not require power supply
- Suitable for high or low pressures

Disadvantages

- Not easily recalibrated
- Not suitable for very low pressures

Problems in practice and safety features

- Each pressure gauge is colour-coded and calibrated for a particular gas or vapour
- The face of the pressure gauge is made of heavy glass as an additional safety feature

Bourdon gauge

Components

- Flexible and coiled tube, which is oval in cross-section. It should be able to withstand the sudden high pressure when the cylinder is switched on
- The tube is sealed at the inner end and connected to a needle pointer, which moves over a dial
- The other end of the tube is exposed to a gas supply

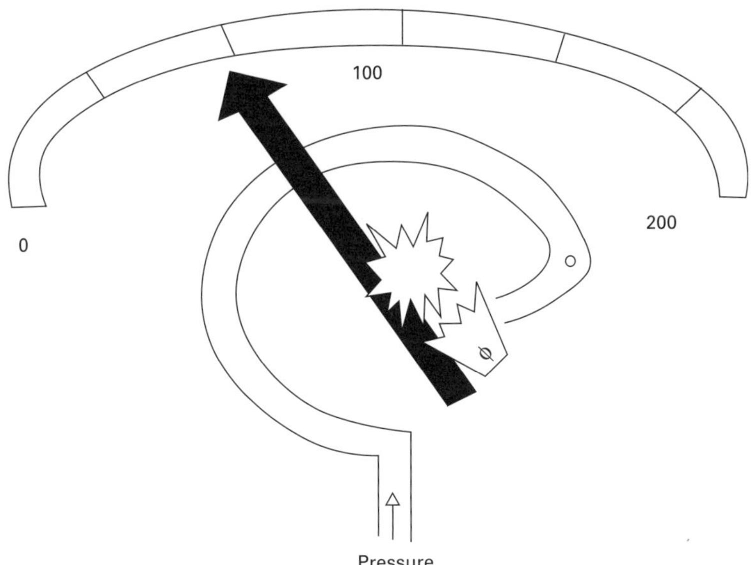

Action

- The high-pressure gas causes the tube to uncoil
- The movement of the tube causes the needle pointer to move on the calibrated dial indicating the pressure

Aneroid gauge

Components

- A bellows, which expands or contracts depending on the pressure across it
- This expansion drives a pointer over a scale

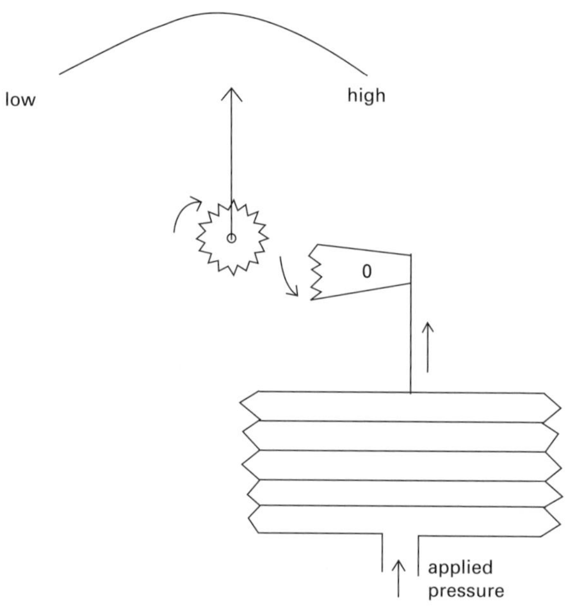

70 (**a**) false (**b**) false (**c**) false (**d**) true (**e**) true

Paramagnetism is used to determine oxygen concentration. Graham's law of diffusion states that the rate of diffusion of a gas is inversely proportional to its density. The Clark cell has a platinum cathode and the fuel cell a gold mesh cathode. At the cathode oxygen combines with water and four electrons to form hydroxyl ions.

$$O_2 + 2H_2O + 4\,e^- \rightarrow 4OH^-$$

The current generated by the reaction is proportional to the concentration of oxygen present. In the mass spectrometer molecules are ionised by bombarding them with a beam of electrons so that each molecule carries a positive charge.

71 (**a**) true (**b**) true (**c**) false (**d**) true (**e**) true

Measurement of aortic cross-sectional area and blood flow allows calculation of cardiac output. Acceleration and peak velocity indicate myocardial performance, while flow time is related to circulating volume and peripheral resistance.

72 (**a**) true (**b**) false (**c**) true (**d**) true (**e**) false

Oxygen is obtained commercially from the atmosphere by the liquefaction and fractional distillation of air. Liquid air is a mixture of liquid nitrogen, boiling point −196 °C, and liquid oxygen, boiling point −183 °C. The nitrogen is more volatile (i.e. it has a lower boiling point) and boils off first during evaporation. Because some oxygen evaporates with the nitrogen, separation of the two gases is brought about by fractionation (i.e. by letting the evolved gas mixture bubble through liquid air rich in oxygen in a tall rectifying column). The oxygen in the gas mixture condenses and almost pure nitrogen gas leaves the top of the column, leaving almost pure liquid oxygen which is then evaporated to give oxygen gas. The oxygen gas is distributed as a compressed gas in high-pressure cylinders.

73 (**a**) true (**b**) true (**c**) false (**d**) true (**e**) false

A pneumotachograph is a fast-response measuring system based on a form of constant-orifice flow meter.

It consists of a pneumatic resistance, across which a pressure difference is generated when gas flow occurs, and a means of measuring that pressure difference.

There are a number of designs of airflow resistance. Most of these are essentially bundles of small-bore tubes placed longitudinally in the gas flow.

These provide a linear resistance so that the pressure drop varies directly with flow rate, in accordance with Poiseuille's law.

Problems

- Temperature change can affect the accuracy of the gas flow by altering viscosity
- Water vapour condensation can block the fine orifices and tubing

74 (**a**) true (**b**) true (**c**) false (**d**) true (**e**) true

- The stimulus should produce a monophasic, rectangular waveform (square wave) because biphasic pulses may cause repetitive firing, thus increasing the response to stimulation
- Length of the pulse should not exceed 0.2–0.3 ms because a pulse width greater than 0.5 ms exceeds the refractory period of the nerve and can induce two separate action potentials. Conversely a pulse width less than 0.1 ms must be used with a very large current to ensure nerve stimulation
- Stimulation at a constant current is preferable to stimulation at constant voltage as the current is the determinant of nerve stimulation

  NB Constant-current nerve stimulators are the safest. As the resistance of the electrodes goes up they compensate by increasing their voltage. As a result the current stays constant. The stimulation of the nerve remains constant
- Should be battery operated
- Should be able to generate no more than 80 mA current
- Polarity of the electrode should be indicated
- A pulse current amplitude appropriate for the particular application. Low amplitude (0.5–5.0 mA) for needle electrodes and higher amplitudes for skin electrodes (10–40 mA)

75 (**a**) true (**b**) true (**c**) false (**d**) false (**e**) false

Serum osmolarity is the number of moles per litre of solution.

Serum osmolality is the number of moles per kilogram of solvent.

Measurement

- Depression of freezing point (osmolality). This is the osmotic effect exerted by the sum of all dissolved molecules and ions across a membrane permeable only to water. NB The depression of the freezing point of a solution is directly proportional to the osmolality, 1 mol of a solute added to 1 kg of water depresses the freezing point by 1.86 °C
- Calculated (osmolarity). Total = $2 \times (Na^+ + K^+)$ + urea and glucose, all units are mmol/l
  - The factor 2 for Na^+ and K^+ is for equal quantities of associated anions and assume complete ionization
  - Normal serum osmolarity is 290 mmol/l

Albumin provides 80% of plasma oncotic pressure. Although albumin is the most abundant serum protein it contributes little to the plasma osmolarity as the concentration is about 0.6 mmol/l when expressed in SI units.

76 (**a**) false (**b**) true (**c**) true (**d**) true (**e**) true

- A Wright's respirometer is a mechanical device which is prone to error at high and low flows

77 (**a**) false (**b**) true (**c**) false (**d**) false (**e**) false

- Mass spectrometry measures agents according to their molecular mass so agents of identical molecular weight can only be identified by their isotopes
- Ultraviolet analyser. Although many gases will absorb ultraviolet radiation, including CO_2 and N_2, a clinical analyser has been developed only for halothane. Its principle is the same as that of infrared analysers
- Infrared analyser. The wavelength of peak absorption is specific to each gas and by the use of variable filters, infrared analysers can be used to measure several gases
- Piezoelectric analysers are not specific to individual anaesthetic agents, and respond to a limited extent to water vapour
- Refractometers are non-specific and may be used for measuring the concentration of a variety of different gases

78 (**a**) false (**b**) true (**c**) true (**d**) false (**e**) false

- The currents used in the TENS stimulator are up to 60 mA
- The pulse durations are between 60 and 380 ms
- The pulse frequency is 2–200 Hz

79 (**a**) true (**b**) true (**c**) false (**d**) true (**e**) true

- An adiabatic change in the volume of a gas involves no transfer of heat to or from the system
- At the boiling point of a substance additional heat does not raise the temperature but provides the latent heat of vaporisation necessary for boiling
- Transfer of heat requires a temperature gradient and therefore no exchange occurs between substances at the same temperature
- As heat capacity increases, the quantity of heat required to raise the temperature of a mass increases, therefore the response time of a thermometer would increase with its heat capacity

80 (**a**) true (**b**) true (**c**) true (**d**) true (**e**) true

- Linear regression is mainly used when there is one measured dependent variable (*X*) and one or more independent variables (*Y*)
- Used when the main purpose is to develop a predictive model; that is, to predict *Y* for a given value of *X*:
  - multiple regressions predict a single dependent variable using a number of independent variables
  - *Y* is a random variable

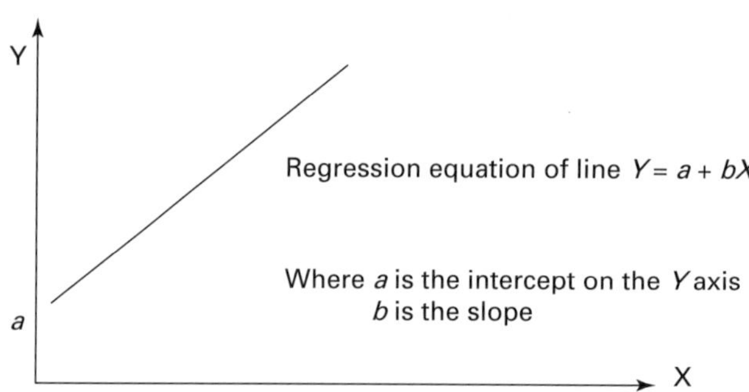

- Y is a dependent variable in a linear regression

$$Y = \alpha + \beta X$$

- Where X is an independent variable capable of measurement without an error. Alpha is a parameter called the intercept of the line; it is the value of Y when $X = 0$.
- Beta is also called the regression coefficient; it is a measure of the slope of the line, i.e the change in Y per unit increase in X

81 (**a**) true (**b**) false (**c**) true (**d**) false (**e**) false

- The forces of attraction, which act on molecules in the surface layer, act in a direction parallel to the surface of the liquid and result in the liquid surface behaving as though a skin were present. This phenomenon is known as surface tension
- Surface tension is expressed in terms of force per unit length (newton per metre)
- Surface tension may influence the readings when narrow capillary tubes are used by
  - increasing the reading in the case of a water manometer
  - decreasing the reading in the case of a mercury manometer
- Laplace's Law states that

$$P = \frac{2T}{R}, \text{ where}$$

  - P is the pressure gradient across the wall of sphere
  - T is the surface tension
  - R is the radius of the sphere
- Therefore, the pressure is inversely proportional to the radius

82 (**a**) true (**b**) true (**c**) true (**d**) false (**e**) false

The spirometer is the standard method for measuring the lung volumes except for residual volume and the capacities involving residual volume. A different approach is required to measure residual volume, functional residual capacity and total lung capacity. Two of the most common methods of obtaining information about these volumes are gas dilution tests and body plethysmography.

In body plethysmography, the patient sits inside an airtight box, inhales or exhales to a particular volume (usually functional residual capacity), and then a shutter drops across their breathing tube. The subject makes respiratory efforts against the closed shutter (this looks, and feels, like panting), causing their chest volume to expand and decompressing the air in their lungs. The increase in their chest volume slightly reduces the box volume (the non-person volume of the box) and thus slightly increases the pressure in the box.

Using the data from the plethysmography requires use of Boyle's law.

83 (**a**) false (**b**) false (**c**) true (**d**) true (**e**) false

The bar is a unit used for high-pressure gas supplies (it is not an SI unit)

$$
\begin{aligned}
1\,\text{bar} &= 100\ \text{Kpa} \\
&= 1\ \text{atm} \\
&= 1\ \text{kg wt/cm}^2 \\
&= 14.5\ \text{pounds(lb)/in}^2 \\
&= 7.5\ \text{torr} \\
&= 750\ \text{mmHg} \\
&= 1000.2\ \text{cmH}_2\text{O}
\end{aligned}
$$

84 (**a**) false (**b**) false (**c**) true (**d**) false (**e**) true

The mol is an SI unit. It is defined as the quantity of a substance containing Avogadro's number of particles (6.022×10^{23}) or the number of atoms in 12 g of carbon-12.

One gram molecule of a substance as a gas occupies 22.4 l and exerts an osmotic pressure of 1 bar at 273 K.

85 (**a**) true (**b**) false (**c**) false (**d**) false (**e**) true

All gases supplied in the pipeline are at 4 bar = 404 kPa or 4×10^5 Pa or 60 psi except for compressed air which is at 700 kPa or 105 psi. Oxygen analysers will test that oxygen leaves the oxygen line but not the pressure or the integrity of the other lines. All the piped medical gases supplied to theatres and other areas finish in special terminal units with a non-interchangeable coupling that has two diameters in each shaft which are gas specific. The terminal outlet into which the Schrader probe fits contains a mechanism to seal off the flow when the probe is withdrawn but not a one-way valve.

86 (**a**) true (**b**) true (**c**) true (**d**) false (**e**) true

Blood passes through a filter of a highly permeable, parallel, flat plate membrane of polysulphone, polyamide or polyacrylonitrile, which is the most efficient. The pore size of the membrane should allow molecules of up to 50 000 Dal to pass through. The extracorporeal pump requires anticoagulation with heparin 200–1000 units/h, monitoring the activated partial thromboplastin time (aPTT). There are two main types of haemofiltration.

(a) Arteriovenous. Blood passes across a highly porous filter membrane by convection, driven by the pressure gradient between the patient's blood pressure and the ultrafiltrate side of the filter. The volume of ultrafiltrate is 10–14 l/day. The water and solutes that are lost are replaced.
(b) Veno-venous. This requires a dual-lumen, large-bore cannula and a peristaltic pump which creates the higher transmembrane pressure. The volume of ultrafiltrate is > 35 l/day.

The ultrafiltrate (UF) volume is determined by a number of factors: the type of membrane; the haematocrit and serum albumin concentration; the type of vascular access; the patient's mean arterial blood pressure; pump flow rate; and suction pressure to the UF port. The transmembrane pressure (TMP) = hydrostatic pressure – oncotic pressure.

The UF contains solutes such as urea, creatinine, electrolytes, drugs and cytokines. Solute clearance is by convection, which increases as the UF volume increases. If a dialysate is passed through the UF side of the filter, chemical gradients increase solute clearance. Glucose can be given to the patient to increase the chemical gradient. Creatinine clearance ranges from 10 ml/min (hollow fibre) to 20 ml/min (parallel plate), increasing to 25 ml/min if a dialysate is used.

Indications

- Acute renal failure
- LVF secondary to volume overload
- Septic shock
- Poisoning
- ECMO

Contraindications

- Inadequate facilities, equipment, trained staff, or medical expertise unavailable

Complications

Related to the vascular access and the extracorporeal circuit: haemorrhage, infection, vascular occlusion, thrombosis, limb ischaemia, air embolism, hypovolaemia, electrolyte disturbances, heparin-induced thrombocytopenia, complement activation, metabolic alkalosis if much lactate is used, removal of drugs and nutrients including elements in parenteral nutrition.

87 (**a**) true (**b**) true (**c**) false (**d**) true (**e**) true

- The Student's *t*-test was invented by W.S. Gosset, a Guinness sampler in Dublin, who signed himself 'student' or 't' for short
- It is the most sensitive test for genuine differences based on the *t*-distribution
- It is used for comparing a single small sample (less than 60) with the general population, or to compare the difference in means between two small samples
- It is inappropriate if more than two means are being compared
- As the sample size increases then the *t* distribution closely resembles the normal distribution and at infinite degrees of freedom the *t* and normal distributions are identical

$$\text{Calculated } t \text{ value} = \frac{\text{observed difference in means}}{\text{standard error of the difference in means}}$$

- The calculated *t* value is compared with a critical *t* value from tables at a predetermined significance level and appropriate degrees of freedom
- The larger the value of *t* (+ or −) the smaller the value of *P* and the stronger the evidence that the null hypothesis can be rejected

88 (**a**) false (**b**) true (**c**) true (**d**) false (**e**) true

Mains electricity passing through the body at 1 mA causes a tingle, 5 mA causes pain, 15 mA is the threshold at which muscle spasm makes it impossible to let go; 50 mA causes respiratory arrest; 75 mA causes cardiac arrest; 100 mA causes ventricular fibrillation. The heart stops in systole if 5 A passes through the body. Class 1 equipment must be fully earthed. Class

III equipment can only work with a low voltage (<24 V). The leakage current from any equipment which can come in contact with the heart must be less than 50 mA to prevent microshock.

89 (**a**) true (**b**) true (**c**) true (**d**) true (**e**) true

Mechano-myography uses a strain gauge to measure the tension generated in a muscle. For light intensity measurements an electrical resistance strain gauge is used.

90 (**a**) true (**b**) true (**c**) true (**d**) true (**e**) false

Doppler ultrasound has many applications and qualitative and quantitative assessment of cardiac function is one of them. The method actually measures velocity, which, when averaged and multiplied by the cross-sectional area of the flow (for example, of the aorta), gives an estimate of cardiac output. The ultrasound probe is positioned behind the aorta, near its origin. The ultrasound waves, which are produced by a piezoelectric crystal, are in the range of 2.5–5.0 MHz. The same transducer alternatively transmits the wave for 1 μs and detects the reflected waves for a period of 250 μs. Some heads use separate transmission and receiving transducers.

MCQ answers primary paper 1

	(a)	(b)	(c)	(d)	(e)
1	F	T	T	F	F
2	F	T	T	T	T
3	F	F	T	T	F
4	T	T	F	F	F
5	T	F	T	T	T
6	T	T	F	F	T
7	F	F	T	T	T
8	F	F	T	T	F
9	T	T	T	T	T
10	F	F	F	T	F
11	F	F	F	F	T
12	F	T	F	T	T
13	F	T	F	F	F
14	T	F	F	F	F
15	F	T	F	T	F
16	T	T	F	T	T
17	T	F	F	F	F
18	T	T	F	F	T
19	T	F	T	F	F
20	T	F	T	F	T
21	T	T	T	F	T
22	T	F	T	F	T
23	F	F	F	F	T
24	T	T	T	F	T
25	F	T	F	F	T
26	F	F	T	T	F
27	T	F	T	T	T
28	T	T	F	T	F
29	F	F	T	T	F

	(a)	(b)	(c)	(d)	(e)
30	F	F	F	T	T
31	F	F	T	T	T
32	F	F	T	T	T
33	F	F	F	F	F
34	F	F	F	T	T
35	F	T	T	T	F
36	T	F	F	F	T
37	F	F	T	F	F
38	F	F	F	T	F
39	F	T	F	T	T
40	T	T	T	F	F
41	F	F	F	F	F
42	F	F	F	F	T
43	F	F	T	T	T
44	F	F	F	T	F
45	F	F	F	F	T
46	T	F	T	F	F
47	T	F	T	F	T
48	F	T	T	T	F
49	T	T	T	T	T
50	T	F	T	F	T
51	F	F	T	F	T
52	T	T	T	F	F
53	T	T	T	F	T
54	T	T	F	T	T
55	T	F	F	F	T
56	T	T	T	F	F
57	T	F	T	F	T
58	F	T	T	T	T
59	T	T	F	T	T
60	T	T	T	F	T

	(a)	(b)	(c)	(d)	(e)
61	F	F	T	T	T
62	T	T	F	F	T
63	T	F	T	F	F
64	T	F	F	F	F
65	F	T	F	T	F
66	T	F	F	F	T
67	T	F	T	T	F
68	T	F	T	T	F
69	F	F	F	T	T
70	F	F	F	T	T
71	T	T	F	T	T
72	T	F	T	T	F
73	T	T	F	T	F
74	T	T	F	T	T
75	T	T	F	F	F
76	F	T	T	T	T
77	F	T	F	F	F
78	F	T	T	F	F
79	T	T	F	T	T
80	T	T	T	T	T
81	T	F	T	F	F
82	T	T	T	F	F
83	F	F	T	T	F
84	F	F	T	F	T
85	T	F	F	F	T
86	T	T	T	F	T
87	T	T	F	T	T
88	F	T	T	F	T
89	T	T	T	T	T
90	T	T	T	T	F

Paper 2 Answers

1 (**a**) false (**b**) true (**c**) true (**d**) false (**e**) false

Myocardial blood supply is derived entirely from the right and left coronary arteries. Blood flows from the epicardium to the endocardial vessels. Blood returns to the right atrium via the coronary sinus and the anterior cardiac veins after perfusing the myocardium. A small amount of blood returns directly into the chambers of the heart by way of the thebesian veins.

Normal coronary blood flow is 250 ml/min (5% of cardiac output at rest).

Factors which determine coronary blood flow are:

(a) Coronary perfusion pressure (CPP)
- Is unique in that it is intermittent rather than continuous
- Is determined by the difference between aortic pressure and ventricular pressure; the left ventricle is perfused almost entirely during diastole, in contrast to the right ventricle that is perfused during both systole and diastole
- CPP = aortic diastolic pressure – LVEDP
- Autoregulation operates over a range of CPP between 60 and 180 mmHg.

(b) Extravascular compression. This is the external compression produced by myocardial contraction during the cardiac cycle.

(c) Duration of diastole, which is inversely related to heart rate.

(d) Metabolic control, under normal conditions changes in blood flow are entirely due to variations in coronary arterial tone (resistance) in response to metabolic demand.
- Oxygen. Hypoxia either directly or indirectly, through the release of adenosine, causes coronary vasodilation.
- Other factors:
  - adenine nucleotide
  - CO_2
  - lactate potassium

- H^+ ions
- prostaglandins
- histamine

(e) Neurohormonal
- Autonomic influences are generally weak
- Both α and β2 adrenergic receptors are present in the coronary arteries
- Sympathetic stimulation generally increases myocardial blood flow because of an increase in metabolic demand and a predomination of β2 receptor activation
- The parasympathetic system plays a minor role as a vasodilator

2 (**a**) false (**b**) false (**c**) true (**d**) true (**e**) true

Parathyroid hormone (PTH) is secreted by the parathyroid glands as a polypeptide containing 84 amino acids. The main physiological actions of parathyroid hormone are:

(a) Mobilisation of calcium from bone by stimulating osteoclasts to reabsorb bone mineral, liberating calcium into blood.

(b) Enhancing absorption of calcium from the small intestine indirectly by stimulating production of the active form of vitamin D in the kidney. Vitamin D induces the synthesis of a calcium-binding protein in intestinal epithelial cells that facilitates efficient absorption of calcium into blood.

(c) Suppression of calcium loss in urine. This effect is mediated by stimulating tubular reabsorption of calcium. Another effect of PTH on the kidney is to stimulate loss of phosphate ions in urine.

3 (**a**) true (**b**) true (**c**) true (**d**) false (**e**) false

The absolute refractory period refers to the time when the cell will not respond regardless of the strength of stimulus.
- Refractory means 'unresponsive' or stubborn
- In physiology, it refers to the period of time when a muscle or nerve cell is unresponsive to stimulation
- The absolute refractory period in skeletal and heart muscle lasts about as long as the action potential (250 ms in heart muscle)
- The relative refractory period refers to the time when the cell will respond only if the stimulus is 'suprathreshold'

4 (**a**) true (**b**) true (**c**) false (**d**) false (**e**) false

Most of the blood from the bronchial circulation drains into the left side of the heart via the pulmonary veins. This deoxygenated blood makes up part of the normal physiological shunt present in the body. The other component of physiological shunt is from the thebesian veins, which drain some coronary blood directly into the chambers of the heart.

The coronary sinus is the main drainage channel of venous blood from the myocardium. It is the main derivative of the left horn of the sinus venosus of fetal life. It is situated within the atrioventricular groove on the posterior surface of the heart between the left atrium and ventricle. It starts towards the left of the groove at the point at which it receives the oblique vein of the left atrium. It passes to the right and inferiorly to terminate by draining into the right atrium at the coronary sinus orifice.

5 (**a**) false (**b**) false (**c**) false (**d**) true (**e**) true

Pulmonary surfactant is a lipid, surface-tension-lowering agent.

Composition

Dipalmitoylphosphatidylcholine (DPPC)	60%
Phosphatidylglycine	5%
Other phospholipids	10%
Neutral lipids	13%
Proteins	8%
Carbohydrates	2%

Synthesis

Type II alveolar epithelial cells produce it. These are pneumocytes regulated by the hypothalamic–pituitary axis. They are cuboidal cells with large nuclei.

Mechanism of action

The molecules of DPPC are:

- hydrophobic at one end
- hydrophilic at the other end

The hydrophilic ends align themselves in the alveolar surface. When this occurs their intermolecular forces repulse one another and oppose the normal attracting forces between the surface molecules, which are responsible for surface tension.

Function

(a) It lowers the surface tension in the wall of alveoli:
- it will increase the compliance of the lung
- it reduces the work of expanding the lung

(b) It promotes alveolar stability
(c) It helps to keep the alveoli dry

Factors that increase the amount of surfactant produced by a fetus or neonate include:
- prolonged rupture of membranes
- maternal hypertension and pre-eclampsia
- steroids given to the mother
- sickle cell disease in the mother
- alcohol abuse by the mother

The amount of surfactant produced by a fetus or neonate is reduced by insulin.

Surfactant's ability to lower surface tension is directly proportional to its concentration within the alveolus; according to the Law of Laplace

$$P = 2T/R$$

Where P = pressure across the wall, T = tension in the wall, R = radius of the alveolus.

6 (**a**) true (**b**) false (**c**) false (**d**) true (**e**) true

The determinants of bronchomotor tone are:

(a) Parasympathetic nerves
- Afferent irritant receptors, especially at the carina
- Efferent vagus fibres with ganglia in the bronchial walls. Postganglionic neurones release acetylcholine which acts on muscarinic receptors

(b) Sympathetic
- There is little direct innervation but they may modulate parasympathetic pathways
- Many beta-2 receptors respond to circulating catecholamines

(c) Non-adrenergic, non-cholinergic (NANC)
  - Both bronchodilator and bronchoconstrictor through NANC neurones

7 (**a**) true (**b**) false (**c**) false (**d**) false (**e**) false

The oxygen content of blood is the volume of O_2 carried in each 100 ml of blood. It is calculated from the sum of the:

- O_2 carried by haemoglobin (Hb)
- O_2 dissolved in solution

$$O_2 \text{ content} = O_2 \text{ carried by Hb} + O_2 \text{ dissolved in solution,}$$

where,

$$O_2 \text{ carried by Hb} = O_2 \text{ saturation} \times O_2 \text{ carrying capacity} \times \text{Hb concentration}$$

- % sat of Hb with $O_2 = SPO_2$
- O_2 carrying capacity: 1 g of Hb can carry 1.39 ml theoretically but 1.34 ml by direct measurement of O_2 when it is fully saturated
- Hb concentration is given in g/100 ml.

and

$$O_2 \text{ dissolved in solution} = \textit{partial pressure } O_2 \times \text{ solubility coefficient of } O_2$$

- partial pressure of $O_2 = PO_2$ (arterial/venous)
- solubility coefficient of $O_2 = 0.023$ (ml/100 ml per kPa)

Normal arterial blood O_2 content (CaO_2) can be calculated using a SPO_2 of 100%

- O_2 carrying capacity $= 1.34$ ml/g Hb
- Hb concentration $= 15$ g/100 ml
- $P_aO_2 = 13.3$ kPa

$$= (1.34 \times 15) + (13.3 \times 0.023)$$
$$= \mathbf{20.4\ ml/100ml}.$$

Normal mixed-venous blood O_2 content (CVO_2)

- $SVO_2 = 75\%$
- O_2 carrying capacity $= 1.34$ ml/g Hb

- Hb concentration = 15 g/100 ml
  - $PVO_2 = 6.0$ kPa

$$= (0.75 \times 1.34 \times 15) + (6.0 \times 0.023)$$
$$= \mathbf{15.2\ ml/100\ ml}$$

Normal arteriovenous O_2 difference

It is the difference between the normal arterial O_2 content (CaO_2) and the normal mixed-venous blood O_2 content:

$$CaO_2 - CVO_2 = 20.4 - 15.2\ \text{ml}/100\ \text{ml}$$
$$= \mathbf{5.2\ ml/100\ ml}$$

8 **(a)** false **(b)** true **(c)** true **(d)** true **(e)** true

Acclimatisation to altitude occurs because of several compensatory mechanisms.

(a) Respiratory changes
- Hyperventilation due to hypoxia. Alveolar ventilation rises by up to 4 times
- Respiratory alkalosis produced by hyperventilation shifts the oxyhaemoglobin dissociation curve (ODC) to the left. But there is a concomitant increase in red blood cell 2,3-DPG, which tends to decrease the O_2 affinity of haemoglobin. The net effect is an increase in P_{50}
- Increased diffusion capacity of the lungs

(b) Cardiovascular changes
- Cardiac output often increases by as much as 30%
- Increased vascularity and capillary density
- Increased pulmonary artery pressure

(c) Haematological changes
- Increased 2,3-DPG concentration
- Increased Hb production
- Increased erythropoietin secretion

(d) Miscellaneous
- Increased number of mitochondria
- Increased cellular use of oxygen

9 (**a**) false (**b**) false (**c**) false (**d**) false (**e**) true

The P_{50} on the oxygen dissociation curve is:

- the O_2 tension at which the Hb is 50% saturated
- normally 3.5–3.9 kPa
- a measure of the shift of the curve to the right or to the left
- increased when the curve shifts to the right.

A shift to the right means more O_2 is given up to the tissues due to a decreased affinity of haemoglobin for O_2. O_2 is more easily displaced from the Hb.

Factors that increase P_{50} are:

- increased H^+
- reduced pH
- increased PCO_2
- increased temperature
- increased 2,3-DPG (by products of glycolysis) accumulated during anaerobic metabolism

Others:

- abnormal haemoglobins
- anaemia

10 (**a**) true (**b**) false (**c**) false (**d**) true (**e**) true

Hyperventilation is an abnormally increased pulmonary ventilation. This results in a reduction of carbon dioxide tension and, if persistent, can lead to the development of an alkalosis. Respiratory alkalosis leads to an increased binding of plasma calcium and reduced ionised calcium (effective hypocalcaemia).

Possible causes of hyperventilation in the presence of a normal chest X-ray and no abnormal lung signs include:

- psychiatric illness, e.g. hysteria
- pulmonary emboli
- initial stages of pulmonary oedema
- an interstitial lung disease
- hyperthyroidism
- fever

- metabolic acidosis, for example diabetic ketoacidosis
- weakness of the respiratory muscles
- lymphangitis carcinomatosis
- stimulation of the central nervous system:
  - drugs, e.g. salicylate poisoning
  - irritative lesions, e.g. cerebral tumours, stroke, infections

Prolonged hyperventilation will lower the PCO_2. This in turn will reduce cerebral blood flow and lactate production. It will also shift the oxygen dissociation curve to the left and may cause vasoconstriction. Renal compensation for this lower PCO_2 will involve reabsorption of bicarbonate and excretion of H^+ in the urine. Active hyperventilation may be associated with a decreased mixed-venous PO_2 since this depends on oxygen demand, oxygen delivery and tissue oxygen extraction.

11 (**a**) false (**b**) false (**c**) false (**d**) false (**e**) true

Glucose is freely filtered by the glomerulus with a fractional excretion of less than 0.1%. Adults excrete about 65 mg of glucose per day. Reabsorption of glucose occurs predominantly on the brush border membrane of the convoluted segment of the proximal tubule. Glucose enters the tubular cells by an active carrier-mediated transport process, which is sodium dependent, and exits via the basolateral membrane by facilitated diffusion by a glucose transporter, which is sodium independent.

Glucose reabsorption is age dependent. In premature infants of less than 30 weeks' gestation, glycosuria is quite common because the filtered load of glucose delivered to the kidney is often too high for the immature nephron to handle. Glycosuria normally occurs when the plasma glucose content is above 300 mg/dl, but some glucose may be seen in the urine at plasma glucose levels as low as 150 mg/dl because there is a great deal of variability in the glucose-handling capacity of individual nephrons. This variability arises from variations in the length of the proximal tubule and differences in glomerular size and location.

Tubular maximum for glucose (Tm glucose, mg/min per 1.73 m^2) corrected for the glomerular filtration rate (GFR) does not vary as a function of age. Tm glucose/GFR (mg/ml) presents as follows

infants	0.9–2.94 mg/ml
children	1.82–2.94 mg/ml
adults	2.31–2.70 mg/ml

The Tm glucose for children expressed in mg/min per 1.73 m^2 is as follows:

premature infants	25–190 mg/ml
term infants	36–288 mg/ml
children	254–401 mg/ml

12 (a) false (b) false (c) true (d) true (e) false

The glomerulus produces a selective ultrafiltrate of blood. The rate of ultrafiltration is called the GFR, which is about 125 ml/min or 756 l/h or 1806 l/24 h.

- It is 10% lower in females than males
- Normally about 99% or more of the filtrate is reabsorbed

NB. At the rate of 125 ml/min the kidneys filter in 1 day an amount of fluid equal to:

- 4 times the total body water
- 15 times the extracellular fluid
- 60 times the plasma volume

The forces required to drive the glomerular filtration are

$$\text{GFR} \times (P_{cap} + \Pi_{BC}) - (P_{BC} + \Pi_{cap})$$

where,

- P_{cap} is the hydrostatic pressure in the glomerular capillary. The mean hydrostatic pressure in the glomerular capillary is 45 mmHg because of the presence of a second resistant vessel, the efferent arteriole
- Π_{BC} is the oncotic pressure in the Bowman's capsule. This pressure is negligible because the ultrafiltrate is virtually protein free
- Π_{cap} is the oncotic pressure in the glomerular capillary. The oncotic pressure in the glomerular capillary rises from 20 mmHg to 35 mmHg as blood flows through it
- P_{BC} is the hydrostatic pressure in Bowman's capsule = 10 mmHg

Inulin is normally used to measure GFR because it:

- is freely filtered; it is not bound to proteins in plasma or sieved in the process of ultrafiltration
- is not reabsorbed or secreted by the kidneys
- is not synthesised or metabolised
- is non-toxic
- is not stored

- does not affect the filtration rate
- is easy to measure in the plasma and urine

Creatinine is also used to measure GFR but a small amount is actively secreted and so measurements overestimate GFR.

Para-aminohippuric acid (PAH) is used to measure renal plasma flow (RPF). The normal filtration fraction is the ratio of the GFR to the RPF:

$$\begin{aligned} FF &= \frac{GFR}{RPF} \quad \left[\frac{C_{in}}{C_{PAH}}\right] \\ &= \frac{120\ \text{ml/min}}{600\ \text{ml/min}} \\ &= 0.2 \end{aligned}$$

normal value = 0.15–0.20.

13 (**a**) false (**b**) false (**c**) true (**d**) false (**e**) true

The liver has a number of functions and so individual tests have less value than consideration of a number of results as a whole. These include plasma bilirubin, albumin, and the enzymes alanine transaminase, aspartate transaminase and alkaline phosphatase. Biochemical measures of liver function commonly assess:

(a) Hepatic anion transport, principally serum bilirubin. Normally less than 5% of serum bilirubin is conjugated.

(b) Abnormal protein synthesis
   - Serum albumin – hypoalbuminaemia in chronic liver injury
   - Prothrombin time (PT), which may be increased due to:
     (a) failure to absorb fat-soluble vitamin K in cholestasis
     (b) factors II (prothrombin), VII, IX and X, which are vitamin K dependent; (c) impaired synthesis of coagulation factors as above plus factor V and fibrinogen. A raised PT due to cholestasis can generally be corrected by the addition of parenteral vitamin K
   - Serum immunoglobulins are usually increased in chronic liver disease. IgM is predominantly increased in primary biliary cirrhosis and IgG in chronic autoimmune hepatitis

(c) Liver enzyme tests
   - Cytoplasmic and mitochondrial enzymes are raised in hepatocellular damage. Alanine amino transperase (ALT) is more liver specific than aspartate aminotransperase (AST) and rises

more than AST in early hepatocellular injury. AST is raised more in chronic injury

- Membrane-associated enzymes such as alkaline phosphatase and gamma glutamyl transferase are anchored to the biliary canaliculus. They are raised in biliary outflow obstruction rather than hepatocellular damage

(d) Miscellaneous – anti-mitochondrial antibodies present in primary biliary cirrhosis; increased plasma lipids in cholestasis; serum urea may be reduced.

14 (**a**) true (**b**) true (**c**) false (**d**) false (**e**) false

The blood–brain barrier reflects the impermeability of capillaries in the CNS, including the choroid plexuses, to circulating substances such as electrolytes and exogenous drugs and toxins. It is composed of a lipid membrane of capillary walls, the endothelial cells of which are joined by tight junctions, and the envelopment of brain capillaries by glial cells.

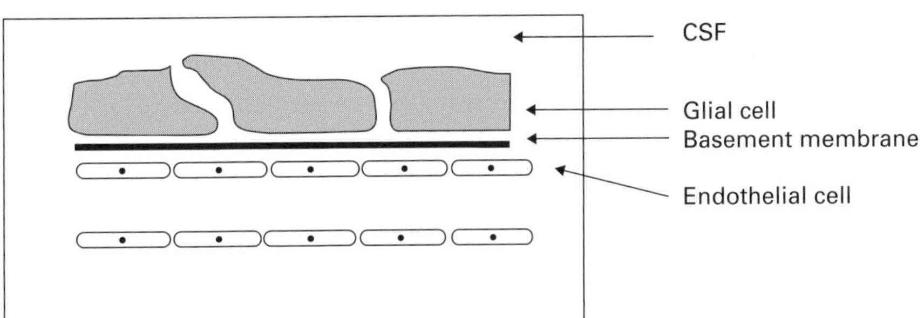

The blood–brain barrier is impermeable to H^+ and HCO_3^-

15 (**a**) false (**b**) false (**c**) false (**d**) false (**e**) true

The parasympathetic component of the autonomic nervous system has a restorative function, returning tone to the basal level after excitation.

Also known as the craniosacral system, the fibres run in cranial nerves III, VII, IX and X, and in the sacral nerves to their respective ganglia.

Relationship of the ganglia to the cranial nerves

Third nerve III	ciliary ganglion
Seventh nerve VII	ganglia pterygopalatine and submaxillary ganglia
Ninth and tenth nerves	otic ganglia
S2, S3, S4	vesical and enteric ganglia

The ganglia are sited peripherally in the viscera. They are distant from the spinal cord close to the innervated viscera. Hence, the preganglionic fibres are long while the postganglionic fibres are short. The effector transmitter from the postganglionic fibres is acetylcholine. The visceral ganglion implies a more refined system, with more local control than the sympathetic nervous system.

Parasympathetic function

Pupil	constriction (greater depth of focal field)
Ciliary muscle	constrict (near focus)
Lacrimal	gland secretion increased
Submandibular gland	secretion released and increased
Parotid gland	secretion increased
Heart	decreased pulse rate and myocardial responsiveness
Lung	constriction of air passages
Gut	increased peristaltic and segmentation motility
Liver, pancreas	reduced blood glucose generation (from starch breakdown) and insulin release
Kidney	no innervation
Urinary bladder	relaxation of sphincter and contraction of bladder wall musculature
Penis	erection plus sensory facilitation
Arterioles in general	no innervation
Arterioles in voluntary muscular system	no innervation
Piloerector muscles (raise hair or goosebumps)	no innervation
Sweat glands	no innervation

16 (**a**) false (**b**) true (**c**) false (**d**) false (**e**) true

The nerve action potential is an all-or-none phenomenon.

An action potential is triggered when successive conductance increases to sodium and potassium ions. This causes a threshold potential of about 50 mV to be reached. The initial, sudden inward rush of sodium ions leads to a positive charge inside the cell, corresponding to the phase of the action potential known as depolarisation. Subsequent increase in the permeability of the cell membrane to potassium allows loss of this positive ion. This leads to a return of the electrical charge inside the cell toward the membrane potential. This phase of the action potential is known as repolarisation.

17 (**a**) true (**b**) false (**c**) true (**d**) false (**e**) false

Active transport is the movement of substances across the cell membrane against an electrochemical gradient.

(a) Characteristics of active transport are:
- substances are moved against their electrochemical gradient
- the exchange of substances requires a transport protein
- the process is rate limiting and saturable
- the breakdown of ATP is required to provide energy

(b) Types of active transport:
- primary active transport requires energy derived directly from the breakdown of ATP
- secondary active transport derives energy secondarily from ionic concentration differences across the membrane.

The sodium/potassium pump is often considered the prototype of active transport.

18 (**a**) true (**b**) true (**c**) true (**d**) false (**e**) false

Activity in the reflex arc starts at a sensory receptor, with a receptor potential whose magnitude is proportional to the strength of the stimulus. The stimulus generates an all-or-none action potential, which is proportionate to the size of the generator potential. In the CNS, the responses are again graded in terms of excitatory (EPSPs) and inhibitory (IPSPs) postsynaptic potentials at the synaptic junctions. All-or-none responses are generated in the efferent nerve. When these reach the effectors, they again set up a graded response.

When the effector is a smooth muscle, responses summate to produce action potentials in the smooth muscle. When the effector is a skeletal muscle, the graded response produces action potentials that bring about a graded muscle contraction.

The simplest reflex arc is one with a single synapse between the afferent and efferent neurones; such arcs are monosynaptic. Reflex arcs in which one or more interneurones are interposed between the afferent and efferent neurones are polysynaptic.

In both types, activity is modified by spatial and temporal facilitation, occlusion and subliminal firing effects.

19 (**a**) false (**b**) true (**c**) false (**d**) false (**e**) true

The main ventilatory response to carbon dioxide is controlled centrally in the medulla of the brain. The peripheral chemoreceptors in the carotid bodies play a much less important role. Alveolar ventilation increases by 1–2 l/min for each 0.1 kPa increase in $PaCO_2$. The ventilation-to-carbon dioxide tension response curve is reduced in gradient and shifted to the right by sleep and by morphine.

20 (**a**) false (**b**) false (**c**) true (**d**) true (**e**) true

The enzymes responsible for protein digestion are:

(a) Endopeptidases, which hydrolyse interior peptide bonds of polypeptides and proteins
   - Trypsin attacks peptide bonds involving basic amino acids
   - Chymotrypsin attacks peptide bonds involving aromatic amino acids, leucine, glutamine and methionine
   - Elastase attacks peptide bonds involving neutral aliphatic amino acids

(b) Exopeptidases, which hydrolyse external peptide bonds of polypeptides and proteins
   - Carboxypeptidase A
   - Carboxypeptidase B.

21 (**a**) true (**b**) true (**c**) true (**d**) true (**e**) false

Hyperkalaemia results from the following.

(a) Decreased or impaired potassium excretion, as observed with:
   - acute or chronic renal failure (most common)
   - potassium-sparing diuretics
   - urinary obstruction
   - sickle cell disease
   - Addison disease
   - systemic lupus erythematosus (SLE)

(b) Addition of potassium into the extracellular space, as observed with:
- potassium supplements (e.g., p.o./i.v. potassium, salt substitutes)
- rhabdomyolysis
- haemolysis (e.g., venipuncture, blood transfusions, burns, tumor lysis)

(c) Transmembrane shifts, when potassium shifts from the intracellular to the extracellular space, as observed with:
- acidosis
- medication (e.g., acute digitalis toxicity, beta-blockers, succinylcholine)

(d) Factitious or pseudohyperkalemia, as observed with:
- improper blood collection (e.g., ischaemic blood, poor venipuncture technique), laboratory error
- leucocytosis
- thrombocytosis

Infusion rates should generally not exceed 10 mmol/hour or 120 mmol daily. The usual daily dose of potassium is 24–63 mmol.

22 **(a)** true **(b)** false **(c)** false **(d)** false **(e)** false

Starling's hypothesis states that the fluid movement due to filtration across the wall of a capillary is dependent on the balance between the hydrostatic pressure gradient and the oncotic pressure gradient across the capillary.

The four Starling's forces are:
- hydrostatic pressure in the capillary (P_c)
- hydrostatic pressure in the interstitium (P_i)
- oncotic pressure in the capillary (p_c)
- oncotic pressure in the interstitium(p_i)

The balance of these forces allows calculation of the net driving pressure for filtration.

$$\text{Net driving pressure} = |(P_c - P_i) - (p_c - p_i)|$$

The net fluid flux is proportional to this net driving pressure. In order to derive an equation to measure this fluid flux additional factors need to be considered:
- the reflection coefficient
- the filtration coefficient (K_f).

Table 2.22 Typical Starling forces

	Typical values of Starling forces in systemic capillaries (mmHg)	
	Arteriolar end of capillary	Venous end of capillary
Systemic capillary hydrostatic pressure	25	10
Interstitial hydrostatic pressure	−6	−6
Capillary oncotic pressure	25	25
Interstitial oncotic pressure	5	5

The net driving pressure is outward at the arteriolar end and inward at the venous end of the capillary. This change in net driving pressure is due to the decrease in the capillary hydrostatic pressure along the length of the capillary.

In the lung the hydrostatic pressure in the pulmonary circulation is low and so the lung has no extracellular water.

23 (**a**) false (**b**) true (**c**) false (**d**) true (**e**) true

(a) Cardiovascular system
- Cardiac output increases by 30%–40% above normal by 32 weeks. Aortocaval compression is sufficient to reduce cardiac output from 20 weeks
- Heart rate increases by 15%, stroke volume increases by 30%. SVR falls resulting in no change in BP
- Cardiac hypertrophy and dilation cause ECG changes of left axis deviation, ST depression and flattening/inversion of T wave in III
- Albumin is diluted, reducing plasma oncotic pressure and predisposing to pulmonary oedema at lower pressures
- Aortocaval compression is significant from mid-pregnancy

(b) Respiratory system
- Increased minute volume by 40%, tidal volume by 15% and respiratory rate. A mild respiratory alkalosis gives a shift of the oxygen dissociation curve to the left. An increase in P_{50} facilitates oxygen unloading across the placenta
- Increased tidal volume with reduced FRC
- Increased closing capacity which may exceed FRC
- Increased O_2 consumption

(c) Gastrointestinal system
- Uterine pressure increases intragastric pressure and distorts lower oesophageal sphincter, causing incompetence of the sphincter
- Delayed gastric emptying and increased acid production

(d) Blood
- Increased red cell mass by 20%–30% and increased plasma volume by 40%–50% at term, causing dilutional anaemia
- Hypercoagulable state with increased fibrinolytic systems

(e) Renal system
- Increase in GFR of 60% reduces plasma urea and creatinine by 40%

(f) Metabolism
- Increased volume of distribution of intravenous agents prolongs their elimination half-lives
- Serum cholinesterase levels fall by 25% during the first trimester and then fall further by 33% during the first 7 days postpartum

24 (**a**) true (**b**) true (**c**) true (**d**) false (**e**) false

Rh disease only occurs if a mother is Rh-negative and her baby is Rh-positive. For this situation to occur, the baby must inherit the Rh factor gene from the father. Most people are Rh-positive. Only 15% of the white population is Rh-negative.

Rh disease and ABO incompatibility disease are caused when a mother's immune system produces antibodies against the red blood cells of her unborn child. The antibodies cause the baby's red blood cells to be destroyed and the baby develops anaemia. The baby's body tries to compensate for the anaemia by releasing immature red blood cells, called erythroblasts, from the bone marrow.

The overproduction of erythroblasts can cause the liver and spleen to become enlarged, potentially causing liver damage or a ruptured spleen. The emphasis on erythroblast production is at the cost of producing other types of blood cells, such as platelets and other factors important for blood clotting. Since the blood lacks clotting factors, excessive bleeding can be a complication.

The destroyed red blood cells release the blood's red pigment (haemoglobin) which degrades into bilirubin. High levels of bilirubin accumulate, causing hyperbilirubinaemia (jaundice).

Other symptoms that may be present include high levels of insulin and low blood sugar, as well as a condition called hydrops fetalis.

25 (**a**) false (**b**) true (**c**) true (**d**) false (**e**) true

Calcium is the most abundant cation in the body, appearing in combination with phosphorus in the ratio 2:1.5. It is essential for the formation of bones and teeth, blood clotting, normal muscle and nerve activity, endocytosis and exocytosis, cellular motility, chromosome movement prior to cell division, glycogen metabolism, and synthesis and release of neurotransmitters.

Some 30%–80% of ingested calcium is absorbed, primarily in the upper small intestine.

Most – 99% – is stored in the bones and teeth. The remainder is stored in muscle, other soft tissues, and blood plasma.

Regulation of plasma levels is by free exchange with body stores, and through the action of hormones such as calcitonin, parathyroid hormone and vitamin D. Excess calcium is mostly excreted in faeces, and in small amounts in urine.

Given the range of roles for calcium within the body, it is important to maintain its free extracellular concentration within narrow limits. Assuming an adequate supply of dietary calcium, this is achieved through:

- efficient gastrointestinal absorption
- free exchange with bone stores; the most important buffer for immediate changes of calcium concentration
- renal excretion of calcium
- hormonal influences on the preceding functions

Additionally, there is a small amount of calcium excretion within sweat, which becomes more significant in extremes of heat and low humidity.

Regulation of calcium homeostasis

Three principle hormones are involved in calcium homeostasis, acting at three target organs, the intestine, bone and the kidneys:

Vitamin D

Vitamin D is a group of closely related sterols produced by the action of ultraviolet light. Vitamin D_3 (cholecalciferol) is produced by the action of sunlight and is converted to 2,5-hydroxycholecalciferol in the liver. The 2,5-hydroxycholecalciferol is converted in the proximal tubules of the kidneys to the more active metabolite 2,5-dihydrocholecalciferol. 2,5-dihydrocholecalciferol synthesis is regulated in a feedback fashion by serum calcium and phosphate. Its formation is facilitated by a parathyroid hormone. The actions of vitamin D are as follows:

- enhances calcium absorption from the intestine
- facilitates calcium absorption in the kidney
- increases bone calcification and mineralisation
- in excess, mobilises bone calcium and phosphate

Parathyroid hormone (PTH)

Parathyroid hormone is a linear polypeptide containing 84 amino acid residues. It is secreted by the chief cells in the four parathyroid glands. Plasma ionised calcium acts directly on the parathyroid glands in a feedback manner to regulate the secretion of PTH. In hypercalcaemia, secretion is inhibited, and the calcium is deposited in the bones. In hypocalcaemia, PTH secretion is stimulated. The actions of PTH are aimed at raising serum calcium.

The actions of PTH are aimed at raising the serum calcium by increasing:

- bone reabsorption by activating osteoclast activity
- renal calcium reabsorption by the distal renal tubules
- renal phosphate excretion by decreasing tubule phosphate reabsorption
- the formation of 2,5-dihydrocholecalciferol by increasing the activity of alpha-hydroxylase in the kidney

A large amount of calcium is filtered in the kidneys, but 99% of the filtered calcium is reabsorbed. About 60% is reabsorbed in the proximal tubules and the remainder in the ascending limb of the loop of Henle and the distal tubule. Distal tubular absorption is regulated by PTH.

Calcitonin

Calcitonin is a 32-amino-acid polypeptide secreted by the parafollicular cells in the thyroid gland. It decreases serum calcium concentration and, in general, has effects opposite to those of PTH. The actions of calcitonin are as follows:

- it inhibits bone reabsorption
- it increases renal calcium excretion.

The exact physiological role of calcitonin in calcium homeostasis is uncertain.

26 (**a**) true (**b**) true (**c**) false (**d**) false (**e**) true

Humans are homeothermic: their core body temperature is controlled within narrow limits.

Control of thermoregulation involves:

(a) Thermal receptors (central and peripheral)

- Peripheral receptors
  - help by providing information on how hot or cold the body part is
  - present in skin, mucous membrane and some viscera
  - types
    - cold thermoreceptors fire maximally over a range of 25–30°C

      Innervated by type Aδ fibres

      Respond both to long-term gradual increase or decrease and sudden changes in environmental temperature.
    - warm thermoreceptors have a maximum discharge rate at 45–50°C

      Innervated by type C nerve fibres
- Central receptors
  - regulate body temperature by influencing neural and hormonal changes
  - sites: hypothalamus, spinal cord, abdominal viscera
  - impulses from
    - peripheral thermoreceptors; fibres ascend in the lateral spinothalamic tract
    - head and neck – V cranial nerve

(b) Central regulation, via hypothalamic pre-optic nuclei

- Heat-sensitive neurones
- Cold-sensitive neurones
- Anterior hypothalamus integrates afferent thermal information, particularly warmth leading to sweating, and vasodilatation
- Posterior hypothalamus controls the descending pathways to effectors in response to cold, leading to shivering

(c) Effectors
- Altered behaviour, quantitatively the most effective mechanism
- Vasomotor response
  - too cold: vasoconstriction and piloerection
  - too hot: vasodilatation and sweating
- Shivering and increased metabolic rate

27 (**a**) false (**b**) false (**c**) false (**d**) false (**e**) true

Atrial natriuretic peptide (ANP) is released by myocytes in response to atrial stretch. There are a variety of forms. The original peptides isolated from the brain are smaller than the forms subsequently isolated from human heart.

Actions:
- reduction of ADH-induced water reabsorption in the collecting ducts
- relaxation of renal arterioles
- modulatory effects on the GFR
- inhibition of aldosterone-mediated sodium reabsorption in the distal tubule (natriuretic effect)

There is massive ANP activity in end-stage renal failure and congestive cardiac failure.

High-affinity binding sites for ANP are present in the renal collecting ducts. Binding results in increased intracellular cyclic guanine monophosphate concentrations and inhibition of sodium transport.

28 (**a**) true (**b**) false (**c**) true (**d**) false (**e**) false

The effects of hypothermia can be categorised by the body system affected.

Cardiovascular system

- Depressed myocardial O_2 uptake
- Depressed myocardial contractility
- Depressed cardiac output by (30%–40% at 34°C)
- Arrhythmias become increasingly common at 32°C
- Ventricular fibrillation at 28°C
- Reduced inotropic effects of catecholamine
- Enhanced negative inotropic effect of volatiles
- Vasoconstriction and increased PVR

- ECG
  - increased P-R interval
  - widen QRS complex
  - increased QT interval
  - J waves
- Increased blood viscosity (4%–6% for each 1°C)
- Diuresis contributes to increased haematocrit
- Platelets/WCC fall (sequestration)
- Increased PT, TT, aPTT (impaired coagulation)

Respiratory system

Reduced oxygen delivery (DO_2), increased oxygen uptake ($\mathring{V}O_2$)

- Apnoea at 24°C
- Reduced respiratory rate
- Loss of hypoxic pulmonary vasoconstriction
- Left shift of oxygen dissociation curve
- Gases become more soluble
- Increased peripheral vascular resistance
- Increased tidal volume

Neurological system

- Impaired short-term memory (confusion) < 35°C
- Unconscious at 30°C
- Pupils become fixed and dilated
- Cold necrosis
- Cerebral blood flow and cerebral metabolic ratio for O_2 (volume of O_2 consumed by the brain) fall by 5% per 1°C
- Protection against cerebral ischaemia
- Cerebral blood flow autoregulation becomes impaired below 32°C
- Reduced MAC

Metabolic

As may happen during a long operation

- Decreased metabolic rate 8% per 1°C
- Shivering increasing $\mathring{V}O_2$ to 800%
- Increased muscle blood flow → more heat loss
- Reduced tissue perfusion → metabolic acidosis
- Hyperglycaemia
- Increased circulatory catecholamines

- Pancreatitis
- Reduced drug metabolism
- Increased resistance to non-depolarising muscle relaxants
- Intracellular shift of potassium
- Increased protein catabolism and decreased synthesis

Hepatic

- Decreased hepatic blood flow
- Decreased drug metabolism

Renal

- Decreased renal blood flow
- Negative resorption of Na
- Negative ADH
- Maintain urinary osmotic pressure unless core temperature $< 20°C$

Others

- Shivering
- Poor wound healing
- Deep vein thrombosis
- Immunosuppression

29 (**a**) true (**b**) false (**c**) true (**d**) true (**e**) true

ACTH is principally responsible for regulating secretions of the adrenal cortex, especially cortisol. It also stimulates the formation of cholesterol in the adrenal cortex. Secretion of ACTH responds most dramatically to stress and is under the control of corticotropin-releasing hormone from the hypothalamus.

Secretory rates of corticotropin-releasing hormone and ACTH are high in the morning and low in the evening.

30 (**a**) false (**b**) true (**c**) false (**d**) true (**e**) true

The gap junction is a specialised channel of transport and communication for small molecules and ions between the cytoplasm of two closely apposed cells.

Electron microscopy reveals the two cell membranes to be separated by only 1–2 nm at the point where the gap junctions are sited. Each membrane has a large number of small protein channels termed connexons. Individual connexons of both cells are joined to each other to create a communicating tunnel, which spans the membrane gap. The internal diameter of the passage is about 2 nm.

Each connexon on each membrane is made up of six polypeptide chain subunits, which span the membrane.

Electrophysiological studies have shown low electrical resistance for the cell when there are abundant gap junctions. Injection of low-molecular-weight dyes results in rapid spread between cells. Therefore, gap junctions provide a pathway by which small molecules and ions can rapidly move down concentration gradients between cells.

Gap junctions are evident in epithelia and smooth muscle. They permit all of the cells to act as a syncytium. However, if continued passive transport is detrimental to the syncytium, individual gap junctions can be rapidly closed.

31 (**a**) false (**b**) true (**c**) false (**d**) true (**e**) false

Most drugs are relatively lipid soluble, with low solubility in plasma water, therefore protein binding is essential for their transport and rapid distribution.

Drugs are usually reversibly bound to plasma proteins. There are considerable differences in the degree of protein binding, even between chemically related drugs. Only the unbound fraction of a drug in plasma is available for diffusion into tissues, and is therefore responsible for the pharmacological effects. Plasma protein binding may restrict the hepatic clearance of extensively bound drugs (>70% bound) with a low intrinsic hepatic clearance (diazepam, phenytoin, warfarin). In these conditions plasma protein binding may limit the access of drugs to hepatic enzymes, decreasing their clearance and prolonging their terminal half-lives. In other circumstances plasma protein binding does not restrict the hepatic or renal elimination of drugs or drug metabolites. The binding of a drug to a protein-binding site is a saturable process governed by the same mass action expression that describes the interaction of a substrate with an enzyme-binding site.

32 (**a**) false (**b**) true (**c**) false (**d**) false (**e**) false

Bioavailability is defined as the fraction of an oral dose reaching the systemic circulation, compared with a standard route of administration.

Drugs with a high bioavailability are stable in the gastrointestinal tract, are well absorbed and undergo minimal first-pass metabolism.

The notable feature of methadone is its relatively low first-pass metabolism resulting in a relatively high oral bioavailability of 75%.

33 (a) false (b) true (c) false (d) false (e) false

The solubility of a gas in a liquid is given by its Ostwald solubility coefficient. This represents the ratio of the concentration in blood to the concentration in the gas phase (the Bunsen coefficient is corrected at standard temperature and pressure and the partial pressure above the liquid is 1 atm or 101.325 kPa). The amount of gas in blood can be independent of pressure, obeying Henry's law, as serum proteins and haemoglobin are major determinants of blood content.

Solubility describes the affinity of the gas for a medium such as blood or fat tissue. The blood/gas partition coefficient describes how the gas will partition itself between the two phases after equilibrium has been reached. Isoflurane for example has a blood/gas partition coefficient of 1.4. Thus if the gas is in equilibrium the concentration in blood will be 1.4 times higher than the concentration in the alveoli. A higher blood/gas partition coefficient means a higher uptake of the gas into the blood and therefore a slower induction time. It takes longer to reach an equilibrium between the alveolar and blood concentrations.

Low blood/gas coefficients are seen with:

- haemodilution
- obesity
- hypoalbuminaemia and starvation

Table 2.33 Blood/gas partition coefficients

Agent	Blood/gas partition coefficient
Nitrous oxide	0.47
Halothane	2.3
Enflurane	1.9
Isoflurane	1.4
Sevoflurane	0.69
Desflurane	0.42

High blood/gas coefficients are seen:

- in adults compared to children
- in hypothermia
- postprandially

34 (**a**) true (**b**) false (**c**) false (**d**) true (**e**) false

Membrane-stabilising drugs were classified by Vaughan Williams.

These are class I antiarrhythmics according to the Vaughan Williams classification. Class I antiarrhythmics have local anaesthetic properties that exhibit membrane-stabilising activity and affect conduction, refractoriness and the action potential.

Class I drugs are subdivided into

(a) Class I a

- slow d*v*/d*t* of phase zero
- prolong repolarisation
- prolong PR, QRS, QT

Examples include:

- quinidine
- procainamide
- disopyramide

(b) Class I b

- limited effect on d*v*/d*t* of phase zero
- shorten repolarisation
- shorten QT
- elevate fibrillation threshold

Examples include:

- lidocaine (lignocaine)
- mexiletine
- tocainamide

(c) Class I c

- markedly slow d*v*/d*t*
- little effect on repolarisation
- markedly prolong PR, QRS

Examples include:

- flecainide
- propafenone

Propranolol has membrane-stabilising activity. This effect is probably of little clinical significance as the dose required to elicit it is higher than those seen in vivo.

35 **(a)** true **(b)** false **(c)** false **(d)** true **(e)** true

Alpha antagonists are classified as

(a) Non-selective
- phenoxybenzamine
- phentolamine
- tolazoline
- ergotamine

(b) $Alpha_1$-receptor antagonists
- prazosin
- doxazosin
- terazosin
- indoramin

(c) $Alpha_2$ receptor antagonists:
- yohimbine

Chlorpromazine has alpha-adrenergic blocking action but it is not classified as an alpha antagonist. We have suggested that D is true.

36 **(a)** true **(b)** true **(c)** false **(d)** false **(e)** false

Cocaine and ephedrine are sympathomimetics. Timolol is a beta-blocker, which may be used as drops in the treatment of glaucoma.

37 **(a)** true **(b)** true **(c)** false **(d)** true **(e)** false

MAC is a measure of potency.
There is a correlation between oil/gas solubility and MAC. This was the basis of the lipid solubility theory of mode of action of anaesthetics. But when the oil/gas solubility is multiplied by the MAC for each volatile agent, the products fall into two groups. One group scatters around 200 and the other around 100. This suggests that the lipid solubility theory of anaesthetic action is not valid. It has been replaced by a theory that involves the proteins in the cell membrane, possibly as well as the phospholipids. Potency increases with increasing molecular weight.

38 (**a**) true (**b**) false (**c**) false (**d**) true (**e**) false

Sevoflurane is a poly-fluorinated isopropyl methyl ether.

Characteristics

- Pleasant odour
- Relatively low blood/gas partition coefficient (0.69)
- Relatively low MAC (2.0)

Metabolism

It undergoes hepatic metabolism by cytochrome P450 (isoform 2E1) to a greater extent than all other commonly used volatile agents except halothane.

39 (**a**) true (**b**) true (**c**) true (**d**) false (**e**) true

Ketamine is a derivative of a phencyclidine and cycloheximide. It is presented as a *racemic mixture* of two enantiomers.

S (+) is 3.5 times more potent than *R* (−).

It is soluble in water.

Mechanisms of action

(a) Non-competitive antagonist of the calcium ion channel operated by the excitatory NMDA glutamate receptor.
(b) Inhibits the NMDA receptor by binding to the phencyclidine binding site.
(c) Interacts with the M, S and K opioid receptors.
(d) Local anaesthetic action medicated by fast sodium channel blockade.
(e) Antagonists at muscarinic acetylcholine receptors.

Pharmacokinetics

Molecular weight	237.5
pH	3.5–5.5
p*K*a	–
Protein binding	20%–50%
Volume of distribution	3.0 l/kg
Clearance	20 ml /kg per min
Elimination half-life	3 h

Elimination

N-Demethylation and hydroxylation by hepatic P450 enzymes to nor-ketamine (30 times as potent as ketamine) then conjugated and excreted in urine.

Effects on uterus

- Ketamine increases uterine tone

Cardiovascular system

- Increases sympathetic tone leading to increases in heart rate, cardiac output, blood pressure, central venous pressure; baroreceptor function is maintained

40 (**a**) false (**b**) true (**c**) true (**d**) true (**e**) true

Methohexitone is a dimethylated oxybarbiturate. It is produced as the sodium salt with sodium carbonate (6% by weight).

Pharmacokinetics

Molecular weight	284
pH	10–11
p*Ka*	7.9
Protein binding	55%
Volume of distribution	2.0 l/kg
Clearance	10 ml /kg per min
Elimination half-life	3–5 h

Elimination

Some 20% is located in the red blood cells, metabolised in the liver and excreted in urine, <1% excreted unchanged.

Differences from thiopentone

- Less soluble
- Less histamine release
- Less cardiovascular depression
- More respiratory depression
- Shorter elimination half-life due to higher hepatic extraction ratio
- High incidence excitatory movement
- More pain on injection
- Greater hypersensitivity reactions

41 (**a**) true (**b**) false (**c**) true (**d**) false (**e**) true

Ester local anaesthetics are rapidly metabolised by plasma cholinesterase and systemic toxicity is relatively a problem.

Amide local anaesthetics are metabolised by the liver.

Lidocaine has a high extraction ratio and metabolism is, therefore, dependent on hepatic blood flow.

42 (**a**) false (**b**) false (**c**) false (**d**) false (**e**) true

Cocaine is a naturally occurring ester local anaesthetic.

Uses

- For topical anaesthesia
- As vasoconstrictor

Action

- Same mechanism of action as other local anaesthetic agents (p*K*a = 8.7)
- Inhibits catecholamine uptake at presynaptic nerve endings and inhibits monoamine oxidase leading to increased synaptic levels of dopamine and noradrenaline resulting in central stimulation

Kinetics

- Well absorbed from mucous membranes
- Protein bound 98%
- Undergoes significant hepatic hydrolysis

Volume of distribution	0.9–3.3 l/kg
Clearance	25–45 ml/kg per min, 10% unchanged
Elimination $t_{1/2}$	25–60 min

Effects

CNS

- Biphasic effect: initially (excitation) due to blockade of inhibitory pathways in the cerebral cortex, which causes secondary depression
- Hyper-reflexia
- Mydriasis
- Increased intra-ocular pressure

CVS

- Increased BP
- Increased HR
- Myocardial depression

Respiratory

- Increased respiratory rate and volume

Metabolic

- Increased body temperature due to:
  - increased motor activity
  - cutaneous vasoconstriction
  - direct effect on hypothalamus

43 (**a**) true (**b**) true (**c**) false (**d**) false (**e**) false

The major metabolic pathway for morphine biotransformation is by phase II conjugation.

- About 70% undergoes conjugation to morphine 3-glucuronide (M3G) This metabolite is a weak analgesic and antagonises the analgesic effect of morphine
- About 5%–10% undergoes conjugation to morphine 6 glucuronide (M6G), which is pharmacologically active and 30 times more potent than morphine
- About 1%–2% is excreted by the kidneys as unconjugated drug
- Extrahepatic metabolism

44 (**a**) true (**b**) false (**c**) false (**d**) false (**e**) false

Tramadol is a centrally acting analgesic. It is a racemic mixture.

Action

- Acts at opioid receptors
- Modifies nociceptive transmission by inhibition of noradrenaline and serotonin uptake
- Stimulates presynaptic serotonin release
- It has a low affinity for opioid receptors, comparable with that of codeine
- It is approximately equipotent to pethidine

- Compared with opioids it is less respiratory depressant and the tolerance and dependence potential are low
- Respiratory depression and analgesia are reversed by naloxone

Side-effects

- Dizziness
- Sedation
- Nausea
- Dry mouth
- Sweating

45 (**a**) false (**b**) true (**c**) true (**d**) true (**e**) true

The lower oesophageal sphincter tone is increased by:

- metoclopramide
- domperidone
- cisapride
- prochlorperazine
- neostigmine
- pancuronium

The lower oesophageal sphincter tone is decreased by:

- atropine
- morphine
- nifedipine
- GTN

46 (**a**) true (**b**) false (**c**) true (**d**) false (**e**) false

The reader is referred to the current *British National Formulary* for current therapies for epilepsy.

47 (**a**) true (**b**) true (**c**) true (**d**) true (**e**) false

Ondansetron is a potent, highly specific $5HT_3$ antagonist.

Kinetics

- Modified bound to plasma proteins
- Relatively large volume of distribution
- Relatively short half-life
- Undergoes hepatic metabolism
- <5% excreted unchanged in urine

Side-effects

- Increased bowel transit time
- Constipation
- Headaches, dizziness, flushing
- Chest pain
- Cardiac arrhythmia

Advantages

- No sedation
- No extrapyramidal side-effects

Disadvantages

Little effect on

- Opioid-induced emesis
- Motion sickness

48 (**a**) false (**b**) false (**c**) false (**d**) true (**e**) true

Edrophonium is a phenolic quaternary amine.

Uses

- Reversal of non-depolarising neuromuscular blockade. (The *British National Formulary* gives a dose of 500–700 μg/kg i.v. over several minutes for "brief" reversal.)
- Diagnosis of suspected phase II block
- Diagnosis of myasthenia gravis (Tensilon test)
- Differentiation of myasthenic from cholinergic crisis. The clinical picture is worsened in the latter

49 (**a**) false (**b**) false (**c**) false (**d**) true (**e**) false

Suxamethonium does not readily cross the placenta because it is

- Fully ionised
- Poorly lipid soluble

50 (**a**) true (**b**) true (**c**) true (**d**) false (**e**) false

Clonidine is an imidazole with alpha-2 adrenergic agonist activity.

It was originally introduced as an antihypertensive but its main clinical role now relates to use as an analgesic, to decrease anaesthetic requirements and to attenuate sympatho-excitatory responses in patients undergoing general anaesthesia.

The action of clonidine on alpha-2 receptors, which are widely distributed throughout the CNS and the rest of the body, results in

- Sedation and anxiolysis
- Antisialogogue effects
- Analgesia (supraspinal and spinal)
- Enhanced conduction blockade by local anaesthetics
- Reduced anaesthetic requirements during surgery (decreased MAC)
- Decrease in intraocular pressure
- Peripheral and central effects on the CVS
  - inhibition of NAD release from prejunctional nerve endings
  - hypotensive and bradycardia, produced centrally
  - antiarrhythmia, mediated vagally
- Diffuse action on hormonal milieu
  - reduced thyroid function
  - reduced sympathetic outflow
  - reduced stress-induced ACTH and cortisol release
  - increased secretion of growth hormone

51 (**a**) true (**b**) false (**c**) false (**d**) false (**e**) false

GTN is an organic nitrate ester of nitric acid and glycerol.

Action

Nitric oxide is released, which activates the enzyme guanylate cyclase leading to increased levels of intracellular cyclic GMP. While the influx of calcium ions into vascular smooth muscle is inhibited, its uptake into smooth endoplasmic reticulum is enhanced so that cytoplasmic levels fall resulting in vasodilatation.

Effects

CVS

- Blood vessels
  - vasodilatation predominantly in the capacitance vessels
  - decrease in preload
  - postural hypotension

- Heart
  - reduced venous return
  - reduced left ventricular end-diastolic pressure
  - reduced wall tension
  - increased coronary blood flow
  - reduced oxygen demand
  - heart rate unchanged

CNS

- Cerebral vasodilatation

GIT

- Sphincter relaxation

Blood

- Methaemoglobinaemia

Kinetics

- Extensive first-pass metabolism. Oral bioavailability is only 5%
- Metabolism by hepatic reductase into glycerol dinitrate and nitrate; 80% of the dose is excreted in the urine

Differences from sodium nitroprusside

- Acts more on venous smooth muscles than arteriolar
- Reduces systolic more than diastolic
- Coronary vasodilator
- No rebound on stopping
- Available in patches
- Does not need to be protected from light
- Tolerance develops within 24 h
- Tachycardia is less prominent
- Less toxic

52 (a) true (b) true (c) true (d) true (e) true

Verapamil is synthetic papaverine derivative class IV antiarrhythmic. It is a racemic mixture.

Action

- *L*-isomer has specific calcium channel blocking action at the sinoatrial (SA) and atrioventricular (AV) node preventing the influx of calcium ions through voltage-sensitive slow (L) channels
- *D*-isomer acts on the fast sodium channels resulting in some local anaesthetic activity

Effects

CVS

- Slows the conduction at SA and AV nodes; reduces heart rate (HR)
- Negative inotropic effect
- Peripheral vasodilatation
- Increases coronary blood flow

CNS

- Cerebral vasodilatation

Others

- Potentiates the effects of depolarising and non-depolarising muscle relaxants with prolonged use

Pharmacokinetics

- Oral bioavailability 20% (extensive first-pass metabolism)
- Protein binding 90%
- Volume of distribution 4.5 l/kg
- Elimination half-time of 5 h

Elimination

- Demethylation to nor-verapamil which retains significant antiarrhythmic properties – 70% excreted in urine, 5% unchanged

53 (**a**) true (**b**) true (**c**) true (**d**) false (**e**) true

Hyoscine compared to atropine:

- more crosses the blood–brain barrier
- has a shorter duration of action
- is a more potent antisialogogue
- is more sedative

- is more potent in preventing motion-induced sickness
- produces less tachycardia
- produces fewer arrhythmias
- is not a good bronchodilator
- has a more marked effect on the eyes
- causes more confusion in the elderly

54 (**a**) true (**b**) true (**c**) false (**d**) false (**e**) true

The following drugs cause prolongation of the QT interval:

- quinidine and other *class Ia* antiarrhythmic drugs
- amiodarone and other *class III* antiarrhythmic drugs
- amitriptyline and other tricyclic antidepressants
- chlorpromazine and other phenothiazine drugs
- terfenadine and astemizole
- erythromycin
- droperidol

55 (**a**) false (**b**) true (**c**) false (**d**) true (**e**) false

Droperidol is a butyrophenone derivative. It is used in the prevention and treatment of postoperative nausea and vomiting (PONV).

Action

- It is an antagonist of D_2 receptors in the chemoreceptor trigger zone

Effects

CNS

- Anxiolysis and induces a placid state
- Sedation is more pronounced
- Extrapyramidal side-effects (oculogyric, opisthotonus)
- Neuroleptic malignant syndrome
- Raised seizure threshold

CVS

- Vasodilatation and decreased arterial pressure due to alpha adrenergic blockade
- Prolongs QT interval

Metabolic

- Hyperprolactinaemia

56 (**a**) true (**b**) true (**c**) true (**d**) false (**e**) true

Factors that increase renal blood flow include:

- parasympathetic stimulation
- prostaglandins
- dopamine
- Ca^{2+} channel block
- dopexamine

57 (**a**) false (**b**) false (**c**) true (**d**) true (**e**) true

Gastrointestinal pressure is increased by:

- cholinergic action – neostigmine
- mu receptor activity
- contraction of the anterior abdominal wall – suxamethonium
- increased in intra-abdominal pressure – laparoscopy

58 (**a**) false (**b**) false (**c**) false (**d**) true (**e**) true

Human albumin solutions (HAS) are derived from human plasma by fractionation.

Table 2.58 Human albumin characteristics

Heat sterilised	
pH	6.4 – 7.1
Osmolality	1500 mosmol/kg
Molecular weight	66.500 Da
Composition 4.5% – 4.5 g and 20% – 20 g protein /100 ml	
Plasma volume increased by 250% for about 24 h	
Metabolism	Interstitial translocation
Excretion	Gut/renal
Allergy	Very low incidence
Na^+	5–120 mmol/l
Cl^-	<40 mmol/l
K^+	<10 mmol/l

59 (**a**) true (**b**) false (**c**) true (**d**) true (**e**) false

Low molecular weight heparins include:

- enoxaparin
- dalteparin
- tinzaparin

These drugs are derived by the depolymerisation of heparin by one of:

- chemical degradation
- enzymatic degradation

Action

- More effective at inhibiting factor Xa
- Less effective at promoting the formation of antithrombin–thrombin complex

Uses

Reduces the incidence of fatal pulmonary embolism, particularly after major surgery

Advantages

- Single daily dose due to a longer half-life
- Less effect on platelets
- Reduced affinity for Willebrand's factor
- Reduced risk of heparin-induced thrombocytopenia
- Reduced need for monitoring

Reversal

Protamine is not fully effective in reversing the effects of low molecular weight heparin

Kinetics

- Subcutaneously once daily (bioavailability 90%)
- Used for extracorporeal circuit in the bypass circuit
- Less protein bound
- Half-life 12 h
- Renal elimination

60 (**a**) true (**b**) true (**c**) true (**d**) true (**e**) false

Metronidazole is a nitro-imidazole, synthetic antimicrobial. It acts by destroying DNA. It is only active when the nitro group is in the reduced form. This is induced by the very low redox values achieved by anaerobic bacteria and some protozoa.

Pharmacokinetics

Bioavailability	60%–80% (rectal)
Protein bound	20%
Elimination half-life	6–10 h
Excretion	60%–80% in urine

Side-effects

CNS

- Headache
- Dizziness
- Confusion
- Depression
- Incoordination
- Peripheral neuropathy

GIT

- Nausea/vomiting
- Abdominal discomfort
- Diarrhoea

Haematological

- Neutropenia
- Thrombocytopenia

Others

- Metallic taste
- Intrauterine mutation
- Disulfiram-type reaction with alcohol
- Enhances warfarin anticoagulant
- Impairs phenytoin and lithium clearance

61 (**a**) false (**b**) false (**c**) false (**d**) true (**e**) false

The Doppler effect is the shift in frequency and wavelength of sound waves that results when the source of the sound moves with respect to the receiver of the sound. The sound waves are reflected back with a shorter wavelength if the source and the reflective surface are moving towards each other.

62 (**a**) false (**b**) false (**c**) true (**d**) false (**e**) false

Viscosity (η) is defined as that property of a fluid which causes it to resist flow. The coefficient of viscosity (η) is defined as:

$$\eta = \frac{\text{force}}{\text{area}} \times \text{velocity gradient}$$

Velocity gradient is equal to the difference between the velocities of different fluid molecules divided by the distance between molecules. The unit of the coefficient of viscosity is the pascal per second.

The practical effects of temperature change on viscosity include:

- increased temperature reduces the viscosity of liquids
- increased temperature increases the viscosity of gases by increasing their molecular activity

63 (**a**) true (**b**) true (**c**) true (**d**) false (**e**) false

The principle of the oscilloscope is that a hot cathode produces an electron beam that passes through two deflecting devices. One device deflects the beam on the *X*-axis and one on the *Y*-axis. The beam then strikes a fluorescent screen where a visible trace is produced. A saw-tooth potential deflects the beam in the *X* direction. The signal then deflects the beam in the *Y* direction.

Advantages

- A very high frequency response
- Continuous display

Disadvantages

- Non-permanent record with the simpler oscilloscope

64 (**a**) false (**b**) true (**c**) false (**d**) true (**e**) false

The characteristics of the audible signal set by British Standards BS 4272 for oxygen failure warning devices are:

- Lasts for at least 7 s
- Powered by the oxygen supply pressure
- Volume 60 db
- Cannot be switched off before the oxygen supply is reconnected
- Alarm should activate as the pressure falls below 250 kPa
- The gas supply should be either progressively reduced as the oxygen fails or replaced with air

65 (**a**) false (**b**) false (**c**) false (**d**) false (**e**) true

Each gas absorbs radiation maximally at a specific wavelength and this absorbance peak is characteristic for each given gas:

CO_2	~428 nm
N_2O	~430 nm
Halogenated agents	~330 nm

Monomolecular gases such as oxygen, nitrogen and helium do not absorb infrared radiation.

66 (**a**) false (**b**) true (**c**) false (**d**) true (**e**) false

The vaporiser inside the circle (VIC) arrangement has a low-resistance vaporiser placed in the inspiratory limb of the circle from which the anaesthetic agent is vaporised by the gases circulating in the system by the patient's breathing. VIC systems are still occasionally used, since they employ an inexpensive vaporiser and provide some degree of autoregulation of the anaesthetic concentration. If the plane of anaesthesia becomes too light, respiration will be less depressed, minute volume will increase, more agent will be vaporised and the plane of anaesthesia will deepen. It is however found that this is not very reliable in practice. It is therefore strongly recommended that an inhalational anaesthetic analyser be used to monitor the inspired concentration whenever such systems are used. In-circuit vaporisers can be used with closed or semi-closed systems. Since water vapour exhaled by the patient condenses in the vaporiser, it is necessary to drain in-circuit vaporisers regularly.

67 (**a**) false (**b**) true (**c**) false (**d**) true (**e**) true

Ideally the natural frequency of the system should *exceed* the maximum frequency of the arterial signal.

The natural frequency of the monitoring system is:

- *directly* related to the catheter diameter
- inversely related to the square root of the system's compliance
- inversely related to the square root of the length of the tube
- inversely related to the square root of the density of the fluid in the system

The natural frequency (resonant frequency) is high in:

- stiff diaphragm
- short tubing
- low density fluid

68 (**a**) true (**b**) true (**c**) false (**d**) true (**e**) false

Chi-squared test is used for discrete or non-continuously variable data (e.g. categorical data) where the observed frequency of measurement is compared with the expected frequency if the null hypothesis were true. As with all tests of significance the null hypothesis should be clearly stated and the level of probability defined at which it may be deemed to be unlikely.

The test is inappropriate for small samples.

69 (**a**) true (**b**) true (**c**) true (**d**) true (**e**) true

Electroconvulsive therapy is delivered as a pulsatile square wave discharge of 35–40 J. A current of 850 mA is passed through the brain through two saline-soaked pads applied to each temple of the anaesthetised patient to induce a major cerebral seizure. The device uses a pulse of 1.25 ms repeated 26 times a second, i.e. 26 Hz, for a total time of 2–5 s.

The potential will depend on the impedance between the electrodes, but could be about 250 V.

Table 2.69 Time constants

Time constant	Amount remaining (%)	% of process completed
One	37	63
Two	13	87
Three	5	95

Paper 2 Answers

70 (**a**) false (**b**) false (**c**) true (**d**) false (**e**) false

The time constant is the time at which the process would have been complete had the initial rate of change been maintained.

After one time constant the concentration has fallen to 37% of its original value. After two time constants the concentration has fallen to 13% of its original value and after three time constants the concentration has fallen to 3% of its original value.

Half-life is the time taken for the concentration being measured to fall to half of its original value.

The time constant is longer than the half-life.

71 (**a**) true (**b**) true (**c**) false (**d**) false (**e**) true

Atoms with a net electrical charge will become aligned parallel to a strong static field. When a second high-frequency pulsating magnetic field force is applied at 90 degrees to the first, these same atoms will deflect causing a release of high-frequency energy. This is used to create the image. Sensitive atoms are hydrogen, carbon, sodium, fluoride and phosphorus. Modern MRI magnets are approximately 1.5 Tesla. Ferric- or iron-containing materials must be removed as they will be attracted into the magnet.

72 (**a**) true (**b**) true (**c**) false (**d**) true (**e**) false

An oxygen concentrator delivers a concentration of argon higher than in air because it works by absorbing nitrogen in zeolite and so concentrates the oxygen and argon that are left, giving a higher concentration of both.

Components

A zeolite molecular sieve is used. Zeolite is made of hydrated aluminium silicates of the alkaline earth metals.

Mechanism of action

- Air is exposed to a zeolite molecular sieve column at a certain pressure
- The sieve selectively retains nitrogen and other unwanted components of air
- These are released into the atmosphere
- The change over between the columns is made by a time switch

- The maximum oxygen concentration achieved is *95% by volume*
- Argon is the main remaining constituent

73 (**a**) true (**b**) false (**c**) false (**d**) true (**e**) true

An electromagnetic flowmeter is an example of the application of an electromagnetic effect. If a conductor is moved through a magnetic field an electrical potential develops and the magnitude of the induced potential is proportional to the rate at which the conductor is moved through the magnetic field.

The electromagnetic flowmeter consists of a C-shaped probe that contains coils to generate the magnetic field, and two electrodes to measure the potential induced as the blood flows. Although the potential is proportional to the rate at which the blood is flowing, the velocity of blood varies across the diameter of the blood vessel and so the electromagnetic flowmeter measures an average velocity.

74 (**a**) false (**b**) true (**c**) false (**d**) true (**e**) false

Infrared analysis can be used to assess any substance that is composed of two or more dissimilar molecules. Each molecule will absorb a maximum of energy at a wavelength that is particular to each molecule. This is 4.28 μm for CO_2. The Beer–Lambert law applies.

The chamber is small to make the response time short, about 100 ms, and continuous. Glass also absorbs infrared radiation so the chamber windows must be made of a crystal of sodium chloride or sodium bromide. The chamber is filled with a CO_2-free gas, or by splitting the incident beam and passing this through a reference chamber for calibration. A reference beam also allows compensation for variations in the output of the infrared source.

75 (**a**) true (**b**) true (**c**) true (**d**) true (**e**) false

Critical pressure is the pressure at which a gas liquefies at its critical temperature.

N_2O	73 bar	36.5°C
N_2O	52 bar	20.0°C
O_2	50 bar	−118°C

76 (**a**) true (**b**) false (**c**) true (**d**) false (**e**) true

Absolute humidity is the mass of water vapour in grams present in a given volume of air (m^3). It is given as mg/l.

Relative humidity is the ratio of the mass of water vapour in a given volume of air to the mass required to fully saturate that volume of air at that temperature.

Fully saturated air at 20°C contains 17 mg/l, at 37°C air contains 44 mg/l.

Relative humidity is expressed in terms of mass but as mass is directly proportional to the number of moles present, then by the ideal gas equation

$$\text{relative humidity} = \frac{\text{actual vapour pressure}}{\text{saturated vapour pressure}}$$

77 (**a**) false (**b**) false (**c**) false (**d**) false (**e**) true

The Bourdon tube is a form of diaphragm pressure gauge for high pressure measurement. The chamber with the diaphragm has been replaced by a flattened tube which is then coiled. As the pressure is increased inside the tube it expands and the flattened tube becomes rounded and so straightens out.

78 (**a**) false (**b**) false (**c**) true (**d**) false (**e**) false

A transducer is a device that is activated by energy from one system and supplies energy usually in another form to a second system. For example, a microphone is a transducer that transforms sound energy into an electrical signal.

A transistor is a device composed of semiconductor material that amplifies a signal or opens or closes a circuit.

A photoelectric cell is a type of transducer which converts light energy to electrical energy.

79 (**a**) true (**b**) true (**c**) false (**d**) false (**e**) true

The boiling point of a liquid is the temperature at which the vapour pressure is equal to the atmospheric pressure.

The lower the atmospheric pressure, the lower the temperature at which a liquid will boil.

Vapour pressure depends only on the liquid and the temperature. It does not depend on the barometer pressure.

80 (a) true (b) true (c) true (d) true (e) false

The ECG frequency range is 0.5–100 Hz.

The beta waves of EEG are in the range of 15–60 Hz.

The potentials detected in the EMG range from about 100 μV to many millivolts. The EMG gives sharp spikes in place of the complex ECG pattern. The potentials detected in the EEG are only about 50 μV.

81 (a) true (b) false (c) true (d) true (e) false

If a distribution is asymmetric it is either **positively skewed** or **negatively skewed**. A distribution is said to be positively skewed if the scores tend to cluster toward the lower end of the scale (that is, the smaller numbers) with increasingly fewer scores at the upper end of the scale (that is, the larger numbers). This might happen with blood glucose or creatinine levels.

A negatively skewed distribution has more values to the right. This might happen with haemoglobin concentrations.

The mean is higher than the median in a positively skewed distribution.

82 (a) true (b) true (c) false (d) true (e) true

The refractometer is non-specific and may be used to measure the concentration of a variety of different gases.

It cannot be used to identify component gases in a mixture and so calibration with known gases in advance is used to check the performance of vaporisers.

83 (a) true (b) true (c) true (d) true (e) true

Methods of measuring cardiac output (CO) are non-invasive or invasive.

Non-invasive

Doppler techniques

These devices transmit an ultrasonic vibration into the body and record the change in the frequency of the signal as it is reflected off the red blood cells. Doppler techniques detect flow as a change in the frequency of the returning ultrasound wave. A measure of the total flow is obtained by integrating the signal over the cross-sectional area of the vessel. Transoesophageal echocardiography (TOE) measures the flow of blood in the ascending aorta in unit time. This is multiplied by the cross-sectional area of the aorta to give the stroke volume. The aorta is not a pure cylinder so the results of these devices are not absolute. Their main value is to show changes or to show whether the frequency shift is within the range found in normal people.

Transthoracic impedance

Impedance can be measured across externally applied electrodes. Impedance changes with the cardiac cycle due to changes in blood volume. The rate of change of impedance is a reflection of cardiac output. It is more useful in estimating changes than for an absolute measurement.

Invasive

The Fick principle

Fick in the nineteenth century realised that the following relationship is true

$$Q = M / (V - A)$$

Where Q is the volume of blood flowing through an organ in a minute; M is the number of moles of a substance added to the blood by an organ in one minute; and V and A are the venous and arterial concentrations of that substance.

This principle can be used to measure the blood flow through any organ that adds substances to, or removes substances from, the blood. The heart does not do either of these but the cardiac output equals the pulmonary blood flow, and the lungs add oxygen to the blood and remove carbon dioxide from it.

The concentration of the oxygen in the blood in the pulmonary veins is 200 ml/l and in the pulmonary artery it is 150 ml/l, so each litre of blood going through the lungs takes up 50-ml. At rest, the blood takes up 250 ml/min of oxygen from the lungs and this 250 ml must be carried away in 50 ml portions; therefore, the CO must be 250/50 or 5 l/min.

Dilution techniques

Dye dilution

A known amount of dye is injected into the pulmonary artery, and its concentration is measured peripherally. Indocyanine green is suitable due to its low toxicity and short half-life. A curve is achieved, which is re-plotted semi-logarithmically to correct for recirculation of the dye. CO is calculated from the injected dose, the area under the curve (AUC) and its duration. (Short duration indicates high CO.)

Thermodilution

First 5–10 ml cold saline is injected through the port of a pulmonary artery catheter. Temperature changes are measured by a distal thermistor. A plot of temperature change against time gives a similar curve to the dye curve (but without the second peak). Calculation of CO is achieved using the Stewart–Hamilton equation.

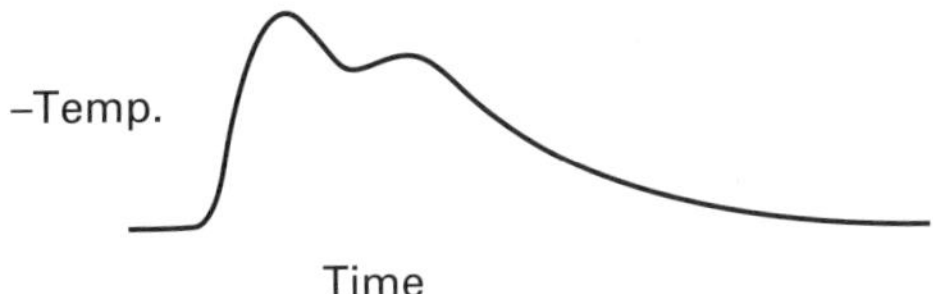

84 (**a**) false (**b**) false (**c**) false (**d**) true (**e**) true

The power of a study is calculated to determine that the null hypothesis will be rejected correctly. This is 1 minus the type II errors (β) or false negatives. A power of 80% (0.8) means an 80% chance of showing a difference when one exists. The power of a study is required to calculate the number of people that are needed to be included in a study to obtain a valid result.

A randomised controlled study is one in which there are two groups: one treatment group and one control group. The treatment group receives the treatment under investigation and the control group receives either no treatment or some standard default treatment. Patients are randomly assigned to the groups. Assigning patients at random reduces the risk of bias and increases the probability that differences between the groups can be attributed to the treatment. In a double-blind experiment, neither the individuals nor the researchers know who belongs to the control group and the experimental group.

A pilot study is a study to test the practical feasibility of the proposed study.

85 (**a**) true (**b**) false (**c**) false (**d**) true (**e**) true

Gas chromatography involves separating a gas mixture into its component parts by passing the mixture through a column.

The system has two phases: a stationary phase and a mobile phase. The stationary phase is a column of fine silica aluminium coated with polyethylene glycol or silicone. An inert carrier gas such as argon or helium is passed through the column. This is the liquid or moving phase. Sample gases are injected into the steam or carrier gas. The speed with which they pass through the column is determined by their differential solubility between the two phases.

The temperature is held constant as the solubility is temperature dependent.

This system is often termed a gas or liquid chromatograph. The column separates the component gases which come out at different times. As the gases leave the column they are detected by: flame ionisation for organic vapours; a thermal conductivity detector for inorganic vapours: and an electron capture detector for a halogenated vapour.

All the detectors have to be calibrated for each gas profile and individual concentration.

86 (**a**) false (**b**) false (**c**) true (**d**) true (**e**) true

Entonox is a 50:50 mixture by volume of O_2 and N_2O. The Poynting effect is the change in critical temperature of one gas, such as nitrous oxide, when it is mixed with another gas, such as oxygen. This gives the nitrous oxide a pseudocritical temperature, which is dependent on the proportion of oxygen. At 50:50 the pseudocritical temperature is −5.5°C.

The cylinders contain gas filled to 137 000 kPa or 2000 psi (137 bar); 1 bar = 100 kPa.

87 (**a**) true (**b**) true (**c**) false (**d**) true (**e**) false

An ideal gas is one which obeys the gas laws under experimental conditions.

Boyle's law states that at constant temperature the volume of a given mass of gas varies inversely with the absolute pressure.

Charle's law states that at constant pressure the volume of fixed mass is proportional to its temperature.

No gas is strictly ideal, because all gases eventually liquefy as they are cooled towards 0 K and some solidify. However, within the range of temperatures and pressures encountered by the anaesthetist, oxygen and nitrogen may be considered ideal gases, whereas nitrous oxide, volatile agents and carbon dioxide may not.

Absolute zero, the zero point of the ideal gas temperature scale, is denoted by zero on the Kelvin and Rankine temperature scales, which is equivalent to –273.16°C and –459.67°F. For most gases there is a linear relationship between temperature and pressure. Gases contract as the temperature is decreased. Theoretically, at absolute zero the volume of an ideal gas would be zero and all molecular motion would cease. Absolute zero cannot be reached.

88 (**a**) true (**b**) true (**c**) true (**d**) true (**e**) true

Surgical diathermy equipment uses the heating effects of an electric current to coagulate blood and to cut tissues.

Cutting diathermy uses current in an alternating sinewave pattern. Coagulation diathermy uses current in a pulsed sine wave pattern and damped wave form.

About 150–500 W of energy can be delivered using unipolar diathermy.

89 (**a**) false (**b**) false (**c**) false (**d**) false (**e**) true

Bispectral analysis (BiS) was first developed using the clinical end points of sedation.

It has been extended to assess the hypnotic effects of a variety of inhalation and intravenous anaesthetic agents. It is used to indicate the potential for awareness and of relative overdose of hypnotic drugs. It does not predict movement or haemodynamic responses to stimulation. It does not predict the exact moment when consciousness returns.

BiS values of 65–85 have been recommended for sedation and of 40–65 for general anaesthesia. Below 40, cortical suppression will be present, correlating with raw EEG traces of burst suppression.

The possibility of postoperative spontaneous recall (awareness) has been shown to be extremely low at BiS <50. Conversely wakefulness is to be expected when the BiS score is >90. Return to consciousness is highly unlikely at BiS <65.

Ketamine anaesthesia and pre-existing neurological disease do not give the typical responses. EMG activity from scalp muscles can give interference and lead to a falsely high BiS score.

90 (**a**) false (**b**) false (**c**) false (**d**) true (**e**) true

Surface tension is a tangential force in newtons per metre.

Laplace's Law

For a tube: $P = T/R$, where P = pressure gradient across the wall of a sphere, T = tension and R = radius.

MCQ answers primary paper 2

	(a)	(b)	(c)	(d)	(e)
1	F	T	T	F	F
2	F	F	T	T	T
3	T	T	T	F	F
4	T	T	F	F	F
5	F	F	F	T	T
6	T	F	F	T	T
7	T	F	F	F	F
8	F	T	T	T	T
9	F	F	F	F	T
10	T	F	F	T	T
11	F	F	F	F	T
12	F	F	T	T	F
13	F	F	T	F	T
14	T	T	F	F	F
15	F	F	F	F	T
16	F	T	F	F	T
17	T	F	T	F	F
18	T	T	T	F	F
19	F	T	F	F	T
20	F	F	T	T	T
21	T	T	T	T	F
22	T	F	F	F	F
23	F	T	F	T	T
24	T	T	T	F	F
25	F	T	T	F	T
26	T	T	F	F	T
27	F	F	F	F	T
28	T	F	T	F	F
29	T	F	T	T	T

	(a)	(b)	(c)	(d)	(e)
30	F	T	F	T	T
31	F	T	F	T	F
32	F	T	F	F	F
33	F	T	F	F	F
34	T	F	F	T	F
35	T	F	F	T	T
36	T	T	F	F	F
37	T	T	F	T	F
38	T	F	F	T	F
39	T	T	T	F	T
40	F	T	T	T	T
41	T	F	T	F	T
42	F	F	F	F	T
43	T	T	F	F	F
44	T	F	F	F	F
45	F	T	T	T	T
46	T	F	T	F	F
47	T	T	T	T	F
48	F	F	F	T	T
49	F	F	F	T	F
50	T	T	T	F	F
51	T	F	F	F	F
52	T	T	T	T	T
53	T	T	T	F	T
54	T	T	F	F	T
55	F	T	F	T	F
56	T	T	T	F	T
57	F	F	T	T	T
58	F	F	F	T	T
59	T	F	T	T	F
60	T	T	T	T	F

	(a)	(b)	(c)	(d)	(e)
61	F	F	F	T	F
62	F	F	T	F	F
63	T	T	T	F	F
64	F	T	F	T	F
65	F	F	F	F	T
66	F	T	F	T	F
67	F	T	F	T	T
68	T	T	F	T	F
69	T	T	T	T	T
70	F	F	T	F	F
71	T	T	F	F	T
72	T	T	F	T	F
73	T	F	F	T	T
74	F	T	F	T	F
75	T	T	T	T	F
76	T	F	T	F	T
77	F	F	F	F	T
78	F	F	T	F	F
79	T	T	F	F	T
80	T	T	T	T	F
81	T	F	T	T	F
82	T	T	F	T	T
83	T	T	T	T	T
84	F	F	F	T	T
85	T	F	F	T	T
86	F	F	T	T	T
87	T	T	F	T	F
88	T	T	T	T	T
89	F	F	F	F	T
90	F	F	F	T	T

Paper 3 Answers

1 (**a**) false (**b**) false (**c**) true (**d**) true (**e**) false

Autoregulation is defined as the intrinsic ability of an organ to maintain a constant blood flow despite changes in perfusion pressure. For example, if the perfusion pressure is decreased to an organ by partially occluding the arterial supply to that organ, blood flow initially falls, then returns to a normal level over the next few minutes. This autoregulatory response occurs independently of neural and hormonal influences and therefore is intrinsic to the organ. When the perfusion pressure (arterial minus venous pressure, $P_A - P_V$) initially decreases, blood flow ($\dot{Q}$) falls. The relationship between pressure, flow and resistance is

$$\dot{Q} = P_A - P_V/R$$

When blood flow falls, arterial resistance (R) falls as the resistance vessels dilate. It is thought that metabolic and myogenic mechanisms are responsible for this vasodilatation. As resistance decreases, blood flow increases despite the presence of a reduced perfusion pressure.

Different organs display varying degrees of autoregulatory behaviour. The renal, cerebral and coronary circulations show excellent autoregulation, whereas skeletal muscle and splanchnic circulations show moderate autoregulation. The cutaneous circulation shows little or no autoregulatory capacity.

The basic mechanism of autoregulation for cerebral blood flow (CBF) is controversial. It is most likely that the autoregulatory vessel calibre changes are mediated by interplay between myogenic and metabolic mechanisms. The influence of perivascular nerves and most recently the vascular endothelium has also been the subject of intense investigation.

2 (**a**) false (**b**) true (**c**) false (**d**) false (**e**) true

The child has a high surface area relative to weight. Tidal volume is 7 ml/kg equal to an adult's but the respiratory rate and minute ventilation are higher due to the dead space being 50% of tidal volume. Lung compliance is 150 ml/5 cmH_2O, which is much less than in an adult. Blood volume is about 80 ml/kg which would be 1600 ml.

3 (**a**) true (**b**) true (**c**) true (**d**) false (**e**) false

The usual mixed-venous oxygen content of blood is 15 ml/dl compared with 20 ml/dl for arterial blood.

Tissues that extract more than 5 ml/dl are the heart and brain. The oxygen content of blood leaving the liver is less than in mixed-venous blood because 65% of the blood supply to the liver is venous blood from the gut, via the hepatic portal vein.

Skeletal muscle and the kidney are relatively well perfused for the metabolic demands of the organs. The venous oxygen content is therefore higher than in mixed-venous blood.

4 (**a**) true (**b**) true (**c**) false (**d**) false (**e**) false

The baroreceptor reflex is made up of afferent information conveyed to the brain via myelinated and unmyelinated fibres in the sinus nerve (a branch of the glossopharyngeal nerve), from the carotid sinus and via the vagus nerve from the aortic arch.

5 (**a**) true (**b**) false (**c**) false (**d**) true (**e**) true

A sea-level native who remains for prolonged periods at high altitude may develop chronic mountain sickness characterised by:

- polycythaemia
- pulmonary hypertension
- right ventricular failure

Tissue perfusion may be impaired if the increased haemoglobin increases the viscosity of blood, leading to thrombus formation. At the same time, widespread pulmonary hypoxaemia causes generalised vasospasm in pulmonary vessels and right heart failure.

Recovery is usually prompt when these individuals are given oxygen to breathe or they return to sea level.

6 (**a**) true (**b**) true (**c**) false (**d**) false (**e**) false

The chemoreceptors that regulate respiration are located both centrally and peripherally. Normal control is exercised by the central receptors located in the medulla, which respond to the CSF hydrogen ion concentration, which in turn determines arterial PCO_2 (P_aCO_2). The carbon dioxide, but not hydrogen ions, diffuses freely across the blood–brain barrier. The response is both quick and sensitive to small changes in $PaCO_2$.

In addition, there are peripheral chemoreceptors located in the carotid and aortic bodies. The carotid bodies are located on the external carotid arteries near to the bifurcation with the internal carotids. Each carotid body is a few millimetres in size and has the distinction of having the greatest blood flow per tissue weight of any organ in the body. Afferent nerve fibres join with the sinus nerve before entering the glossopharyngeal nerve. A decrease in carotid body perfusion results in cellular hypoxia, hypercapnia and decreased pH. This leads to an increase in receptor firing. The threshold PO_2 for activation is about 8 kPa. Any elevation of PCO_2 above a normal value of 5.3 kPa, or a decrease in pH below 7.4 causes receptor firing. If respiratory activity is not allowed to change during chemoreceptor stimulation (thus removing the influence of lung mechanoreceptors), then chemoreceptor activation causes bradycardia and coronary vasodilatation (both via vagal activation) and systemic vasoconstriction (via sympathetic activation).

7 **(a)** true **(b)** true **(c)** true **(d)** false **(e)** false

The amount of oxygen delivered to the tissues is referred to as the oxygen flux (DO_2):

- It is the amount of O_2 in ml/min available to the peripheral tissue
- It is the product of
  - arterial O_2 content (CaO_2) and
  - cardiac output (CO)

$$O_2 \text{ delivery} = \text{arterial } O_2 \text{ content} \times \text{cardiac output}$$

- Normal arterial O_2 content = 20.4 ml/100 ml
- Normal cardiac output = 5 l/min or 5000 ml/min.
- Thus O_2 delivery $= \frac{20.4}{100} \times 5000 = 1020$ ml/min
- Normal O_2 delivery is 1020 ml/min of which the body usually extracts 250 ml
- The minimum DO_2 compatible with survival is in the region of 300–400 ml/min and is dependent on factors such as
  - cardiac output
  - Hb concentration
  - Hb saturation

8 (**a**) false (**b**) true (**c**) true (**d**) true (**e**) true

The alveolar–arterial PO_2 gradient is the difference between the observed O_2 tension in arterial blood and the calculated ideal alveolar O_2 tension, from the alveolar air equation.

$$P_AO_2 = FiO_2 - \frac{PaCO_2}{R}$$

Normal gradient 2 kPa; this may be up to 5 kPa in the elderly. It increases to 15 kPa when breathing 100% oxygen.

Causes of an increased alveolar–arterial gradient

This is the commonest cause of arterial hypoxaemia.

(a) Diffusion defects

(b) Ventilation defects

- Reduced FRC
- Pneumonia
- Anaesthesia

(c) Perfusion defects

- Reduced mixed-venous O_2 tension due to
  - reduced CO
  - anaemia
  - increased O_2 consumption
  - hypovolaemia

(d) Increased right-to-left shunt

(e) Hormones

- Pregnancy and progesterone
- Hepatic failure

(f) Drugs

- Volatile anaesthetics
- Vasodilators

9 (**a**) false (**b**) true (**c**) true (**d**) false (**e**) true

Functional residual capacity (FRC) is the volume of air (about 3 l in an adult) that is present in the lungs at the end of normal expiration, i.e. when the elastic recoil of the lung is balanced with the elastic recoil of the chest and the diaphragm.

It is the sum of two volumes

- Residual volume
- Expiratory reserve volume

It is the resting volume of the lung where gases are exchanged.

Factors affecting the FRC

(a) Factors which increase FRC
- Height – FRC is directly proportional to height
- Position – maximum when upright
- CPAP
- PEEP

(b) Factors which decrease FRC
- Sex (10% less in females)
- Obesity
- Supine position
- Rest

10 (**a**) false (**b**) false (**c**) false (**d**) true (**e**) true

The intrapulmonary shunt can be calculated using the shunt equation:

$$\text{Shunt fraction} = \frac{(\text{pulmonary end} - \text{capillary } O_2 \text{ content} - \text{arterial } O_2 \text{ content})}{(\text{pulmonary end} - \text{capillary } O_2 \text{ content} - \text{mixed-venous } O_2 - \text{content})}$$

The oxygen content of a given blood volume comprises both oxygen bound to haemoglobin and that dissolved in plasma. This requires the partial pressure of oxygen, oxygen saturation and the haemoglobin concentration to be known. Since pulmonary end-capillary O_2 tension cannot be measured directly it can be estimated from the alveolar oxygen tension.

11 (**a**) true (**b**) false (**c**) true (**d**) false (**e**) true

The normal urine specific gravity is 1003–1030. In diabetes mellitus the glucose in the urine raises the specific gravity. In physiological oliguria there is production of small amounts of concentrated urine.

In impaired tubular function small amounts of poor-quality urine are produced.

12 (**a**) false (**b**) true (**c**) true (**d**) true (**e**) false

At 2 atm ambient pressure breathing is still controlled by the tension of carbon dioxide and minute ventilation will remain the same or increase to take into account the extra energy demanded from working at depth.

13 (**a**) false (**b**) false (**c**) true (**d**) true (**e**) false

The sympathetic nerves leave the spinal cord from the thoracic and lumbar regions (T1 to L1). The preganglionic nerves are short and synapse in paired ganglia adjacent to the spinal cord.

The synapses in the sympathetic ganglion use acetylcholine as a neurotransmitter. The synapses of the postganglionic neurones with the target organ use noradrenaline as the neurotransmitter. There is one exception: the sympathetic postganglionic neurones that terminate on the sweat glands use acetylcholine.

14 (**a**) false (**b**) false (**c**) true (**d**) false (**e**) true

Smooth muscle does not contain troponin, and regulation of contractile forces occurs at the level of the thick filament.

Initiation of contraction in response to an increase in cytoplasmic Ca^{2+} concentration in smooth muscle cells occurs as a result of the binding of Ca^{2+} ions to calmodulin.

15 (**a**) false (**b**) false (**c**) true (**d**) true (**e**) true

The effects of spinal shock

(a) Initially

- All spinal reflex responses are profoundly depressed (flaccid). This effect usually lasts for a minimum of 2 weeks up to 4 weeks. This leads to:
  - hypotension; the effect increases if the lesion is above T6
  - hypothermia
  - bradycardia; the effect increases if the lesion is above T1
  - bladder stasis
  - paralytic ileus

- oedema
- flaccid paralysis

(b) Recovery

- New nerve endings may sprout in the cord. This leads to
  - spasticity as the stretch reflex is first to return
  - autonomic hyper-reflexia; most if the lesion is above T5
  - increased blood pressure
  - increased heart rate
  - increased sweating

16 (**a**) true (**b**) true (**c**) false (**d**) false (**e**) true

Depolarisation potentials are produced at the postsynaptic motor end plate of the neuromuscular junction by the binding of acetylcholine to receptors.

The size and duration depend on the amount of acetylcholine released, the number of acetylcholine receptors that are free and the activity of acetylcholinesterase. Miniature end-plate potentials of under 1 mV are thought to be produced by random release of acetylcholine from single vesicles (quantal theory), and are too small to initiate muscle contraction.

17 (**a**) true (**b**) false (**c**) true (**d**) false (**e**) false

The rate of transfer of drugs across the placenta is dependent on the following

- Lipid solubility
- Degree of ionisation (only the non-ionised fraction of a partly ionised drug crosses the placenta membrane)
- Protein binding, which is influenced by
  - pH (acidosis reduces protein binding of local anaesthetics)
  - concentration of plasma proteins
- pH of maternal blood
- Maternal–fetal concentration gradient (the rate of transfer is determined by Fick's law of diffusion)

$$Q/T = kA \quad \frac{C_m - C_f}{D}$$

Where

Q/T = rate of diffusion per unit time
k = diffusion constant
A = surface area available for exchange

C_m = maternal concentration of free drug
C_f = fetal concentration of free drug
D = thickness of diffusion membrane

- Placental blood flow
- Molecular weight of the drug

18 **(a)** false **(b)** false **(c)** false **(d)** true **(e)** true

The withdrawal reflex is a typical polysynaptic reflex, which occurs in response to a noxious and usually painful stimulation of the skin, subcutaneous tissues or muscle.

The response is flexor muscle contraction and inhibition of extensor muscles, so that the part stimulated is flexed and withdrawn from the stimulus.

19 **(a)** true **(b)** true **(c)** false **(d)** true **(e)** true

Normal blood lactate is 0.6–1.2 mmol/l and levels above 5 mmol/l cause a significant acidosis. Concentrations greater than 1 mmol/l carry an 80% mortality rate.

Lactate is made in skeletal muscle and red blood cells. When oxygen supplies are limited pyruvate is reduced to NADH to form lactate. The reaction is catalysed by lactate dehydrogenase.

The importance of this reaction is that it produces two molecules of ATP. It generates NAD^+, which sustains continued glycolysis in skeletal muscle and erythrocytes under anaerobic conditions.

The limiting factor is the liver, which must oxidise lactate back to pyruvate for subsequent gluconeogenesis in the Cori cycle. This pathway merely buys time during the period of anaerobic metabolism.

20 **(a)** false **(b)** true **(c)** false **(d)** true **(e)** false

Platelets are formed in the bone marrow from cells called megakaryocytes. Production is regulated by the colony-stimulating factors that control the production of megakaryocytes. Platelets have no nucleus but can secrete a variety of substances.

Platelets have membranes which contain receptors for collagen, vessel wall Von Willebrand factor and fibrinogen.

Paper 3 Answers

Platelet cytoplasm contains actin, myosin, glycogen, lysosomes, and two types of granules (dense granules and alpha granules).

The normal concentration in the blood is about 250 000 platelets per cubic millimetre.

Platelets remain functional for about 7–10 days (after which they are removed from the blood by macrophages in the spleen and liver). They play an important role in haemostasis (preventing blood loss).

Cell fragment components are cytoplasm, cell membrane but no nucleus.

21 (**a**) true (**b**) false (**c**) true (**d**) false (**e**) false

An estimation of the serum osmolarity is made from the osmolar concentration of plasma derived from the measured Na, K, and urea and glucose concentrations. This value for the osmolarity is unreliable in various conditions, e.g. pseudohyponatremia, hyperlipidaemia in nephrotic syndrome, or hyperproteinaemia.

Osmolarity is the number of particles per litre of solution (i.e. in the case of plasma, per litre of whole plasma). This contrasts with osmolality, which is the number of particles per kg of solvent.

Units of osmolarity are mosmol/l.

Osmolality is a colligative property and is the number of particles per kg of solvent – in the case of plasma, per kg of plasma water.

The normal osmolality of extracellular fluid is 280–295 mosmol/kg. The osmolality is monitored through osmoreceptors in the hypothalamus, which can detect a 1% change in osmolality. Antidiuretic hormone (ADH) is secreted from the posterior pituitary and acts on the collecting duct to increase the reabsorption of water. The level of ADH is increased at osmolalities above 295 mosmol/kg, and is undetectable at less than 280 mosmol/kg.

22 (**a**) false (**b**) false (**c**) true (**d**) false (**e**) false

Vasopressin is a hormone synthesised in the hypothalamus and transported along axons bound to neurophysin carrier proteins. Antidiuretic hormone is also called ADH, vasopressin or arginine vasopressin (AVP). It descends the pituitary stalk to the posterior pituitary gland. It is secreted by the posterior pituitary gland in response to:

- hypovolaemia
- high plasma osmolality
- decreased tension in the great veins
- emotional stress
- raised temperature at the hypothalamus
- pain
- various drugs, e.g. carbamazepine, clofibrate, morphine

Normal plasma vasopressin or ADH is approximately 4 pg/ml.

There are several mechanisms regulating the release of AVP. Hypovolaemia, as occurs during haemorrhage, results in a decrease in atrial pressure. Specialised stretch receptors within the atrial walls and large veins (cardiopulmonary baroreceptors) entering the atria decrease their firing rate when there is a fall in atrial pressure. Afferent nerve fibres from these receptors synapse within the nucleus tractus solitarius of the medulla, which sends fibres to the hypothalamus, a region of the brain that controls AVP release by the pituitary. Atrial receptor firing normally inhibits the release of AVP by the posterior pituitary. In hypovolaemia or decreased central venous pressure, the decreased firing of atrial stretch receptors leads to an increase in AVP release. Hypothalamic osmoreceptors sense extracellular osmolarity and stimulate AVP release when osmolarity rises, as occurs with dehydration. Angiotensin II receptors located in the hypothalamus regulate AVP release. An increase in angiotensin II simulates AVP release.

ADH acts at two types of receptors. V1 (for vasopressin receptor 1) is found in vascular smooth muscle while V2, which works by adenylate cyclase activation, is found in the kidney. ADH binding to V2 receptors in the kidney increases cyclic adenosine monophosphate (cAMP) levels, which in turn increase the water permeability of the renal tubule. The increased resorption of water by the renal tubule decreases urine volume and increases urine osmolality. ADH binding to the V2 receptor in the smooth muscle in the gastrointestinal tract causes peristalsis (contractile waves). ADH agonists, such as desmopressin and DDAVP, increase blood pressure. Desmopressin is an analogue of ADH that is more potent and longer acting. It has little vasoconstrictor activity. DDAVP is the commercial name for desmopressin acetate. ADH agonists are indicated for use only during abdominal surgery. Drugs that act on the sympathetic nervous system to increase peripheral resistance without decreasing coronary blood flow are better choices for the treatment of low blood pressure.

23 (**a**) true (**b**) false (**c**) false (**d**) false (**e**) false

In utero, the placenta acts as the fetal lung, and oxygenated blood saturated with oxygen leaves the placenta and passes through a single umbilical vein to the fetus. This blood then flows predominantly through the ductus venous and into the inferior vena cava, so by-passing the liver. Most of the oxygenated blood entering the right atrium from the inferior vena cava preferentially passes through the foramen ovale into the left atrium, so by-passing the lungs. Passage of this oxygenated blood directly to the left atrium allows perfusion of the fetal brain with maximal available concentrations of oxygen.

Blood entering the right atrium from the superior vena cava is mainly oxygenated blood from the fetal head regions. This blood enters the right ventricle for delivery into the pulmonary artery and then to the descending thoracic aorta via the ductus arteriosus.

As a result, this deoxygenated blood is delivered distal to the blood vessels that supply the fetal brain.

Blood is returned to the placenta by two umbilical arteries for oxygenation.

Fetal circulation oxygen saturated (SPO_2%) and oxygen tension (PO_2 kPa) values are given in Table 3.23.

The pressure gradient across the foramen ovale causes the flag like valve to occlude the opening.

Flow through the ductus arteriosus decreases after birth due to constriction of the muscular wall of this vessel on exposure to higher concentrations of oxygen.

Table 3.23 Fetal oxygen levels

	Saturation (%)	Oxygen tension (kPa)
Umbilical vein	80	5.3
Inferior vena cava	67	4.4
Superior vena cava	30	2.5
Rt atrium and ventricle	52	3.2
Lt atrium and ventricle	62	4.0
Ductus arteriosus	52	3.2
Descending aorta	58	3.5

24 (**a**) true (**b**) true (**c**) true (**d**) true (**e**) true

The total blood calcium consists of ionised (free) calcium and protein bound calcium.

The ionised calcium is affected by pH and serum albumin. The binding of calcium to albumin is pH dependent such that a rise in pH leads to a reduction in the ionised fraction.

As calcium is bound to albumin the serum calcium has to be adjusted by adding 0.2 mmol/l for every gram that the albumin is below 45 g/l.

25 (**a**) true (**b**) true (**c**) false (**d**) false (**e**) false

Cerebral blood flow (CBF) affects cerebral volume, oxygen delivery and removal of products of metabolism. The adult brain weighs 1500 g and receives a blood flow of 750 ml min^{-1}. This represents 15%–20% of cardiac output. Normal CBF values are:

whole brain	50 ml 100 g^{-1} min^{-1}
grey matter	80 ml 100 g^{-1} min^{-1}
white matter	20 ml 100 g^{-1} min^{-1}

Regulation of cerebral blood flow

The control of CBF to the brain is primarily dictated by its metabolic needs and is mediated through chemical changes. Changes in arterial PCO_2 produce the most marked change in CBF. Neurogenic control through the sympathetic nervous system is of much less significance.

- Metabolic. CBF increases with an increase in metabolism. On a global level, the highest level of CBF will be seen during epileptic seizures when brain metabolism is maximal; low levels of CBF occur in coma. On a regional level an increase in CBF can be demonstrated in the contralateral cortex during muscle contraction, coincident with an increase in oxygen demand
- CO_2 is a potent vasodilator. Small increases in $PaCO_2$ produce a significant increase in CBF. Over the normal range the relationship between $PaCO_2$ and CBF is almost linear with an increase in $PaCO_2$ of 1 kPa increasing CBF by 30%. At $PaCO_2$ above 10 kPa or below 4 kPa the changes in CBF become less marked

- Oxygen. Changes in PaO_2 have little effect on CBF over the normal range. Only if the PaO_2 falls below 7 kPa will cerebral vasodilatation occur
- Autoregulation. In the healthy brain CBF remains constant despite changes in arterial blood pressure. In normotensive subjects flow remains constant between mean arterial pressures of 50 and 150 mmHg. In chronic hypertension the autoregulatory curve is shifted to the right, protecting small capillaries from a rise in perfusion pressure
- Neurogenic. The cerebral vessels have a sympathetic nerve supply originating from the superior cervical ganglion and a parasympathetic supply from the facial nerve
- Other factors such as hypothermia reduce cerebral metabolism, which in turn reduces CBF. Metabolism falls approximately 5% for each degree centigrade fall. Blood viscosity also affects CBF. Increased viscosity reduces and decreased viscosity increases CBF

26 (**a**) true (**b**) true (**c**) true (**d**) false (**e**) false

Oedema is the accumulation of interstitial fluid in abnormally large amounts. The composition of interstitial fluid is similar to plasma except for proteins.

Composition of CSF

Constituent	Concentration (mmol/l)
Na	141
CL	124
Mg	1.2
HCO_3	23
K^+	1.9

Composition of intracellular fluid

Constituent	Concentration (mmol/l)
Na	10–35
K^+	150
Mg	12–18
HCO_3	10–20
CL	5
Po_4	3

Composition of saline in dextrose 4%/saline 0.18%

Constituent	Concentration (mmol/l)
Na	31
Cl	31

27 (**a**) true (**b**) false (**c**) true (**d**) false (**e**) true

There are three types of sweating, each with their own neurological control:

- thermoregulatory sweating
- emotional sweating
- gustatory sweating

Sweat is formed by active secretion deep within the dermis. Its initial composition is near to that of plasma but with minimal protein. During passage along the sweat duct, reabsorption of sodium and chloride ions occurs until their concentrations are less than half of the plasma values, e.g. 60 mmol/l and 50 mmol/l respectively. Conversely, potassium is secreted to give a value of 7–8 mmol/l in sweat.

The control mechanism for sweat secretion is both neural (cholinergic fibres of the thoracolumbar sympathetic nervous system descending from the anterior hypothalamus) and hormonal (adrenaline). If the rate of production is high, excessive amounts of solute may be lost and so aldosterone stimulation is triggered. As well as its renal reabsorption role, it also enhances sodium and chloride reabsorption along the duct of the sweat gland. Sweating, along with vasodilatation, is one of the body's means of losing heat. The signal to increase the rate of sweating arises from the hypothalamic sympathetic outflow to exocrine sweat glands.

Heat is lost from the surface of the skin as the energy used to evaporate sweat. The evaporation of 1 g of water uses 2.4 kJ of heat. Normally, every hour there is a basal, insensible evaporative loss of water of about 20–30 g from both skin and lungs.

The rate of sweating is dependent upon core as well as surface body temperature. It occurs at a higher core temperature if the surface temperature is lowered, and vice versa.

The capacity of sweating to lose heat is dependent upon external humidity. Hence, in high humidity environments such as the rainforest, a lower temperature is tolerated than in low-humidity settings, e.g. desert.

28 (**a**) true (**b**) false (**c**) true (**d**) true (**e**) false

Thyroid-releasing hormone (TRH) is a tripeptide that is released by the hypothalamus. It stimulates the production of thyroid-stimulating hormone (TSH) a polypeptide from the anterior pituitary. TSH in turn stimulates the release of the thyroxines (T4 and the more potent T3) from the thyroid gland.

The thyroid gland produces predominantly T4 with a small amount of T3. About 85% of circulating T3 is the result of mono-deiodination of T4 in the tissues, especially the liver, muscle and kidney. T3 is about five times more active than T4. Most of the T3 and T4 is carried in the plasma bound to thyroxine-binding globulin (TBG), thyroxine binding pre-albumin (TBPA) and albumin. However, unbound T3 and T4 are the active forms and gain entry into the cell by an ATP dependent process.

Production of T3 and T4 is controlled primarily by the circulating concentrations of free thyroid hormone, which exert a negative feedback on TSH release. However, dopamine, somatostatin and glucocorticoids may reduce plasma TSH and so affect TSH release. Both T3 and T4:

- increase cell metabolism
- facilitate normal growth
- facilitate normal mental development
- increase the local effects of catecholamines

The half-life of T3 is approximately 24 hs whereas the half-life of T4 is about 7 days.

29 (**a**) true (**b**) true (**c**) true (**d**) true (**e**) true

Vomiting is the process by which the contents of the stomach are expelled through the mouth.

When the effort of vomiting is made but nothing is expelled the process is called retching. Retching is a common symptom of alcoholism.

The vomiting centre in the brain coordinates the contraction of the abdominal wall and the opening of the cardiac sphincter of the stomach. The vomiting centre is found in the floor of the fourth ventricle.

Vomiting can lead to:

- hypokalaemia

- hypochloraemia
- alkalosis
- Mallory–Weiss syndrome
- aspiration

30 (**a**) false (**b**) true (**c**) false (**d**) true (**e**) false

The complement system is activated by invading organisms but more often triggered by antibodies. It 'complements' the action of antibodies.

Complement consists of 11 plasma proteins produced by the liver.

Functions

- Membrane attack complex proteins form a channel in the membrane of the invading cell. The resulting influx of water causes lysis (or bursting) of the invading cell
- Chemotaxins
- Opsonins bind with microbes and thereby enhance their phagocytosis
- Cause vasodilatation and increase vascular permeability to increase blood flow to the invaded area
- Stimulate release of histamine from mast cells, which enhances the vascular changes characteristic of inflammation
- Activate kinins, which reinforce the vascular changes induced by histamine and act as powerful chemotaxins

31 (**a**) true (**b**) false (**c**) true (**d**) false (**e**) false

There are about five dopamine receptors identified on molecular biological grounds. D_1 and D_2 are the most important.

D_1 receptors

(a) Gs-coupled adenylate cyclase; when activated leads to an increase in cAMP

(b) Peripheral effects
   - Vasodilatation of renal and mesenteric coronary vasculature
   - Natriuresis and diuresis
   - Renin release

D_2 receptors

(a) G_1-coupled adenylate cyclase; inhibited decreases cAMP
(b) Central effects
- Chemoreceptor trigger zone (nausea & vomiting)
- Nigrostriatal pathway (movement)
- Mesocorticolimbic pathway (emotion)
- Tuberoinfundibular pathway (prolactin secretion)

(c) Peripheral
- inhibits release of noradrenaline and acetylcholine

32 (**a**) true (**b**) true (**c**) true (**d**) false (**e**) true

The physical properties of inhalational anaesthetics include:
- fluoride ions are lighter than chloride and bromide ions
- solubility is reduced when the molecular weight is reduced
- potency increases with increasing molecular weight
- increasing the fluorination of the carbon skeleton increases the stability and SVP, but it reduces boiling point, flammability, and toxicity

33 (**a**) true (**b**) false (**c**) true (**d**) true (**e**) false

Two major types of hepatotoxicity are associated with halothane administration. The two forms appear to be unrelated and are termed type I (mild), possibly due to hepatic hypoxia, and type II (fulminant), which includes antibody formation.

Type I hepatotoxicity characteristics

- Benign
- Self-limiting
- Relatively common (up to 25%–30% incidence)
- Marked by mild, transient increases in serum transaminase and glutathione *S*-transferase concentrations and by altered postoperative drug metabolism
- Not characterised by jaundice or clinically evident hepatocellular disease
- Probably the result of reductive (anaerobic) biotransformation of halothane rather than the normal oxidative pathway

- Absent following the administration of other volatile anaesthetics because they are metabolised to a lesser degree and by different pathways than halothane

Type II hepatotoxicity characteristics

- Is associated with massive centrilobular liver cell necrosis, which leads to fulminating liver failure
- Has no specific histopathologic findings
- Is characterised clinically by fever, jaundice and grossly elevated serum transaminase levels
- Appears to be immune mediated and is initiated by oxidative halothane metabolism to an intermediate compound. This compound then binds to trifluoroacetylate proteins in the hepatic endoplasmic reticulum. It is thought to occur in genetically predisposed individuals. The potential for volatile anaesthetics to cause type II hepatotoxicity is directly related to the relative degree of their oxidative metabolism to acetylated protein adducts. Approximately 20% of halothane undergoes oxidative metabolism compared to only 2% of enflurane and 0.2% of isoflurane

Risk factors

- Multiple exposures (especially at intervals of <6 weeks): this is the single greatest risk factor for halothane hepatitis
- Prior history of postanaesthetic fever or jaundice
- Obesity
- Female sex
- Middle age
- Genetic predisposition
- Enzyme induction
- Pre-existing liver disease itself is not a risk factor for halothane hepatitis

Sex: the male: female ratio is 1:1.6.

Age: halothane hepatotoxicity is more common in middle age. Although children were once thought to be immune, the incidence has been demonstrated to be 1 case per 100 000–200 000 patients.

34 **(a)** true **(b)** false **(c)** false **(d)** false **(e)** true

Table 3.34 Recommendations for dosage regimen adjustment (DRA) in renal-impairment

	Comments
Antimicrobial agents	
Aminoglycosides	Contraindicated because of nephrotoxicity
Penicillins	Accumulation, but high therapeutic index. For dicloxacillin and oxacillin, no change. For others, when GFR <0.5 ml/kg per min, divide the dose by 2 or multiply the dosage interval by 2
Cephalosporins	Potentially nephrotoxic (especially cephaloridine)
Sulphonamides	DRA recommended: for sulfisoxazole, multiply the dosage interval by 2–3 when GFR< 1 ml/kg per min.
Tetracyclines	Severe accumulation, potentially nephrotoxic, exacerbation of azotemia; contraindicated, except doxycycline, which has substantial non-renal elimination
Fluoroquinolones	DRA recommended in humans
Lincosamides and macrolides	No DRA required for erythromycin and clindamycin
Metronidazole	No DRA required
Anti-inflammatory drugs	
NSAIDs	Nephrotoxic risk. No accumulation observed with tolfenamic acid
Corticosteroids	Worsen azotemia
Cardiovascular drugs	
Digitalis glycosides	Accumulation of digoxin, but not digitoxin. Therapeutic drug monitoring highly recommended.
ACE inhibitors	Enalapril and captopril are extensively cleared by the kidney
Antiarrhythmic drugs	Hepatic elimination, but active metabolites are most often cleared by the kidney and the therapeutic index is low
Diuretics	Decreased elimination and diuretic response for frusemide

Anaesthetics	
Barbiturates	Adverse renal haemodynamic effects and potential increase in sensitivity of the central nervous system
Ketamine	Reduced risk of adverse effects in renal impairment
Volatile anaesthetics	Isoflurane should be preferred to halothane and methoxyflurane

35 (**a**) true (**b**) true (**c**) true (**d**) false (**e**) true

Ranitidine is a competitive and specific antagonist of H_2 receptors at parietal cells.

Differences from cimetidine include:
- it is more potent
- it does not inhibit hepatic cytochrome P450
- it has no antiandrogenic effects
- it undergoes a greater degree of first-pass metabolism (oral bioavailability = 50%)

36 (**a**) false (**b**) true (**c**) false (**d**) true (**e**) false

Therapeutic blood concentration for salicylate is 250–300 mg/l. An increase in urinary pH is used when the salicylate level is >750 mg/l or >500 mg/l with a metabolic acidosis; also with phenobarbitone or phenoxyherbicide poisoning.

The objective is to maintain a urine pH between 7.5 and 8.2 by an IV infusion of sodium bicarbonate.

37 (**a**) false (**b**) true (**c**) false (**d**) true (**e**) false

The most important route for elimination of inhalational anaesthetics is the alveolus.

Many of the factors that speed induction also speed recovery for example:
- elimination of rebreathing
- high fresh gas flow
- low anaesthetic circuit volume
- low absorption by the anaesthetic circuit
- decreased solubility
- increased ventilation

Paper 3 Answers

38 (**a**) true (**b**) true (**c**) false (**d**) false (**e**) true

Isoflurane is a halogenated ethyl-methyl ether.

Only 0.2% is metabolised and none of the products has been linked to toxicity.

39 (**a**) true (**b**) true (**c**) false (**d**) false (**e**) false

The mechanism of action of propofol is unclear but it is thought to be due to a reduction in Na^+ channel opening times.

Effects

(a) Cardiovascular
- Reduced SVR resulting in a drop in blood pressure
- Bradycardia
- Reduced myocardial contractility
- Reduced sympathetic activity

(b) Respiratory
- Respiratory depression leading to apnoea

(c) CNS
- Excitatory measurement as a manifestation of subcortical excitatory – inhibitory centre imbalance

(d) Gut
- It may possess anti-emetic properties

(e) Pain
- Is probably due to a direct irritant effect, while delayed pain occurring 10–20 s after the start of injection is probably the result of activation of the kinin system

(f) Metabolic
- Prolonged infusion may result in fat overload syndrome with hyperlipidaemia

(g) Genitourinary
- May turn urine green

NB Its clearance exceeds hepatic blood flow, suggesting some extrahepatic metabolism.

40 (**a**) false (**b**) true (**c**) true (**d**) false (**e**) false

Etomidate is a carboxylated imidazole with a chiral carbon atom and an ester linkage.

It is metabolised by non-specific hepatic esterases and possibly plasma cholinesterase to ethyl alcohol and its carboxylic acid metabolite. It may inhibit plasma cholinesterase. It is 87% excreted in urine, 3% unchanged.

Side-effects include

- Pain on injection in up to 25% of patients
- PONV (2%–10%)
- Excitatory movements
- Inhibition of steroidogenesis, which lasts 3–6 h after a single dose, by inhibition of the enzymes 11β-hydroxylase and 17α-hydroxylase
- Histamine release is minimal
- The therapeutic index – effective dose/lethal dose (ED_{50}/LD_{50}) – is reported as 16 (in dogs)

41 (**a**) false (**b**) false (**c**) false (**d**) true (**e**) false

If the fetus becomes acidotic there will be an increase in the ionised fraction and local anaesthetic will accumulate in the fetus in significant amounts due to their rapid metabolism.

42 (**a**) false (**b**) true (**c**) true (**d**) true (**e**) true

Ropivacaine is the *S*-enantiomer of the propyl (C_3H_7) derivative of *N*-alkyl pipecoloxylidine.

Pharmacokinetics of amide local anaesthetic agents

Mol.wt.	274 Da
p*ka*	8.1
Partition coefficient	2.9
Protein binding	94%
Volume of distribution	0.8 l/kg
Clearance	10 ml/min
Half-life	110 min

Differences between bupivacaine and ropivacaine, are such that ropivacaine:

- is 2–3 times less lipid soluble
- has a smaller volume of distribution
- has greater clearance
- has a shorter elimination half-life
- is slightly less potent

The two drugs have a similar
- p*K*a
- Plasma protein binding

43 (**a**) false (**b**) true (**c**) false (**d**) true (**e**) true

Diamorphine is a *semi-synthetic* derivative of morphine.

Mechanism of action

Diamorphine is diacetylmorphine; it is a pro drug. The initial metabolic product is 6-monoacetylmorphine, which is then deacetylated again to the active from of morphine, so its analgesic effect is the same as morphine's. The acetylation makes it more water soluble, so it has a quicker onset of action and is more likely to lead to addiction in susceptible patients.

Differences between diamorphine and morphine. Diamorphine has:
- greater analgesic potency (1.5 times)
- greater lipid solubility
- a more rapid onset of action
- a shorter duration of action
- a more sedative effect
- a high potential for addition
- induces more sedation
- has a high potential for addition

44 (**a**) true (**b**) false (**c**) true (**d**) true (**e**) false

Peripheral sensitisation of the nociceptors occurs due to chemical, mechanical and thermal stimulation.

The chemical mediators released from the tissue include: bradykinin, serotonin, histamine, potassium ions, adenosine triphosphate, protons, prostaglandins, nitric oxide, leukotrienes and cytokines.

Altered pH is important in inducing mechanical sensitisation and pain due to ischaemia. Protons cause a reduction in pH.

Central sensitisation occurs with *N*-methyl-D-aspartate (NMDA) and release of amino acids such as glutamate and the neuropeptides substance P and neurokinin. These are not inflammatory mediators. These lead to a cascade of G-protein-mediated activation of phospholipase C.

45 **(a)** true **(b)** true **(c)** false **(d)** false **(e)** false

Tricyclic antidepressants are used in the treatment of a variety of adult conditions including depression and chronic pain disorders, as well as paediatric conditions including enuresis, attention deficit and hyperactivity disorder.

Action

(a) Competitively block neuronal uptake (uptake 1) of noradrenaline and serotonin (5-HT), as a result of which they increase the concentration of transmitter in the synapse

(b) Also block
- Muscarinic receptors
- Histaminergic
- Adrenoreceptors

Effects

(a) CNS
- Sedation
- Seizures in epileptic patients

(b) CVS
- Postural hypotension in the elderly
- Tachycardia/arrhythmia

(c) Anticholinergic effects
- Dry mouth
- Blurred vision
- Constipation

46 **(a)** true **(b)** true **(c)** false **(d)** false **(e)** true

The anti-emetics can be classified into

(a) Anti-serotogenic ($5HT_3$)
- Ondansetron
- Granisetron

(b) Anti-dopaminergic (D_2 receptors)
- Phenothiazines
  - prophylamines, e.g. chlorpromazine
  - piperazine, e.g. prochlorperazine, perphenazine
  - piperidine

- Butyrophenones
  - droperidol
  - haloperidol
- Benzamide
  - metoclopramide

(c) Antihistaminic (H_1 receptors)
- Cyclizine

(d) Anticholinergic (M_3 receptors)
- Hyoscine

(e) Neurokinin receptor antagonist

(f) Cannabinoid receptor
- Dronabinol

(g) Opioid receptors
- They have both emetic and antiemetic effects

Others: steroids, propofol, ginger root

47 (**a**) true (**b**) false (**c**) false (**d**) false (**e**) false

Methyldopa is a phenylalanine derivative.

Action

- Crosses blood–brain barrier – decarboxylated to alpha-methyl noradrenaline, which is stored in adrenergic nerve terminals within the CNS
- Alpha-methyl noradrenaline is a potent agonist at α2 (presynaptic) nerve terminals (α2: α1 10)
- It reduces central sympathetic discharge
- It reduces BP

Side-effects

CVS	Orthostatic hypotension
	Bradycardia
	Peripheral oedema
CNS	Sedation
	Depression
	Dizziness
	Paraesthesia
	Weakness

GI	Thrombocytopenia
	Positive Coomb's test (20%)
	Haemolytic anaemia
Miscellaneous	Dry mouth
	Impotence
	Fluid retention
	Constipation

Approximately 50% is excreted unchanged in the urine.

48 (**a**) false (**b**) true (**c**) false (**d**) false (**e**) true

Suxamethonium-induced bradycardia is often more severe after the second dose but may be prevented by atropine.

This phenomenon is often more pronounced in children. The initial depolarising block is described as phase I block; however, if further doses are given it may become a phase II block.

49 (**a**) false (**b**) false (**c**) false (**d**) false (**e**) false

Medetomidine is an alpha 2 agonist. It is a racemic mixture but only the D-stereoisomer is active, so it has been developed as dex-medetomidine.

Action

It stimulates alpha 2 receptors in the lateral reticular nucleus resulting in reduced central sympathetic flow, and in the spinal cord where it augments endogenous opiate release and modulates the descending noradrenergic pathway involved (a spinal nociceptive processing).

Differences from clonidine include

- Medetomidine is more potent
- Medetomidine has a higher affinity for the alpha 2 receptors
- Medetomidine has a shorter elimination half-life

50 (**a**) true (**b**) true (**c**) false (**d**) true (**e**) true

The drugs which release histamine can precipitate bronchospasm.

(a) Opioids – morphine
(b) Muscle relaxants
  - depolarising, e.g. suxamethonium
  - non-depolarizing, e.g. atracurium, mivacurium
(c) Anticholinesterases drugs – neostigmine
(d) IV induction agents – thiopentone, methohexitone

Paper 3 Answers

51 (**a**) false (**b**) false (**c**) true (**d**) true (**e**) false

Sympathomimetics exert their effect via adrenoreceptors or dopamine receptors

- Directly acting – sympathomimetics attach to and act directly via these receptors
- Indirect acting – sympathomimetics cause the release of noradrenaline to produce their effects via these receptors

Sympathomimetics can be classified into:

(a) Naturally occurring catecholamines
  - Epinephrine (adrenaline)
  - Norepinephrine (noradrenaline)
  - Dopamine

(b) Synthetic non-catecholamines
  - Directly acting
    - phenylephrine
    - methoxamine
  - Indirectly acting
    - ephedrine
    - amphetamine
    - metaraminol

52 (**a**) true (**b**) true (**c**) false (**d**) false (**e**) true

Anti-arrhythmics may be divided on the basis of their clinical use in the treatment of:

(a) Supraventricular tachyarrhythmias (SVT)
  - Digoxin
  - Adenosine
  - Verapamil
  - Beta blockers
  - Quinidine

(b) Ventricular tachyarrhythmias
  - Lidocaine (lignocaine)
  - Mexiletine

(c) Both SVT and VT
  - Amiodarone
  - Procainamide
  - Flecainide

- Disopyramide
- Sotalol

(d) Digoxin toxicity
- Phenytoin

53 (**a**) true (**b**) true (**c**) true (**d**) true (**e**) false

Pyridostigmine is a quaternary amine used mainly in the treatment of myasthenia gravis.

Compared with neostigmine, pyridostigmine:
- has one-quarter of the potency
- has a slower onset of action (15 min)
- has a longer duration of action (3–6 h)
- is less arrhythmogenic
- relies on renal elimination more than neostigmine (75% excreted unchanged)

54 (**a**) false (**b**) true (**c**) true (**d**) false (**e**) true

Amiodarone is a benzofuran derivative.

Action
- Traditionally designated as a Class III antiarrhythmic
- Amiodarone also demonstrates Class I, II and IV activity
- By blocking K^+ channels, it slows the rate of depolarisation thereby increasing the duration of the action potential
- The refractory period is also increased

Pharmacokinetics

Bioavailability	20%–85%
Protein binding	97%
Half-life	1300 h

Side-effects
(a) Skin
- Photosensitivity
- Rashes
- Aloplecia
- Dermatitis

(b) Eye
- Corneal micro deposit
- Optic neuritis

(c) Neurological
- Peripheral neuropathy

(d) Cerebellar dysfunction
- Thyroid – hypo or hyper with abnormal TFT

(e) Lungs
- Fibrosis
- Alveolitis
- Pneumonitis

(f) Heart
- Prolongation of Q-T interval

55 **(a)** true **(b)** false **(c)** true **(d)** true **(e)** true

Mechanism of action

- Acetazolamide is a carbonic anhydrase inhibitor
- Non-competitive inhibitor of carbon anhydrase enzyme
- Carbonic anhydrase is present in the brush border and cytoplasm of proximal tubule cells
- HCO_3 must be converted to CO_2 via carbonic acid before it can be absorbed into the cell where it is converted back into carbonic acid
- Carbonic acid then dissociates into bicarbonate and hydrogen ions. The H^+ is then exchanged with Na^+ in lumen and bicarbonate leaves the cell and is exchanged with chloride ions in the bloodstream
- When the enzyme is inhibited Na^+ accompanies the non-absorbed H^+
- H^+ excretion is inhibited
- K^+ is enhanced (distal convoluted tubule) due to increased Na^+ delivery

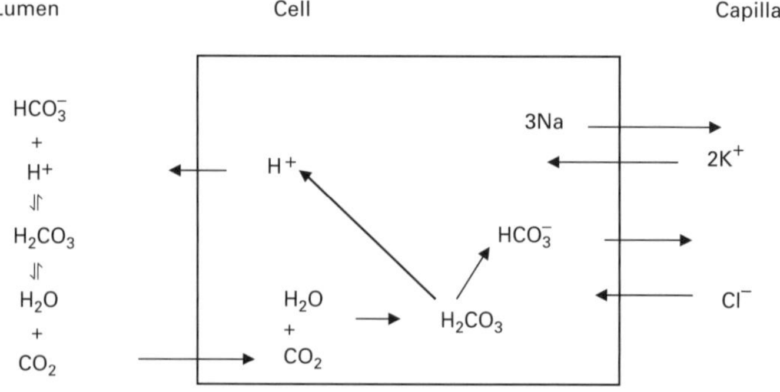

Effects
- Hyperchloraemic acidosis
- Alkaline urine
- Hypokalaemia

Pharmacokinetics
- Bioavailability is 95%
- Highly protein bound
- Is excreted unchanged in the urine

Uses
- Glaucoma
- Epilepsy

56 (**a**) false (**b**) false (**c**) false (**d**) false (**e**) true

Left ventricular end-diastolic pressure (normally <12 mmHg) is proportional to left ventricular end-diastolic volume in an exponential way. It reflects the preload on the left ventricle.

An increase occurs with:
- reduced myocardial contractility either intrinsically or due to drugs with a negative inotropic action
- increased venous return and increased blood volume

A decrease will occur with a reduced preload, as will occur with a vasodilator or with inotropic drugs, or with a sympathetically mediated increase in cardiac contractility. Halothane has a direct, negative inotropic effect to reduce myocardial contractility and reduce cardiac output.

Isoflurane acts as a vasodilator with no effect on myocardial contractility to increase venous return.

Thiopentone causes a dose-related myocardial depression and little effect on SVR but reduces venous return.

Ketamine, by its sympathomimetic effect, will increase myocardial contractility.

57 (**a**) true (**b**) true (**c**) true (**d**) true (**e**) true

Characteristics
- Is a chlorinated procainamide derivative
- Is used as an antiemetic/prokinetic

- Approximately half of the clinical studies have demonstrated that placebo is as effective as metoclopramide
- Is soluble and stable in water

Action

- It is a non-specific antagonist at central and peripheral D_2 receptors (risk of Parkinson-like effects)
- Selective stimulation of gastric muscarinic receptors; this acetylcholine effect promotes gastric motility (prokinetic) and increases lower oesophageal tone
- High doses: a 5-HT_3 antagonist
- Antagonist at 5-HT_4 receptors

Effects

(a) CNS – crosses the blood–brain barrier
- Extrapyramidal side-effects
- Neuroleptic malignant syndrome
- Sedation (long-term use)
- Neuroleptic and anti-psychotic

(b) CVS
- Hypotension (brady/tachycardia after rapid IV injection)

(c) Metabolic
- Increases aldosterone
- Hyperprolactinaemia
- Should be avoided in porphyria
- Inhibits pseudocholinesterase

(d) Gastrointestional
- Increase lower oesophageal sphincter (LOS) tone
- Relaxation of pylorus
- Accelerates gastric emptying
- Accelerates amplitude of concentration

Side-effects

- Dizziness/drowsiness/faintness
- Diarrhoea
- Extrapyramidal side-effects
  - Akinesia
  - Oculogyric
- Renal impairment, especially in high doses and the elderly

58 **(a)** false **(b)** false **(c)** true **(d)** true **(e)** true

Recommendations for dosage regimen adjustment (DRA) in renal impairment:

(a) Antimicrobial agents
- Aminoglycoside
- Pencillins
- Cephalosporins
- Sulphonamides
- Tetracyclines
- Fluoroquinolones

(b) Anti-inflammatory drugs
- NSAIDS
- Steroids

(c) Cardiovascular drugs
- Digoxin
- ACE inhibitors
- Antiarrhythmics
- Diuretics

(d) Anaesthetics
- Barbiturates
- Halothane

59 **(a)** false **(b)** false **(c)** true **(d)** true **(e)** false

Sumatriptan is a 5-HT_{1D} agonist. The specific receptor subtype is present in the cranial and basilar arteries. Activation of these receptors causes vasoconstriction of those dilated arteries. Sumatriptan is also shown to decrease the activity of the trigeminal nerve.

Pharmacokinetics

Mol.wt.	295.4
Bioavailability	15% (oral)
	96% (s.c.)
Elimination half-life	2.5 h
Excretion	60% urine, 40% faeces

Indications

- Migraine headache
- Cluster headache

Contraindications

- Coronary artery disease
- Monoamine oxidase inhibitor

Side-effects

- Coronary artery vasospasm
- Transient myocardial ischaemia
- Myocardial infarction
- Ventricular tachycardia/fibrillation
- Hypertensive crisis

60 (**a**) true (**b**) true (**c**) false (**d**) false (**e**) true

Penicillinase-resistant penicillins include:

- methicillin (dimethoxy benzylpenicillin)
- oxacillin
- cloxacillin
- dicloxacillin
- flucloxacillin

These penicillins are not susceptible to hydrolysis by staphylococcal penicillinase, which would otherwise hydrolyse the cyclic amide bond of the beta lactam ring and render the antimicrobial inactive.

61 (**a**) true (**b**) true (**c**) false (**d**) false (**e**) false

Flow is defined as the quantity of a fluid, i.e. a gas or liquid, passing a point in a unit time.

$$\text{Mean flow} = \frac{\text{Quantity (mass or volume)}}{\text{time}}$$

Flow can be measured in gases by:

- flow meter
- Wright spirometer
- pneumotachograph
- bubble flow meter
- Bourdon gauge
- mass spectrometry

Several methods exist for measurement of flow in liquids:

- visually
- infusion controllers and pumps

- infrared infusion rate detector
- volumetric pump
- ultrasonic
- electromagnetic

62 (**a**) true (**b**) false (**c**) true (**d**) true (**e**) true

Static electricity is defined as the imbalance of positive and negative charges. Protons and neutrons in the nucleus are held together very tightly. Some of the outer electrons are held very loosely. They can move from one atom to another. An atom that loses electrons has more positive charges (protons) than negative charges (electrons) and it is positively charged.

An atom that gains electrons has more negative than positive particles; it has a negative charge.

Static charges are produced on non-conductive materials.

Materials are classified as *insulators* or *conductors*

Insulator characteristics
- Hold electrons very tightly
- Electrons do not move through them very well

Conductor characteristics
- Contain some loosely held electrons
- Electrons move through them very easily

Electrons can be moved from one place to another by rubbing two objects together if they are
- made of different materials
- both insulators

Electrons may be transferred or mixed from one material to another.

The more the rubbing, the more the electrons move and the larger the charges that are built up.

Although the quality of static electricity generated in the operating theatre is relatively small, there is sufficient energy in the spark when it is rapidly discharged to ignite flammable vapours.

Arrangements should be made not only to prevent the generation of static electricity but also to discharge slowly to earth any that does occur.

Prevention of static charges

(a) Antistatic *conducting material* should be used in place of non-conductors.
(b) Resistance of antistatic material should be between 50 KΩ/cm and 10 MΩ/cm.
(c) All materials should be allowed to leak static charges through the floor of the operating theatre.
(d) The floor of the operating theatre is designed to have a resistance of 25 KΩ when measured between two electrodes placed 1 cm apart. This allows the gradual discharge of static electricity to earth. If the conductivity of the floor is too great there is a risk of electrocution.
(e) Keep the relative humidity of the atmosphere above 50% because:
   - Moisture encourages the leakage of static charges along surfaces to the floor
   - The risk of sparks from accumulated static electricity charge is reduced.

63 (**a**) true (**b**) false (**c**) false (**d**) false (**e**) true

A Patient's peak expiratory flow rate is measured by a Wright's peak flow meter.

The normal value for peak expiratory flow rate (PEFR) is 500–600 l/min. A peak flow meter is a variable-orifice, constant-pressure meter.

Components

- Inlet and outlet
- A rotating vane surrounded by fixed slits to allow the escape of gas
- Vane is attached to a pointer

Action

- One-way system
- As the patient blows, gas flow onto the vanes
- The vanes move and a slot is opened to allow the expired gas to escape
- The movement of the vane is resisted by the force of a coiled spring which produces a constant resistance
- The coil is connected to a pointer that indicates the volume of gas that has passed through

Measurement of a patient's PEFR

- Explain to the patient the procedure
- Check the meter is zeroed and re-set
- Should be held horizontally
- Apply nose clips
- The patient is asked to take a full inspiration to total lung capacity
- The lips must be placed tightly around the mouth piece

Problems with Wright's peak flow meters

- Moisture, which causes the pointer to stick
- It under-reads at low flows
- It over-reads at high flows
- Inertia
- Friction

64 (**a**) true (**b**) true (**c**) true (**d**) true (**e**) false

Gases cannot be compressed into a liquid at room temperature, whereas a vapour can. If the critical temperature of a substance is less than the surrounding temperature then it is a gas and cannot be compressed into a liquid.

Gases at room temperature include:

- oxygen (critical temperature is $-118°C$)
- air
- Entonox
- xenon
- helium

65 (**a**) false (**b**) false (**c**) false (**d**) true (**e**) true

The boiling point of a liquid is the temperature at which the vapour pressure is equal to the atmospheric pressure. The lower the atmospheric pressure, the lower the boiling point.

66 (**a**) false (**b**) false (**c**) true (**d**) true (**e**) true

A pressure gauge indicates the pressure within each cylinder. In the case of oxygen and other gases, which do not liquefy at normal temperatures (air, Entonox), this enables the volume of the contents to be estimated, since the amount of gas contained in the cylinder is proportional to the pressure (Boyle's law).

This is not the case for vapours such as N_2O and CO_2, which are liquefied by the high pressure within the cylinder. The pressure remains relatively constant until all the liquid is evaporated, after which the pressure drops rapidly as the remaining gas is removed. The contents of these cylinders can only be estimated by weighing the cylinder.

67 (**a**) false (**b**) false (**c**) true (**d**) false (**e**) true

Air flows to the operating theatre should have the following characteristics:

- pressure gradient about 35 Pa
- air changes 20–40 times per hour
- air flow 45–60 m^3/min
- temperature 21–24°C
- humidity about 50%

NB The oxygen content of 100 ml of arterial blood with 15 g haemoglobin is 19.8 ml/100 ml. Air contains 20.9% oxygen or 20.9 ml/100 ml.

68 (**a**) false (**b**) false (**c**) true (**d**) true (**e**) false

The measures of scatter or dispersion (variation or spread) are as follows:

- Sample range: the difference between the highest and the lowest values
- Percentile: the level, below or above which a specific proportion of the distribution falls
- variance and standard deviation: these measure the spread of observations about the mean
  - variance is a measure of dispersion calculated by taking the sum of the differences between individual data points and the overall mean, squaring this value, and then finding their average value by dividing this by the number of observations.
  - standard deviation (SD) is the square root of the variance.
- The coefficient of variation is the ratio of the SD of a series of observations to the mean of the observations expressed as a percentage; coefficient of variation is the (SD/mean) × 100%.

69 (**a**) true (**b**) true (**c**) false (**d**) false (**e**) false

Damping is the tendency of a system to resist oscillations.

Some of the energy of an oscillation is absorbed, and its amplitude is reduced. The damping factor is an index of the system's ability to resist oscillation. Factors that affect the resonant frequency inversely affect damping.

Damping is low in:
- short wide tube
- low-viscosity fluid

Damping is high in:
- long narrow tube
- viscous fluid

The effect of damping is to:
- reduce the maximum amplitude
- reduce the resonant frequency of the system
- increase the flat range of the system

70 (**a**) true (**b**) true (**c**) false (**d**) false (**e**) false

The characteristic of both TEC 4 and 5 are:
- locking lever so that the vaporiser cannot be turned on unless the lever is engaged
- interlocking extension rods
- only one vaporiser can be switched on at a time
- splitting ratio is controlled by a temperature-sensitive bimetallic valve situated outside the vaporising chamber
- anti-tip mechanism

The changes specific to the TEC 5 are:
- improved surface area available for vaporisation because the wick assembly is constituted using a hallow cloth tube
- improved keyed filling action
- an easier mechanism for switching on the rotary valve and locking it (now single handed)

71 (**a**) false (**b**) false (**c**) false (**d**) true (**e**) false

Pulse oximetry errors and problems arise as follows:

(a) A reduction in peripheral pulsatile blood flow produced by
  - Peripheral vasoconstriction
    - hypovolaemia
    - severe hypotension
    - cold

- cardiac failure
  - arrhythmias
- Peripheral vascular disease

(b) Significantly high levels of
- Carboxyhaemoglobin (CoHb): some, but not all, of the CoHb is read as reduced Hb so the oximeter will overestimate the saturation of oxyhaemoglobin
- Methaemoglobin (metHb): as the concentration increases the oximeter readings will tend towards 85% but not lower, regardless of the true oxygen saturation

(c) Circulating dyes: a short-lived reduction in saturation is recorded
- Methylene blue
- Iodocyanine green

(d) Intense ambient light: this is compensated for by a pulsed beam from the probe, rather than a continuous light beam

(e) Excessive movement (e.g. shivering) may cause difficulties in picking up an adequate signal

(f) Electrical device (diathermy): the signal may be interrupted

(g) Increased pulsatile, venous components, e.g. tricuspid incompetence

(h) Cannot detect acute desaturation for 10–20 s.

(i) Nail varnish may cause falsely low readings

(j) The newer units are not affected by:
- hyperbilirubinaemia
- anaemia
- pigmented or oil-covered skin

72 (**a**) true (**b**) true (**c**) true (**d**) false (**e**) false

The boiling point of a liquid is the temperature at which the vapour pressure is equal to the atmospheric pressure.

The lower the atmospheric pressure, the lower the boiling point.

Vapour pressure depends only on the liquid and the temperature. It does not depend on the barometric pressure.

73 (**a**) true (**b**) true (**c**) true (**d**) true (**e**) false

There is an indirect increase in the splitting ratio with a fall in temperature. Temperature compensated vaporisers possess a mechanism that produces an increase in flow through the vaporising chamber as the temperature of liquid anaesthetic decreases.

Methods

A Bimetallic strip

This consists of two metals with different coefficients of thermal expansion joined together along their length as a strip. As the temperature changes one metal expands or contracts more than the other so the strip bends one way or the other.

This bending is used to open or close an opening.

It is positioned inside the vaporisation chamber in the Tec MK 2.

It is positioned outside the vaporisation chamber in the Tec MK 3, Tec MK 4 and Tec MK 5.

Bellows

These are small flexible bellows containing some fluid that has a high coefficient of expansion. As the temperature changes the bellows expand or contract and thus open or close an opening.

Metal rod

Expansion of a metal rod acts to open or close an orifice to modify flow in the vaporising chamber according to the temperature.

By adding the liquid anaesthetic directly to the gas stream

The anaesthetic agent is delivered into the gas stream through a fine nozzle. The rate of delivery depends on the pressure difference across the nozzle, which is adjusted by the throttle valve.

74 (**a**) false (**b**) false (**c**) true (**d**) true (**e**) false

Only gases that have two or more different types of atom in the molecule will absorb infrared light.

If there are only two atoms, absorption only occurs if the two atoms are dissimilar.

Paper 3 Answers

75 (a) true (b) true (c) false (d) false (e) true

pH is a measure of the hydrogen ion activity in a liquid. pH is defined as the negative logarithm to the base 10 of the H^+ concentration. Each decrease of one pH unit is equivalent to a tenfold increase of $[H^+]$.

pH of 7.4 = 40 nmol l^{-1} $[H^+]$ or $10^{-7.4}$ mol l^{-1}.

There is a rise in pH as the temperature of blood falls. The reason for the change in pH is that the degree of ionisation of protein elements in blood is reduced as the temperature falls.

76 (a) false (b) true (c) false (d) true (e) true

The likelihood of the onset of turbulent flow is predicted by

$$\text{Reynold's number (Re)} = \text{pvd}/\eta$$

where,

- D = the diameter of the tube
- v = the velocity of flow
- p = rho, the density of the fluid in $kg.m^{-3}$
- η = eta, the viscosity of the fluid in pascal seconds

Empirical studies show that, for cylindrical tubes, if Re > 2000 turbulent flow becomes more likely. For a given set of conditions there is a critical velocity at which Re = 2000. The effect of turbulent flow may be reduced by reducing the gas density, i.e. O_2 density 1.3, helium density 0.16.

77 (a) false (b) false (c) true (d) false (e) false

Mechanism of action

A microprocessor controls the sequence of inflation and deflation of the cuff. The cuff is inflated to a pressure above the previous systolic pressure; it is then deflated incrementally. A transducer senses the pressure changes in the cuff, which are processed by the microprocessor. It is accurate to ± 2%. The mean arterial pressure (MAP) corresponds to the maximum oscillation at the lowest cuff pressure. The systolic pressure corresponds to the onset of rapidly increasing oscillations. Diastolic pressure corresponds to the onset of rapidly decreasing oscillations. It is also calculated from the systolic pressure and MAP (MAP = diastolic + one-third pulse pressure).

Sources of error

- If the cuff is too small, the blood pressure is over-read
- If too large, then the blood pressure is under-read; the greatest error is seen with an undersized cuff
- Systolic pressure is over-read at low pressures (<60 mmHg)
- High systolic pressures may be under read
- Arrhythmias such as atrial fibrillation affect the accuracy
- External pressure on the cuff can cause inaccuracies

78 (**a**) false (**b**) false (**c**) true (**d**) true (**e**) true

The sample is passed into a chamber where the particles are ionised. The ionised particles are then accelerated as a beam into an arc, which passes though a strong magnetic field. The magnetic field separates the particles which fall out into the detector according to their weight. The lighter ones fall out of the arc first. The position where they fall out is used to tell their size.

By varying the accelerating voltage, molecules of different masses can be made to describe the same arc in one detector. Alternatively, multiple detectors can be used.

An alternative means of manipulating the accelerated beam is the quadrupole. Four electrically charge rods are positioned around the beam such that only a molecule of a given charge/mass ratio will remain undeflected.

When a mixture of gases with similar molecular weights is present, an isotope fragment of the compound is analysed to allow differentiation between molecules of the same charge/mass ratio. This occurs with N_2O and CO_2, both of which have a molecular weight of 44; however, the nitrous oxide fragments into nitric oxide, which is used for the differentiation.

Advantages

- Rapid response time < 100 ms
- Highly accurate
- Incorporates a correction for the presence of water vapour

Disadvantages

- Very bulky
- Expensive

- Noisy in operation
- Gases cannot be returned to the breathing system
- Susceptible to damage from water vapour and other drugs
- Needs calibration

79 (**a**) false (**b**) true (**c**) false (**d**) false (**e**) true

(a) In vitro CO_2 measurement
  - Astrup technique
  - CO_2 electrode, Severinghaus electrode

(b) In vivo measurement
  - Intravascular probe
  - Transcutaneous electrodes
  - Optodes

(c) Measuring CO_2 concentration in respiratory gases
  - Capnography (infrared spectrography)
    - side stream
    - main stream
  - Mass spectrography (MW)
  - Raman spectrography
  - Photoacoustic spectrography
  - Fenem CO_2 detector

80 (**a**) false (**b**) true (**c**) false (**d**) false (**e**) false

The absolute pressure equals the gauge pressure plus the atmospheric pressure. In the mercury barometer a vacuum is present above the mercury so that the absolute pressure is recorded. In many manometers a disc of material permeable to air is placed at the top of the tube to prevent spillage of the mercury.

A full O_2 cylinder has a gauge pressure of 137 bar.

81 (**a**) false (**b**) false (**c**) false (**d**) true (**e**) true

Oxygen is paramagnetic and is therefore attracted into a magnetic field; this is due to the unpaired outer shell electrons of the oxygen molecule. Most other gases, such as N_2, are weakly diamagnetic and are repelled from a magnetic field. The paramagnetic analyser measures oxygen concentration.

82 (**a**) true (**b**) true (**c**) false (**d**) true (**e**) false

An alpha particle is a combination of two protons and two neutrons. An isotope of an element can be described by the total number of neutrons and protons which the nucleus contains.

83 (**a**) true (**b**) true (**c**) true (**d**) true (**e**) true

A radiofrequency lesion is caused by a form of electromagnetic energy similar to a diathermy lesion. It requires a large, well-applied earth electrode that makes a good electrical contact with the skin.

84 (**a**) true (**b**) false (**c**) false (**d**) false (**e**) true

The Bunsen Solubility Coefficient is the volume of gas (corrected to STP) that dissolves in one unit volume of the liquid at the temperature concerned, where the partial pressure of the gas concerned is 1 atm.

The Ostwald Solubility Coefficient as the volume of gas which dissolves in 1 unit volume of the liquid at the temperature concerned.

- The temperature must be specified
- It is independent of pressure: as the pressure rises the number of molecules of gas in the liquid phase increases; however, when measured at the higher pressure the volume is the same

The Partition Coefficient is the ratio of the amount of a substance present in one phase compared to the amount present in a second phase, the two phases being of equal volume and in equilibrium, and the temperature must be specified.

85 (**a**) false (**b**) false (**c**) false (**d**) true (**e**) true

Methods of preventing electrical accidents include:

- Whenever possible patients should be insulated from electrical earth
- Installation of an isolating transformer
- A pair of conductors that share a common magnetic core use the electronic magnet principle. They prevent accidents associated with unwanted currents returning to earth. The isolated transformers are included in the circuitry of each item of mains-operated electromedical equipment that can be connected to a patient; the patient circuit is earth free and said to be fully floating
- Earth leakage detectors are a current-operated earth leakage circuit breaker (COELCB) also known as an earth trip or residual current

circuit breaker. They detect unwanted current passing to earth, and either sound a warning or automatically switch off the supply

86 (**a**) false (**b**) false (**c**) false (**d**) false (**e**) true

Electrical burns are due to

- Poor contact between the neutral plate and the patient. Prevented by an audible warning if the plate is not plugged in or the lead is broken
- In advertent depression of the foot switch. Prevented by
  - keeping the forceps in a protective quiver
  - installation of a buzzer which is activated when the switch is depressed
- The electrical circuit being completed via the operating table or other points through which the patient may be earthed

Risks are reduced by the use of

- Isolating capacitors in diathermy equipment. This is due to the fact that capacitors have a high impedance to low frequency (50 Hz) current, but a low impedance to high-frequency (1 MHz) current, so the damaging effects of all stray mains currents are minimised
- Isolated transformer. The design of the circuit prevents the flow of current to earth by any alternative earth-linked path from a fault in the generator; should the circuit be broken, the diathermy is deactivated
- Infarction of an organ with a thin vascular pedicle. For example, the risk of infarction when unipolar diathermy is used on an organ that has been temporarily raised on its vascular pedicle (testis): the current density is greatly increased in the vas thus causing its destruction

87 (**a**) true (**b**) true (**c**) true (**d**) true (**e**) false

Rebreathing alveolar gas conserves heat and humidity. CO_2 in exhaled gas must be eliminated to prevent hypercarbia. CO_2 chemically combines with water to form carbonic acid:

$$CO_2 + H_2O \rightarrow H_2CO_3 \text{(carbonic acid)}$$

Carbon dioxide absorbents (soda lime or barium hydroxide lime) contain hydrogen salts that are capable of neutralising carbonic acid.

$$H_2CO_3 + 2NaOH \rightarrow Na_2CO_3 + 2H_2O + \text{Heat}$$
$$Na_2CO_3 + Ca(OH)_2 \rightarrow CaCO_3 + 2NaOH$$

The end products of the reaction include:

- heat (the heat of neutralisation)
- water
- calcium carbonate

All volatile agents react with soda lime but only trichloroethylene is known to produce a toxic product.

88 (**a**) true (**b**) true (**c**) false (**d**) false (**e**) false

Oxygen is paramagnetic and is therefore attracted into a magnetic field.

This is due to the unpaired outer shell electrons of the oxygen molecule. Most other gases, such as N_2, are weakly diamagnetic and are repelled from a magnetic field. A paramagnetic analyser actually measures oxygen *concentration.* Most common systems use deflection of nitrogen-containing glass spheres, arranged in a dumbbell shape or similar. These indicate either by direct rotation of a pointer or deflection of light, or they may be arranged in a null deflection system.

They require calibration before use with 100% N_2 and 100% O_2.

The presence of water vapour biases the result, therefore gases should be dried through silica gel before analysis.

89 (**a**) true (**b**) true (**c**) false (**d**) false (**e**) false

By convention a gas is above its critical temperature at the ambient temperature but a vapour is below its critical temperature at ambient temperature.

A gas cannot be compressed into a liquid above its critical temperature whatever the pressure applied.

At room temperature nitrous oxide (N_2O), which has a critical temperature of 36.5 °C, is a vapour but when exhaled at the body temperature of 37 °C it is a gas; the same holds for carbon dioxide (CO_2), which has a critical temperature of 31°C.

Paper 3 Answers

90 (**a**) true (**b**) true (**c**) false (**d**) true (**e**) true

A transducer is a device which converts one form of energy into another for the purposes of measurement. The second form of energy is normally electrical.

Examples include:

- a microphone converts sound into an electrical signal
- a thermistor converts temperature variation into an electrical signal
- a piezo electrical signal converts a pressure variation into an electrical signal

	(a)	(b)	(c)	(d)	(e)
1	F	F	T	T	F
2	F	T	F	F	T
3	T	T	T	F	F
4	T	T	F	F	F
5	T	F	F	T	T
6	T	T	F	F	F
7	T	T	T	F	F
8	F	T	T	T	T
9	F	T	T	F	T
10	F	F	F	T	T
11	T	F	T	F	T
12	F	T	T	T	F
13	F	F	T	T	F
14	F	F	T	F	T
15	F	F	T	T	T
16	T	T	F	F	T
17	T	F	T	F	F
18	F	F	F	T	T
19	T	T	F	T	T
20	F	T	F	T	F
21	T	F	T	F	F
22	F	F	T	F	F
23	T	F	F	F	F
24	T	T	T	T	T
25	T	T	F	F	F
26	T	T	T	F	F
27	T	F	T	F	T
28	T	F	T	T	F
29	T	T	T	T	T

Paper 3 Answers

	(a)	(b)	(c)	(d)	(e)
30	F	T	F	T	F
31	T	F	T	F	F
32	T	T	T	F	T
33	T	F	T	T	F
34	T	F	F	F	T
35	T	T	T	F	T
36	F	T	F	T	F
37	F	T	F	T	F
38	T	T	F	F	T
39	T	T	F	F	F
40	F	T	T	F	F
41	F	F	F	T	F
42	F	T	T	T	T
43	F	T	F	T	T
44	T	F	T	T	F
45	T	T	F	F	F
46	T	T	F	F	T
47	T	F	F	F	F
48	F	T	F	F	T
49	F	F	F	F	F
50	T	T	F	T	T
51	F	F	T	T	F
52	T	T	F	F	T
53	T	T	T	T	F
54	F	T	T	F	T
55	T	F	T	T	T
56	F	F	F	F	T
57	T	T	T	T	T
58	F	F	T	T	T
59	F	F	T	T	F
60	T	T	F	F	T

	(a)	(b)	(c)	(d)	(e)
61	T	T	F	F	F
62	T	F	T	T	T
63	T	F	F	F	T
64	T	T	T	T	F
65	F	F	F	T	T
66	F	F	T	T	T
67	F	F	T	F	T
68	F	F	T	T	F
69	T	T	F	F	F
70	T	T	F	F	F
71	F	F	F	T	F
72	T	T	T	F	F
73	T	T	T	T	F
74	F	F	T	T	F
75	T	T	F	F	T
76	F	T	F	T	T
77	F	F	T	F	F
78	F	F	T	T	T
79	F	T	F	F	T
80	F	T	F	F	F
81	F	F	F	T	T
82	T	T	F	T	F
83	T	T	T	T	T
84	T	F	F	F	T
85	F	F	F	T	T
86	F	F	F	F	T
87	T	T	T	T	F
88	T	T	F	F	F
89	T	T	F	F	F
90	T	T	F	T	T

Paper 4 Answers

1 (**a**) false (**b**) true (**c**) false (**d**) true (**e**) true

There is a progressive reduction in all enzyme activity with cooling but it is not until 30°C that life-threatening changes start to appear.

Below 35°C cognitive impairment begins, leading to loss of consciousness at 30°C.

At 30°C cardiac output has been reduced by about one-third and J waves start to appear on the ECG.

Bradycardia and prolonged conduction in nerve tissue will occur with longer PR, QT and QRS complexes.

Life-threatening ventricular arrhythmias appear at 30°C and ventricular fibrillation at 28°C, which is difficult to reverse unless the heart is re-warmed.

Causes of death are asystole and ventricular fibrillation at temperatures below 30°C and apnoea at 24°C.

2 (**a**) false (**b**) false (**c**) true (**d**) false (**e**) false

Pulse pressure reflects the intermittent ejection of blood flow from the heart into the aorta. The pulse pressure is the difference between the systolic and diastolic pressures.

The main factors that alter pulse pressure in the arteries either increase systolic pressure or reduce diastolic pressure.

Increased systolic pressure

(a) Left ventricular stroke volume: the larger the stroke volume the greater is the volume of blood that must be accommodated in the arterial vessels with each contraction.
(b) Velocity of blood flow: pulse pressure increases when the flow of blood from arteries to veins is accelerated, such as in patent ductus

arteriosus and aortic regurgitation, reflecting rapid run-off of blood into the pulmonary circulation or left ventricle.

(c) Heart rate: an increase in heart rate while cardiac output remains constant causes the stroke volume and pulse pressure to decrease.

(d) Compliance of the arterial tree: pulse pressure is inversely proportional to compliance (distensibility) of the arterial system.
- For example, with aging the distensibility of the arterial walls often decrease and pulse pressure increases
- A reduced oxygen tension will increase sympathetic activity and increase cardiac output
- A raised LVEDV is normally associated with heart failure and a falling cardiac output

Reduced diastolic pressure

(a) Systemic vascular resistance (SVR): pulse pressure increases when SVR decreases.

3 **(a)** false **(b)** true **(c)** true **(d)** true **(e)** true

The pulse pressure wave gets larger as it passes down the aorta and the main arteries, and then it dies out in the smaller arteries. The veins are not pulsatile. The pressure wave is a function of the heart beating, not blood flowing.

Exercise increases heart rate, which shortens diastole and so raises the diastolic pressure and reduces the pulse pressure.

With age the systolic pressure rises with increased aortic stiffness and reduced compliance of the main arteries due to atherosclerosis.

4 **(a)** false **(b)** true **(c)** false **(d)** true **(e)** true

Inotropy is the term applied to changes in heart muscle performance (changes in force generation) independent of alterations in preload and afterload.

Changes in inotropy alter the rate of force and pressure development by the ventricle, and therefore change the rate of ejection (i.e. ejection velocity). For example, an increase in inotropy shifts the Frank–Starling curve up and to the left. This causes a reduction in end-systolic volume and an increase in stroke volume.

Increasing inotropy leads to an increase in ejection fraction (EF), while decreasing inotropy decreases EF. Therefore, EF is often used as a clinical index for evaluating the inotropic state of the heart. In heart failure, for example, there is often a decrease in inotropy that leads to a fall in stroke volume as well as an increase in preload, thereby decreasing EF. The increased preload, if it results in a left ventricular end-diastolic pressure greater than 20 mmHg, can lead to pulmonary congestion and oedema.

5 (**a**) true (**b**) true (**c**) true (**d**) true (**e**) false

Factors affecting the oxygen dissociation curve

Rightward shift

- Means more O_2 is given up to the tissues due to a decreased affinity of haemoglobin for O_2 (O_2 is more easily displaced from Hb)
- Increase in *P*50

Factors

- Acidosis:
  - increased H^+
  - reduced pH
- Increased PCO_2
- Increased temperature
- Increased 2,3-DPG (byproduct of glycolysis) accumulated during anaerobic metabolism
- Others
  - abnormal haemoglobins
  - anaemia

Leftward shift

- Means increased affinity of haemoglobin for O_2 and reduces the availability of oxygen to the tissues
- Reduced *P*50

Factors

- Alkalosis
  - reduced H^+
  - increased pH
- Reduced PCO_2
- Reduced temperature
- Reduced 2,3-DPG
- Others

- COHb – carbon monoxide has 300 times more affinity than oxygen for Hb so it displaces the oxygen
- MetHb – ferrous iron in the molecule is converted to ferric which cannot combine with O_2
- HbF (2α, 2γ)
- Pulmonary capillary blood
- Ammonia (combines with Hb at O_2-binding sites and displaces O_2)

6 (**a**) true (**b**) true (**c**) true (**d**) true (**e**) false

Hypercarbia produces cerebral vasodilatation and can lead to raised intracranial pressure and cerebral oedema.

Normal carbon dioxide partial pressure is 5.3 kPa or 40 mmHg. This is in equilibrium with an intracellular pH of 7.4. It is only the carbon dioxide that crosses the cell membrane and not hydrogen ion. Hypercapnia is defined as >6 kPa or 45 mmHg.

The effect of a raised $PaCO_2$ is to stimulate sympathetic activity.

This leads to increased cardiac output, which increases organ perfusion including an increase in cerebral blood flow.

Other changes include a rise in intracranial pressure, reduced cognitive function at about 13 kPa and anaesthesia at 25 kPa. Hickman, in 1822, is credited with the idea of the first anaesthetic when he put a donkey to sleep using carbon dioxide. Unfortunately he chose the wrong gas and died soon afterwards of tuberculosis. If he had lived longer and chosen a different gas the world might have had anaesthesia before 1842.

7 (**a**) true (**b**) true (**c**) true (**d**) true (**e**) false

Total physiological dead space can be calculated from the Bohr equation.

Expired carbon dioxide = (alveolar carbon dioxide × alveolar ventilation) + inspired carbon dioxide

$$P_ECO_2 \times V_T = P_ACO_2 \times (V_T - V_D) + P_ICO_2 \times V_D$$

Inspired carbon dioxide can be ignored

By changing the variables around we can derive the Bohr equation to give a measure of physiological dead space or total dead space:

$$V_D/V_T = (Pa_{co2} - P_{ECO2})/Pa_{co2}$$

Breathing needs to be slow and deep, as rapid shallow breathing will reduce alveolar ventilation at the same minute ventilation. This happens in children who compensate with a higher respiratory rate.

This equation is for the total dead space, or physiological dead space, made up of anatomical dead space and alveolar dead space. Alveolar dead space is lung that contains varying concentrations of carbon dioxide due to suboptimum blood flow. Alveolar dead space is a concept that gives a hypothetical volume of alveolar lung that should have contained carbon dioxide if the lung were functioning normally. The calculation is made to represent all the suboptimum area of lung as a volume that contains no carbon dioxide.

In a healthy lung end-tidal carbon dioxide partial pressure equates with arterial partial pressure.

8 **(a)** true **(b)** false **(c)** false **(d)** false **(e)** false

For individual lung units (each alveolus and its capillary) the ventilation/perfection ($\dot{V}/\dot{Q}$) ratio can range from 0 (no ventilation) to infinity (no perfusion). The normal range is 0.3–3.0, with the majority of lung areas being close to 1.0.

Distribution of $\dot{V}/\dot{Q}$ ratios

- In the normal upright lung, from apex to base
- Increased ventilation 3 times
- Increased perfusion 12 times

So, the $\dot{V}/\dot{Q}$ ratio varies from a high value at the apex to a low value at the base.

Ideal $\dot{V}/\dot{Q}$

Since alveolar ventilation ($\dot{V}$) is normally about 4 l/min and pulmonary capillary perfusion ($\dot{Q}$) is 5 l/min the overall $\dot{V}/\dot{Q}$ ratio is ~ 0.8.

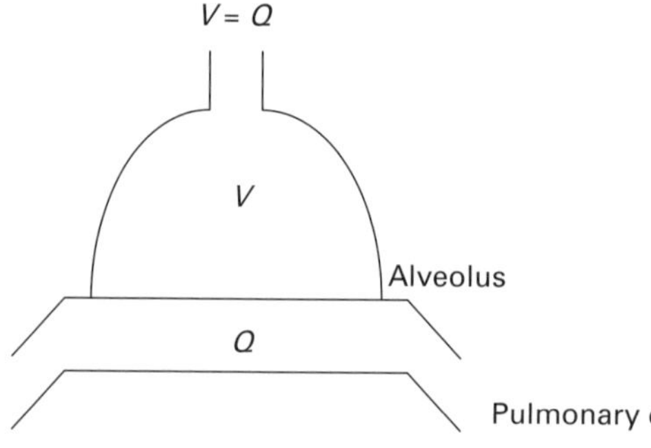

High $\dot{V}/\dot{Q}$ ratio

- $R > 0.8$
- Ventilation in excess of perfusion
- Contributes to alveolar dead space
- Alveolar gas tensions approach those of inspired air
  - PaO_2 increased
  - $PaCO_2$ reduced
- High $\dot{V}/\dot{Q}$ regions lead to a reduction in $PaCO_2$ which causes regional bronchoconstriction and diversion of ventilation to better perfused regions of the lung

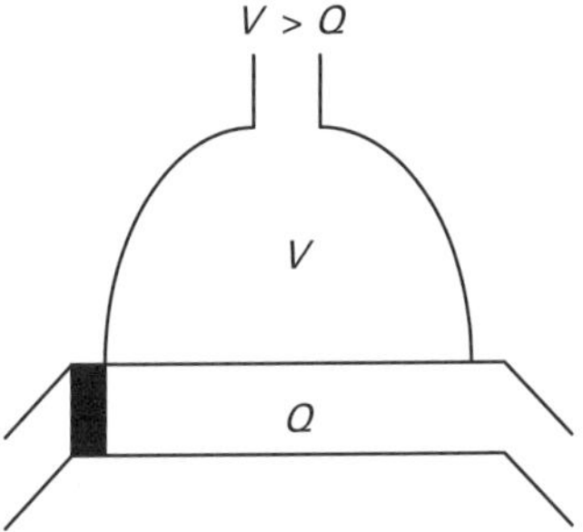

Low $\dot{V}/\dot{Q}$ ratio

- $R < 0.8$
- Ventilation below perfusion requirements
- Contributes to physiological shunt
- Alveolar gas tensions approach those of mixed-venous blood
  - PaO_2 decreased
  - $PaCO_2$ increased
- Low $\dot{V}/\dot{Q}$ regions lead to a fall in PaO_2, which causes pulmonary vasoconstriction and diversion of blood to better ventilated regions of the lung

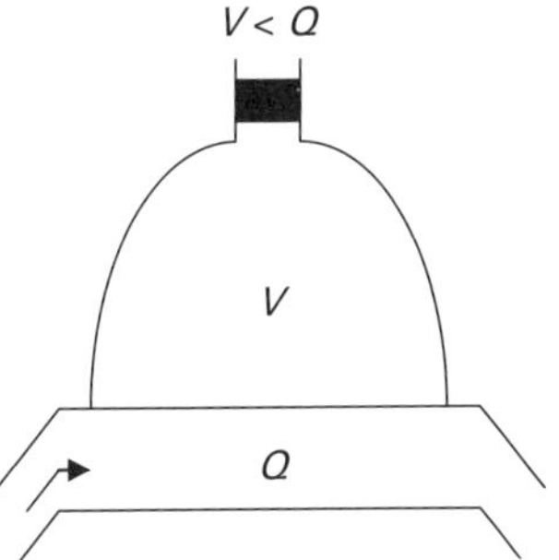

9 **(a)** true **(b)** true **(c)** true **(d)** false **(e)** false

Compliance is defined as the volume change caused by unit pressure change $= \frac{\text{Volume}}{\text{Pressure}}$

There are two components to total compliance: (a) lung compliance and (b) chest wall compliance.

Lung compliance

Lung compliance reflects the *elastic recoil of the lung*. Lung compliance is a change in lung volume caused by a unit change of transmural pressure. This is the pressure difference between the alveolar pressure measured at the mouth with no flow, i.e. breath held, and the intrapleural pressure measured by a balloon in the oesophagus, across the lung wall.

$$C_{lung} = \frac{\text{Change in lung volume}}{\text{Change in transmural pressure}}\ \text{ml/cmH}_2\text{O}$$

Normal lung compliance in a conscious erect man is 1.5–2.0 l/kPa (150–200 ml/cmH_2O).

Dynamic loop of pressure-volume

Note the difference between inspiration and expiration. Compliance is measured from maximum expiration to maximum inspiration.

Slope = static compliance

It can be seen from the graph that compliance is lowest at the extremes of lung volumes.

Elastance is the reciprocal of compliance.

- Small lung volume

Factors reducing lung compliance include:
- increased pulmonary blood volume
- increased extravascular lung water
- inflammation, ARDS, pneumonia
- fibrosis, emphysema
- extremes of age, e.g. neonatal compliance 20 ml/cmH_2O

Factors increasing lung compliance include:
- surfactant improves lung compliance especially at low lung volumes

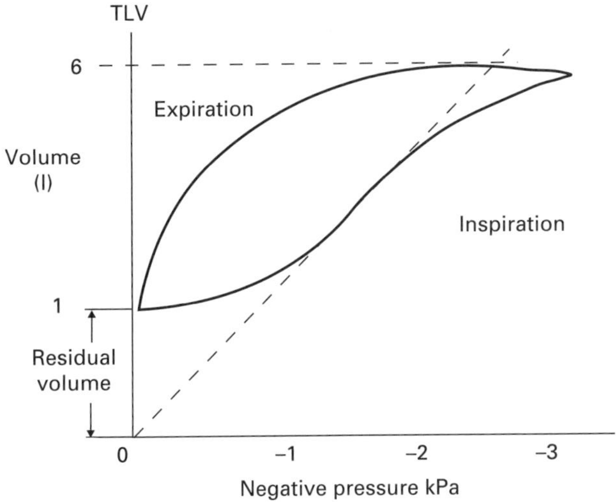

Chest wall compliance

Chest wall compliance is a change in chest volume caused by a unit change in transthoracic pressure. Transthoracic pressure equals alveolar pressure minus intrapleural pressure. This is difficult to measure due to the effect of muscle

$$C_{chest} = \frac{\text{Change in chest volume}}{\text{Change in transthoracic pressure}}$$

Normal chest wall compliance is 2 l/kpa or 200 ml/cmH_2O.

Total lung compliance

Total lung compliance is the change in lung volume that occurs with a unit change in the alveolar/ambient pressure.

Total compliance (lung and chest together) is 0.85 l/kpa (85 ml/cmH_2O)

Total compliance is expressed as

$$\frac{1}{C_{total}} = \frac{1}{C_{chest}} + \frac{1}{C_{lung}}$$

Static and dynamic lung compliance

Static compliance is:

- a measure of the stiffness of lung and chest wall
- usually due equally to lung and chest wall compliance
- measured when all gas flow in the lung has ceased (equilibrium)

Dynamic compliance includes the extra pressure needed to overcome:

- resistance to air flow
- inertia of chest wall
- viscoelasticy of the tissues

Dynamic compliance is measured when gas flow is zero at the mouth but during rhythmic breathing.

Dynamic compliance is reduced in bronchitis, at extremes of lung volumes, and at the bases and apices of the erect lung.

Specific compliance

$$\text{Equals compliance divided by FRC} = \frac{\text{Compliance}}{\text{FRC}}$$

It compensates for compliance varying with different body sizes.

10 (**a**) true (**b**) true (**c**) true (**d**) false (**e**) true

Dead space is that part of tidal volume which does not participate in alveolar gas exchange.

Total dead space is the sum of

- Anatomical dead space – gases in the non-respiratory airways
- Alveolar dead space – alveoli gas that is wasted due to inadequate perfusion

Physiological dead space

- The functional measurement that combines anatomical and alveolar dead space

$$\text{physiological dead space} = \text{anatomical dead space} + \text{alveolar dead space}$$

- It is equal to 2 ml/kg
- The weight of the individual in pounds is roughly equivalent to their dead space in millilitres
- It is measured by the dead space equation (Bohr equation)

$$\frac{V_{\text{D physiological}}}{V_{\text{T}}} = \frac{P_{\text{a}}CO_2 - P_{\text{E}}CO_2}{P_{\text{a}}CO_2}$$

- It is expressed as:
  - dead space/Tidal volume
  - normally 150/500 ml during resting breathing

- The reason it is expressed as the V_D/V_T ratio is because the dead space can alter with the characteristics of the inspiratory flow

Dead space equation (Bohr equation)

This is used to derive the total dead space or physiological dead space. Based on the fact that the dead space (V_D) does not contribute to expired CO_2, therefore by the principle of conservation of mass:

$$V_T \cdot F_ECO_2 = V_A \cdot F_ACO_2,$$

where V_T is tidal volume, F_ECO_2 is fractional CO_2 in expired gas, V_A is alveolar volume and F_ACO_2 is fractional concentration of CO_2 in alveolar gas.

Remember $V_A = V_T - V_D$, where V_D is total dead space volume. Therefore, by substitution

$$V_T \cdot F_ECO_2 = (V_T - V_D) \cdot F_ACO_2$$

Expanding gives

$$V_T \cdot F_ECO_2 = V_T \cdot F_ACO_2 - V_D \cdot F_ACO_2$$

Dividing by V_T gives

$$F_ECO_2 = F_ACO_2 - (V_D/V_T) \cdot F_ACO_2$$

Giving

$$V_D/V_T = (F_ACO_2 - F_ECO_2)/F_ACO_2$$

which is the Bohr equation (1891).

Anatomical dead space

Increased in:

- neonates and old age
- standing
- neck extension
- jaw protrusion
- increased tidal volume
- catecholamines
- anticholinergics

Decreased by:

- sitting
- neck flexion
- hypoventilation
- anaesthesia
- intubation/tracheostomy
- 5-HT
- histamine

Alveolar dead space

Usually has a volume that is close to zero in normal awake, spontaneous breathing humans.

Increased by:

- most lung diseases
- pregnancy
- pulmonary emboli
- anaesthesia
- hypovolaemia and hypotension
- IPPV
- PEEP

11 (**a**) false (**b**) true (**c**) true (**d**) true (**e**) true

Glomerular filtration and ultrafiltrate (GFR)

GFR in an average-sized normal man is approximately

- 125 ml/min
- 7.5 l/h
- 180 l/day
- 10% lower in females

About 99% or more of the filtrate is normally reabsorbed. At the rate of 125 ml/min the kidneys filter in 1 day an amount of fluid equals to:

- 4 times total body water
- 15 times extracellular fluid volume
- 60 times plasma volume

Control of GFR

Is achieved in three main ways:

- hydrostatic and osmotic pressure gradients across the capillary wall

- permeability of the glomerular capillary
- the size of the capillary bed

Hydrostatic and osmotic pressure gradients across the capillary wall

Also known as glomerular filtration forces. These are the forces required to drive the glomerular filtration:

$$\text{GFR}\ (P_{\text{cap}} + \pi_{\text{Bc}}) - (\text{P}_{\text{Bc}} + \pi_{\text{cap}})$$

Where,

P_{cap} = hydrostatic pressure in the capillary
P_{Bc} = hydrostatic pressure in the Bowman's capsule
π_{cap} = oncotic pressure in the capillary
π_{Bc} = oncotic pressure in the Bowman's capsule

- Mean arterial blood pressure in the glomerular capillary is 45 mmHg, because of the presence of a second resistance afferent arteriole
- Oncotic pressure in Bowman's capsule is negligible because the ultrafiltrate is virtually protein free
- Oncotic pressure in the capillary is increased as the fluids pass through the glomerulus, because, as the fluid leaves, the plasma protein concentration increases and hence the oncotic pressure

$$\text{GFR} = K_{\text{T}}(P_{\text{cap}} - P_{\text{Bc}} - \pi_{\text{cap}})$$

where,
K_{T} = Sieving coefficient (resistance to flow)

The net filtration pressure

- At the afferent arteriole

  $P_{\text{cap}} = 45$ mmHg
  $P_{\text{BC}} = 10$ mmHg
  $\pi_{\text{cap}} = 20$
  Net pressure = (45–10–20) = 15 mmHg

The net filtration pressure

- At the efferent arteriole

  $P_{\text{cap}} = 45$ mmHg
  $P_{\text{Bc}} = 10$ mmHg
  $P_{\text{cap}} = 35$
  Net pressure = (45–10–35) = 0 mmHg

An increase in intravascular (extracellular) volume will tend to increase glomerular capillary pressure and filtration.

Permeability of the glomerular capillary

Permeability of the glomerular capillary is 100 times greater than that of the capillaries in the skeletal muscles due to

- Size = 4–8 nm: filtration is inversely proportional to the diameter
- Charge
  - sialoproteins in the glomerular capillary wall are negatively charged
  - they repel negatively charged substances in the blood
- Molecular weight: cut-off is 70000 Da
- Shape: change in the shape may facilitate the passage

Note:
Albumin

- Molecular diameter less than 7 nm
- Molecular weight is less than 70000 Da
- Negatively charged
- Repelled by negatively charged sialoproteins
- (normally 120 mg/24 h)

The size of the capillary bed

K_F, resistance to flow through the capillary basement membrane, is altered by the size of mesangial cells.

Contraction of mesangial cells decreases K_F and GFR. Causes of contraction include:

- norepinephrine (noradrenaline)
- angiotensin II
- vasopressin
- histamine
- thromboxane A2
- prostaglandin f_2 (PGf_2)

Relaxation of mesangial cells increases the K_F and GFR. Causes of relaxation include:

- atrial natriuretic peptide (ANP)
- cAMP
- dopamine
- PGE_2

12 (**a**) true (**b**) false (**c**) false (**d**) false (**e**) true

Antidiuretic hormone (ADH) is a nonapeptide synthesised in the supraoptic nucleus of the hypothalamus. It is transported via the hypothalamic–hypophyseal nerve tract to the posterior pituitary. It is released from the posterior pituitary to the circulation by the nerve cells. It has a half-life of 18 min.

Types of vasopressin receptors

- V1a receptors: located in the blood vessels; causing vasoconstriction when stimulated
- V1b receptors: located in the anterior hypothalamus, causing increased ACTH secretion when stimulated
- V2 receptors: located in the kidneys (peritubular capillary side of the collecting duct), causing antidiuresis when stimulated.

These are G-protein-coupled receptors.

13 (**a**) true (**b**) false (**c**) false (**d**) false (**e**) false

EEG

The dominant waves that occur with the eyes closed but awake are alpha waves recorded over the parietal-occipital area of the brain.

Alpha waves are associated with partial eye closing.

Beta waves are recorded from the frontal area and occur normally in infants, to be replaced by alpha waves in the adult.

Delta waves are slow and found in children and during sleep.

Theta waves are large, regular waves found normally in children.

Fast low-voltage activity occurs when the eyes are open.

Ketamine is unique in causing loss of alpha waves and mostly theta wave activity.

Deep sleep is associated with large irregular delta waves. Rapid eye movement (REM) is associated with arousal during sleep.

During anaesthesia alpha rhythm is replaced by high-frequency rhythm. Deeper anaesthesia is associated with a slow-frequency rhythm with increased amplitude. This is followed by bursts of activity with periods of no activity, then there are no more bursts and only an iso-electric line.

Hypoxia is associated with an initial increase in amplitude followed by a fall in amplitude and slow waves.

14 (**a**) true (**b**) true (**c**) true (**d**) false (**e**) true

There is an electric charge across the resting cell membrane with the inside of the cell being 70–80 mV negative compared to the outside of the cell. This membrane potential is caused by (a) the differential permeability of the cell membrane to different ions, e.g. most cell membranes are not permeable to sodium ions, (b) different concentrations of ions on the inside and the outside. Active pumps help to maintain this uneven distribution.

For a typical cell, intracellular: sodium 10 mmol/l, potassium 156 mmol/l, extracelluar sodium 140 mmol/l, potassium 3.7 mmol/l.

Only a very small number of potassium ions have to move from outside to inside to produce the resting potential.

The action potential is an all-or-nothing event which occurs when there is an increase in membrane conductance for sodium. If the external sodium decreases the action potential is smaller or does not occur.

Transmission of a nerve impulse across a synapse occurs when an action potential depolarises the terminal membrane which opens voltage-sensitive calcium channels. Hyperkalaemia and hypokalaemia are both associated with reduced muscle and nerve function as repolarisation is slowed.

15 (**a**) false (**b**) true (**c**) true (**d**) true (**e**) true

The liver glycogen stores are depleted within 24 h. Muscle, protein and fat are mobilised as energy sources in the process of gluconeogenesis. Gluconeogenesis takes place in the liver and a small amount in the kidney. Other organs can utilise lactate. Ketoacidosis occurs in starvation and diabetes mellitus when the breakdown of fats exceeds the breakdown of carbohydrates. Then the supply of acetyl coenzyme from β oxidation exceeds the rate at which oxaloacetic acid can be formed in the tricarboxylic acid cycle. So the acetyl-coenzyme A that cannot enter the cycle is formed into ketone bodies. These ketone bodies, acetone, acetoacetic acid and beta-hydroxyl butyric acid, are used for energy in cardiac muscle and the renal cortex where they are converted back into acetyl coenzyme A.

16 (**a**) true (**b**) true (**c**) true (**d**) false (**e**) false

Cerebrospinal fluid is produced by the choroid plexus in the lateral ventricles.

Table 4.16 Composition of CSF and blood

	CSF	Blood
Glucose	2.7–4.2 mmol/l (lower)	3.0–5.0 mmol/l
Protein	200–400 mg/l (lower)	60–80 g/l
Sodium	144–150 mmol/l (higher)	136–145 mmol/l
Potassium	2.0–3.0 mmol/l (lower)	3.8–5.0 mmol/l
Bicarbonate	22–30 mmol/l	22–30 mmol/l
Chloride	115–125 (higher)	95–105 mmol/l
Calcium	1.1–1.3 mmol/l (lower)	2.3–2.6 mmol/l
Lymphocytes	$<5/mm^3$	$(1–2) \times 10^9/l$
pH	7.3–7.5 (slightly lower)	7.4
Specific gravity	1007 (higher)	1000
Osmolarity	300–320 mosmol/l (slightly higher)	280–300 mosmol/l

The higher chloride ion concentration is because glial cells contain carbonic anhydrase, which facilitates the combination of carbon dioxide with water to then form bicarbonate ions. The resulting increase in bicarbonate ions means that more can be exchanged for chloride, which passes into the CSF.

Total CSF volume is 100–150 ml of which about half is in the spinal canal.

17 (**a**) true (**b**) true (**c**) true (**d**) true (**e**) true

The parasympathetic nervous system has nerve fibres in cranial nerves 3, 7, 9 and 10 and sacral roots S2–4.

The effects of stimulation are: bradycardia; vasodilatation of coronary and skeletal muscle; increased perfusion of coronary, pulmonary and renal circulations; relaxation of sphincters and sweating.

18 (**a**) true (**b**) true (**c**) true (**d**) true (**e**) true

Thoracio-lumbar sympathetic nerve stimulation produces

- Eye: pupil dilatation
- Bronchodilatation
- Increased chronotropy (heart rate), ionotropy (rate of conduction and force of contraction) and vasoconstriction of visceral blood vessels but dilatation of muscle blood vessels
- GI: increased sphincter tone and reduced gut motility
- Relaxation of bladder
- Skin: piloerection, vasoconstriction and secretion by sweat glands

19 (**a**) false (**b**) false (**c**) true (**d**) false (**e**) false

Fetal haemoglobin has two alpha and two gamma chains. It is 80% of the Hb at birth but drops to nil by 6 months.

The arch of the aorta has the highest saturation, 60%, due to blood coming through the patent atrial septum between the atria. This blood supplies the brain. The pulmonary artery has a lower saturation of 50%, which enters the aorta through the ductus arteriosus after the carotid arteries.

20 (**a**) true (**b**) false (**c**) true (**d**) false (**e**) true

Corticotrophin is the releasing factor secreted by the hypothalamus that stimulates adrenocorticotrophin hormone (ACTH) secretion from the anterior pituitary. It is released in response to physical or emotional stress. Like many body functions there is a diurnal variation. ACTH controls the production and release of corticosteroids, glucocorticoids and aldosterone from the adrenal gland. Glucocorticoids have a negative feedback on ACTH production. Long-term steroid therapy has the potential for long-term suppression of ACTH but this is probably rarer than thought in the past.

21 (**a**) true (**b**) true (**c**) false (**d**) false (**e**) false

See also question 13.

Slow, high-amplitude waves are seen in deep anaesthesia. High amplitude waves are seen in hypoxia but as the hypoxia continues slow waves with reduced amplitude are seen.

22 (**a**) false (**b**) false (**c**) true (**d**) true (**e**) false

Pregnancy has many effects on the respiratory system.

It increases minute ventilation by an increased tidal volume of 200 ml. $PaCO_2$ falls to 4 kPa and PaO_2 rises to 14.5–15 kPa.

The functional residual capacity (FRC) falls due to pressure on the diaphragm from the uterus. There is a reduction in both residual volume and expiratory reserve volume of 200–300 ml or 20%–45%.

Closing capacity is closing volume plus residual volume. In health it is less than FRC. The closing capacity is increased by age, it is position dependent, being higher when lying, smoking and in obesity. It might be expected that as the residual volume decreases so the closing capacity would fall in pregnancy but studies have shown that in the sitting pregnant patient closing capacity remains unchanged hence (c) is marked true.

23 (**a**) true (**b**) false (**c**) true (**d**) false (**e**) false

When you touch a hot object, you quickly pull your hand away using the withdrawal reflex.

These are the steps

- The stimulus is detected by receptors in the skin.
- These initiate nerve impulses in sensory neurones leading from the receptors to the spinal cord.
- The impulses travel into the spinal cord where the sensory nerve terminals synapse with interneurones.
    - Some of these synapse with motor neurones that travel out from the spinal cord entering mixed nerves that lead to the flexors that withdraw your hand.
    - Others synapse with inhibitory interneurones that suppress any motor output to extensors whose contraction would interfere with the withdrawal reflex.

24 (**a**) true (**b**) true (**c**) false (**d**) false (**e**) false

The effects of pregnancy on the cardiovascular system include an increased blood volume and red cell mass, but by dilution the packed cell volume (PCV) is lower. Heart rate and stroke volume increase as cardiac output increases. Smooth muscle relaxation leads to a fall in systemic vascular resistance.

At term there is virtually no pseudocholinesterase in the blood. The blood glucose is not changed but the renal threshold for retaining glucose is reduced and glycosuria is common.

25 (**a**) true (**b**) true (**c**) true (**d**) false (**e**) false

Gastric emptying is reduced by food, most by fat, less by protein and least by carbohydrate. A high-protein meal and amino acids delay gastric emptying but not as much as fat so we mark this true.

Stress, pain, trauma and alcohol all delay emptying.

The drugs that delay emptying include opioids, anticholinergics by reducing vagal activity, and sympathomimetics.

Iron preparations are associated with gastric irritation and diarrhoea.

26 (**a**) false (**b**) true (**c**) true (**d**) true (**e**) false

The passage of ions across cell membranes can be passive, as in the case of sodium and potassium reaching osmotic equilibrium, or active requiring energy as in the Na/K pump. Channels in the cell membrane are not permanently open and require energy to open and to pump ions against a concentration gradient.

Ions pass through voltage-sensitive channels, such as the passage of calcium at a synapse, when an action potential opens the channel.

Drugs and hormones act at specific protein sites on the cell membrane known as receptors. Each receptor recognises specific neurotransmitters called ligands which can be an agonist or an antagonist.

27 (**a**) false (**b**) true (**c**) false (**d**) false (**e**) false

The Bohr equation is used to derive the total or physiological dead space. It is based on the premise that the amount of carbon dioxide expired equals the inspired carbon dioxide and the carbon dioxide given out by the lungs. Certain assumptions are made. First that inspired carbon dioxide is negligible and can be ignored. Then that concentration can be calculated from partial pressure and haemoglobin concentration using the carbon dioxide dissociation curve, and that end-tidal carbon dioxide tension equals arterial carbon dioxide tension. So the final equation is often written as:

$$V_A/V_T = (P_ACO_2 - P_ECO_2)/P_ACO_2$$

28 (**a**) true (**b**) false (**c**) true (**d**) false (**e**) true

The interior of a resting muscle fibre has a resting potential of −80 to −90 mV. Note that nerve has a resting potential of −70 mv and cardiac muscle −60 mv. The influx of sodium ions reduces the charge, creating an end plate potential. If the end-plate potential reaches the threshold voltage (approximately –50 mV), sodium ions flow in with a rush and an action potential is created in the fibre. The action potential sweeps down the length of the fibre just as it does in an axon.

No visible change occurs in the muscle fibre during (and immediately following) the action potential. This period, called the latent period, lasts 3–10 ms.

Calcium ions (Ca^{2+}) link action potentials in a muscle fibre to contraction.

- In resting muscle fibres, Ca^{2+} is stored in the endoplasmic (sarcoplasmic) reticulum

- Spaced along the plasma membrane (sarcolemma) of the muscle fibre are in-pockets of the membrane that form tubules of the 'T system'. These tubules plunge repeatedly into the interior of the fibre
- The tubules of the T system terminate near the calcium-filled sacs of the sarcoplasmic reticulum
- Each action potential created at the neuromuscular junction sweeps quickly along the sarcolemma and is carried into the T system
- The arrival of the action potential at the ends of the T system triggers the release of Ca^{2+}
- The Ca^{2+} diffuses among the thick and thin filaments where it binds to troponin on the thin filaments
- This turns on the interaction between actin and myosin and the sarcomere contracts
- Because of the speed of the action potential (milliseconds), the action potential arrives virtually simultaneously at the ends of all the tubules of the T system, ensuring that all sarcomeres contract in unison

When the process is over, the calcium is pumped back into the sarcoplasmic reticulum using a Ca^{2+}-ATPase.

29 (**a**) false (**b**) false (**c**) true (**d**) false (**e**) true

A block of the cervical sympathetic chain can be due to a therapeutic block or by tumour in the superior mediastinum or lung apex.

A Horner's syndrome results in: miosis, ptosis, anhidrosis, enophthalmos (and nasal stuffiness, which is not defined within Horner's syndrome).

Dilatation of the pupil is due to sympathetic stimulation. Salivation is due to parasympathetic stimulation.

30 (**a**) true (**b**) false (**c**) true (**d**) true (**e**) true

Muscarinic receptors are G-protein-coupled receptors and mediate their responses by activating a cascade of intracellular pathways. Muscarine is the prototypical muscarinic agonist and derives from the fly agaric mushroom *Amanita muscaria.* Like acetylcholine, muscarine contains a quaternary nitrogen important for action at the anionic site of the receptor (an aspartate residue in transmembrane domain III).

Muscarinic receptors are found in the parasympathetic nervous system. Muscarinic receptors in smooth muscle regulate cardiac contractions, gut motility and bronchial constriction. Muscarinic receptors in exocrine glands stimulate gastric acid secretion, salivation and lacrimation. Muscarinic receptors also are found in the superior cervical ganglion where they can produce at least two physiologically distinct responses. In addition, muscarinic receptors are found throughout the brain, including the cerebral cortex, the striatum, the hippocampus, thalamus and brainstem.

Subtypes of muscarinic receptors

- M_1 receptors are found in the forebrain, especially in the hippocampus and cerebral cortex.
- M_2 receptors are found in the heart and brainstem.
- M_3 receptors are found in smooth muscle, exocrine glands and the cerebral cortex.
- M_4 receptors are found in the neostriatum.
- M_5 receptor mRNA is found in the substantia nigra, suggesting that M_5 receptors may regulate dopamine release at terminals within the striatum.

31 (**a**) false (**b**) false (**c**) true (**d**) true (**e**) false

Rapid onset of CNS action is favoured by non-ionised drugs at blood pH, with high lipid solubility to cross the blood–brain barrier. Lipid solubility

Table 4.31 Characteristics of thiopentone and propofol

	Thiopentone	Propofol
pH	10.5	
p*K*a	7.6	11
Non-ionised	60%	Very lipid soluble
Clearance	3.4 ml/kg per min	20 ml/kg per min
Volume of distribution	2.5 l/kg	12 l/kg
Effect limited by redistribution	Yes	Yes
Metabolism	Zero-order 10%–15% each hour in liver, 1% in urine unchanged	Liver to glucoronides and sulphates, 0.3% in urine unchanged
Distribution half-life	Minutes	Minutes
Elimination/ terminal half life	5–10 h	1.5 h
Stays in body	Over 24 h	
Accumulation	Yes on repeated dosage	None, elimination equals administration

is favoured when the p*Ka* is equal to the blood pH. The high lipid solubility will give a large volume of distribution. The volume of distribution relates the blood concentration of a drug to the amount of the drug in the body. Anything which increases the amount in the body increases the volume of distribution, e.g. lipid solubility, tissue binding. The half-life equals 0.7 × volume of distribution/clearance. The half-life will be low because the clearance from the blood is high. The half-life cannot be high if the clearance is high.

The blood concentration will be high if the drug has low protein binding, and there is a low cardiac output.

Thiopentone and propofol are compared in this context.

32 (**a**) true (**b**) false (**c**) true (**d**) true (**e**) false

Metabolic acidosis is associated with paracetamol poisoning. Hepatic toxicity occurs when glutathione is used up. Sodium nitroprusside releases cyanide ions and ammonium chloride is adding acid to the body.

33 (**a**) true (**b**) false (**c**) true (**d**) false (**e**) false

Clearance of a drug is defined as the theoretical volume of plasma in millilitres that is completely cleared of the drug in 1 min by an organ or by the body.

Drug clearance usually depends on liver metabolism and renal excretion.

Most drugs are eliminated by more than one route. If the clearance is greater than glomerular filtration rate it implies the drug is secreted into the tubular cells or metabolised by another organ. Metabolism may be the main path of elimination, in which case it may be rate limited.

34 (**a**) false (**b**) false (**c**) true (**d**) false (**e**) false

Alkalinisation increases the rate of excretion of salicylates.

Acid diuresis helps eliminate amphetamine.

35 (**a**) false (**b**) false (**c**) false (**d**) true (**e**) true

The factors that determine the uptake of an inhalational anaesthetic agent are: blood solubility, cardiac output and concentration across the alveoli/capillary membrane.

The speed of uptake of an anaesthetic agent from the lung is proportional to the alveolar ventilation and the vapour concentration. A high coefficient of blood/gas solubility is proportional to the amount taken up to reach a particular alveolar concentration. This means that more agent must be taken up to reach an anaesthetic concentration. The temperature affects solubility – as the temperature falls the solubility increases; temperature affects vaporisation and the delivery to the lung. A high cardiac output increases the rate of uptake. The minimum alveolar concentration (MAC) is a measure of the potency of the agent.

This question is asked in a number of slightly different ways regarding the different factors affecting: alveolar concentration, speed of induction and time to reach MAC.

Solubility increases uptake but slows the time to reach an alveolar concentration for anaesthesia (MAC), high cardiac output increases uptake from the alveolus but slows the time to reach MAC and the onset of anaesthesia. The higher the inspired concentration the higher the alveolar concentration. Changes in ventilation are proportional to the alveolar concentration of the soluble agents.

36 (**a**) true (**b**) true (**c**) false (**d**) false (**e**) true

The drugs that relax uterine muscle are either direct-acting smooth muscle relaxants or beta-2 agonists.

Terbutaline is a beta-2 agonist. Volatile agents cause dose-related relaxation, and alcohol directly relaxes uterine muscle.

Prostaglandin F2α stimulates contraction.

37 (**a**) false (**b**) false (**c**) false (**d**) false (**e**) true

Comparison of volatile agents

Table 4.37 Comparison of volatile agents

	Isoflurane	Enflurane	Sevoflurane
Oil/gas solubility	97	98	53
Blood/gas solubility	1.4	1.9	0.6
Boiling point (°C)	49	56	58
Metabolism	<0.2% minimum fluoride ions	2.5%	5% metabolised inorganic fluoride
MAC (%)	1.2	1.8	2
SVP(kPa)	33	24	21

38 (**a**) true (**b**) false (**c**) true (**d**) true (**e**) false

See answer to question 37.

More compound A is formed the higher the temperature of the soda lime and the higher the concentration of sevoflurane.

Sevoflurane reduces blood pressure by vasodilatation with a possible compensatory tachycardia.

39 (**a**) true (**b**) false (**c**) true (**d**) true (**e**) true

Barbiturates – long side groups are related to greater potency. Sulfur at position 2 in thiopentone reduces its duration of action and increases its anti-epileptic potency. Methyl at position 1 in methohexitone is associated with excitation; methyl substitutes increase excitatory phenomena. An aromatic nucleus in an alkyl group at position 5 is a convulsant.

40 (**a**) true (**b**) false (**c**) true (**d**) false (**e**) true

Propofol is an alkyl phenol. It is mainly metabolised to glucuronides, only 0.3% is excreted in the urine unchanged. The clearance is 25–30 ml/kg per min. It significantly reduces blood pressure by reducing myocardial contractility or reducing SVR, or a combination of both. The use of the word significant may be important in deciding true or false.

It has been used to treat status epilepticus.

41 (**a**) true (**b**) false (**c**) false (**d**) false (**e**) false

The CSF volume is reduced by dilated epidural veins. Spinal cord blood flow is increased, metabolism is increased, and turnover of CSF is increased.

42 (**a**) true (**b**) false (**c**) false (**d**) true (**e**) true

Local anaesthetics act by blocking membrane depolarisation in all cells. The ionised portion occupies the sodium channel and prevents any movement of sodium and so no action potential can occur. They inhibit propagation of the action potential.

Local anaesthetics are usually acidic solution (hydrochloride salts pH 5). They are water soluble. A proportion of the drug dissociates to form the free base which is lipid soluble. This crosses the lipid capillary membrane into the axon where it re-ionises.

43 (a) false (b) false (c) true (d) true (e) true

Alfentanil is derived from fentanyl. It is less potent and more protein bound. Its smaller volume of distribution means a high plasma level. It has a shorter duration of action than fentanyl, which is more lipid soluble than alfentanil and so more potent, rapidly reaching the receptors. Its duration of action is limited by redistribution. (Some animals such as the rabbit rapidly metabolise fentanyl.)

The clearance of alfentanil is lower but due to the smaller volume of distribution the elimination half-life is shorter and the time for elimination is shorter.

Table 4.43 Comparison of opioids

	Elimination half-life (min)	Distribution half-life (min)	Volume of distribution (l/kg)	Clearance (l/min)	Lipid solubility	% Protein bound
Morphine	3	25	3	1	1	30
Pethidine	3	8	3	1	30	50
Fentanyl	4	3	4	1	810	80
Alfentanil	1.5	2	0.5	0.3	120	90
Sulfentanil	2.5	1	1.5	2.5	1800	92
Remifentanil	0.1		0.4	3	3	

44 (a) true (b) true (c) true (d) true (e) true

This generation of non-steroidal anti-inflammatory drugs (NSAIDs) was introduced as being less likely to lead to peptic ulceration. Their effect on asthma, renal blood flow and platelets was thought to be the same as other NSAIDs. Recent reports of side-effects have led to doubts about their safety regarding cardiac effects. A single dose peri-operatively may still have beneficial effects and be less likely to develop bronchospasm in asthmatics, less renal vessel constriction and fewer platelet effects.

45 (a) false (b) false (c) true (d) true (e) true

Phenothiazines are a group of drugs with actions as anticholinergic, antihistaminergic (H_1), antidopaminergic (D_1 and D_2), and α-adrenergic antagonists. They are divided into three groups, those with: an aliphatic side-chain, a piperidine side-chain and those with a piperazine side chain.

Their action is on the chemoreceptor trigger zone, hypothalamus, ascending reticular system, limbic system and basal ganglia.

They act as antiemetics and sedatives and they stop shivering. Trimeprazine is said to potentiate opioid analgesia. Side-effects include extrapyramidal movement and vasodilatation leading to postural hypotension.

46 (**a**) false (**b**) false (**c**) false (**d**) true (**e**) false

Dopexamine is an analogue of dopamine. Dopamine is a precursor of noradrenaline. It causes renal and peripheral vasodilatation through d type-1 receptors.

Table 4.46 Dopamine, dobutamine and dopexamine compared

	Dopamine	Dobutamine	Dopexamine
Strong agonist	Inotropic β_1, α_2, dopaminergic receptors in kidney	Inotropic β_1	Dopamine receptors Inotropic
Weak agonist	α_1	β_2 and α	β_1, β_2
HR	Increased	Less tachycardia than dopamine	Mild tachycardia
LVEDP		Reduced if raised	
SVR			Reduced
Renal blood flow	Increased but this is the effect of increased cardiac output		
Plasma half-life	1 min	2 min	
Excretion	Metabolised	Urine	

47 (**a**) false (**b**) true (**c**) false (**d**) false (**e**) false

See answer to question 43.

Remifentanil is a phenylpiperidine derivative, metabolised by red cell cholinesterase. It does not act at the kappa receptor (OP2). Remifentanil is rapidly broken down by non-specific plasma and tissue esterases. Unlike morphine and pethidine, remifentanil has very little potential for histamine release.

Table 4.47 Opioid receptors

	Opioid receptor		
	OP3 mu	OP2 kappa	OP1 delta
Effect	Mu 1, supraspinal analgesia; Mu 2, other effects	Act at spinal level; analgesia, meiosis, respiratory depression sedation,	Analgesia
Morphine	Yes	Weak	Yes
Fentanyl and alfentanil	Yes	No	
Pethidine	Yes	Yes	
Buprenorphine	Partial agonist		
Pentazocine		Yes	

48 **(a)** true **(b)** true **(c)** false **(d)** true **(e)** false

Table 4.48 Mechanism of antibiotic action

DNA	mRNA	Translation – affect protein synthesis	Outer cell membrane	Cell wall
Bactericidal Inhibit DNA replication 4 – quinolones ciprofloxacin	Inhibit RNA – metronidazole	Streptomycin	Polymyxins – attach to ionic sites	Bactericidal Glycopeptides Teicoplanin vancomycin
Bind to DNA – proflavine	Bind to RNA – Rifamycins	Bactericidal aminoglycosides neomycin	Imidazoles – bind to fungal membranes increasing permeability	Bactericidal Beta lactams – penicillins, cephalosporins – block cross linkage of pentapeptide chains
Bacteriostatic Inhibit synthesis sulphonamides Inhibit folic acid synthesis – trimethoprim		Bacteriostatic Erythromycin		
		Bacteriostatic Tetracyclines Fusidic acid		

Antibiotics work by inhibiting (a) DNA or RNA structure or function, (b) protein formation in the cell, (c) cell wall integrity and synthesis. When a sulphonamide is combined with trimethoprim as co-trimoxazole the mixture is bactericidal.

49 (**a**) false (**b**) true (**c**) false (**d**) false (**e**) false

Agonists have a high affinity for a receptor and produce a maximum effect. The dose–response curve is sigmoid in shape. At low doses there is no response, then as the dose increases the response rises steeply until a maximum 100% response when the curve plateaus. By taking the $\log_{10}$ of the dose a straight line graph is obtained.

The nearer the curve is to zero and the left, the lower the dose required and so the greater the potency of the agonist. Curves to the right but of the same shape are drugs occupying the same receptors but with less potency.

The slope of the curve is affected by the number of receptors and the number of organs that need to be occupied to give the effect.

A competitive antagonist is a drug that combines reversibly with the receptor. An increased dose of agonist is required for the same effect as the full agonist so the curve is shifted to the right.

An agonist cannot overcome the full effect of a non-competitive antagonist. A non-competitive antagonist inactivates the receptor so that a maximum effect cannot be obtained by a full agonist. The normal curve is cut short and the plateau reached before 100%. The curve is also shifted to the right as antagonism is taking place, requiring a bigger dose, and the curve is less steep indicating the different mechanism of action. A non-competitive antagonist may be reversible or non-reversible.

A partial agonist will not have the same maximum response as the agonist and so the sigmoid curve will plateau before 100% response.

When a partial agonist and a full agonist are given together the effect is to reduce the full effect of the full agonist.

50 (**a**) true (**b**) false (**c**) true (**d**) true (**e**) true

See answer to question 46.

Dopamine is a precursor of adrenaline and noradrenaline. Its main effect is inotropic at β 1 receptors to increase cardiac output. This, with vasodilatation, causes an increase in blood flow in the renal and mesenteric blood vessels.

The effects of adrenergic receptors are mediated by intracellular substances or second messengers that link the extracellular adrenaline to the cellular response.

For $\alpha 1$ receptors the second messenger is an increase in calcium ions; $\alpha 2$ reduces intracellular cAMP; and $\beta 1$ and $\beta 2$ increase intracellular cAMP.

Dopamine receptors are activated by cAMP. High doses activate alpha receptors leading to vasoconstriction.

Dopamine crosses the blood–brain barrier to suppress the release of oxytocin and other pituitary hormones.

51 (**a**) false (**b**) true (**c**) false (**d**) true (**e**) false

Nifedipine is a calcium channel blocker most effective in dilating coronary blood vessels. The small negative inotropic effect may cause a baroreceptor-induced increase in heart rate, occasionally causing palpitations. Due to its vasodilator properties it can cause headache, dizziness and flushing. Other effects include inhibition of platelet aggregation, reduced bronchospasm, vessel dilation in Reynaud's phenomenon and improved lower oesophageal sphincter function.

52 (**a**) false (**b**) false (**c**) true (**d**) true (**e**) false

Clonidine is an imidazole with alpha-2 adrenergic agonist activity. It was originally introduced as an antihypertensive. Its main clinical role is now related to use as an adjuvant to analgesics and anaesthetics, to decrease anaesthetic requirements and to attenuate sympathetic excitatory responses in patients undergoing general anaesthesia.

The action of clonidine on alpha-2 receptors, which are widely distributed throughout the CNS and the body, results in:

- sedation and anxiolysis
- antisialogogue effects
- analgesia – supraspinal and spinal
- enhanced conduction blockade by local anaesthetics
- reduced requirement for general anaesthetic agents
- decreased intraocular pressure
- no shivering postoperatively

Peripheral and central effects on the CVS

- Inhibition of noradrenaline release from prejunctional nerve endings
- Hypotensive and bradycardic effects produced centrally
- Antiarrhythmic effects mediated by the vagus nerve

Diffuse action on hormone function

- Reduces thyroid function
- Reduces sympathetic outflow
- Reduces the stress-induced ACTH and cortisol release
- Increases secretion of growth hormone

53 (**a**) false (**b**) true (**c**) false (**d**) true (**e**) false

Bumetidine is a frusemide-like diuretic that acts by inhibiting Na/K reabsorption. The main side-effect is hypokalaemia and myalgia in high doses.

54 (**a**) true (**b**) true (**c**) true (**d**) true (**e**) true

Hyoscine is an anticholinergic which crosses the blood–brain barrier, to cause sedation, reduce vomiting and confusion in the elderly.

55 (**a**) true (**b**) false (**c**) true (**d**) false (**e**) true

Thiazide diuretics act at the proximal part of the distal convoluted tubule to inhibit sodium reabsorption. They also act on the proximal tubule to inhibit carbonic anhydrase and to increase bicarbonate and potassium loss.

They lower plasma sodium, potassium, magnesium and create a hypochloraemic alkalosis. They raise plasma uric acid, glucose and cholesterol.

Frusemide is derived from the sulphonamides.

56 (**a**) true (**b**) true (**c**) true (**d**) false (**e**) false

Renal clearance is a calculated volume of plasma cleared of a substance as it passes through the organ.

Renal clearance is increased by higher renal blood flow, higher glomerular filtration rate and passive and active secretion into the tubules.

57 (**a**) false (**b**) true (**c**) true (**d**) false (**e**) false

Most drugs given enough time will cross the placenta.

Paper 4 Answers

The rate of transfer is dependent on:

(a) Lipid solubility
- Lipophilic molecules diffuse readily across lipid membranes, of which the placenta is one

(b) Degree of ionisation
- Only non-ionised drugs cross the placental membrane
- Most drugs used in anaesthesia, analgesia and sedation are poorly ionised in the blood and their placental transfer is almost unrestricted
- Muscle relaxants are highly ionised and their transfer is almost negligible

(c) Protein binding
- The diffusibility of protein-bound drugs is negligible compared with that of the free drug
- Protein binding is influenced by
  - blood pH: acidosis reduces protein binding of local anaesthetics; more unbound drug promotes greater transfer
  - concentration of plasma proteins: a low serum albumin, as in pre-eclampsia, increases the amount of unbound drug and increases transfer

(d) pH of maternal blood
- The pH alters the degree of ionisation of the drug
- This effect is dependent on the p*K*a of the drug
- If the p*K*a is near to the pH of the blood then small changes in the blood pH produce a large change in the drug ionisation

(e) Materno–fetal concentration gradient
- When a drug is transferred by simple diffusion the rate of transfer is determined by Fick's law of diffusion which states that the rate of diffusion of a substance across a unit area of a membrane is proportional to the concentration gradient:

$$\text{Flow of gas } \alpha \ \frac{A}{T} \cdot D(P_1 - P_2)$$

A = lung area (50–100m^2); T = lung thickness (0.3 μm); (P_1–P_2 = partial pressure gradient across the membrane; D = diffusion of gas constant α solubility/$\sqrt{\text{molecular weight}}$.

$$Q/T = kA\,(C_M - C_F)/D$$

(f) Placental blood flow

- With poorly diffusible drugs the concentration in maternal and fetal blood changes little during placental transit hence blood flow has little impact on the trans-placental gradient
- With highly diffusible drugs the drug concentration falls significantly as a result of transfer; hence, blood flow has a marked effect on the gradient

(g) Molecular weight of drug

- Drugs with a molecular weight of 600 Da or less readily diffuse across the placenta

58 (**a**) false (**b**) true (**c**) false (**d**) true (**e**) false

- Lithium is used in the long-term management of mania (plasma levels 0.8–1.2 mmol/l). It acts by inhibiting the release and increasing the uptake of cellular noradrenaline
- Lithium acts like sodium ions and potentiates both depolarising and non-depolarising muscle relaxants
- Toxic effects are seen in hyponatraemia when both sodium and lithium are reabsorbed:
  - in toxic doses <1.5 mmol/l: hyper-reflexia, weakness, tremor, hypokalaemia followed by convulsions and coma
- It reduces the dose of anaesthetic drugs
- Hypothyroidism occurs as lithium is taken up and concentrated by the thyroid gland leading to reduced thyroxine release
- Lithium interferes with ADH control leading to a nephrogenic diabetes insipidus
- Hyperparathyroidism is induced with elevated plasma calcium and magnesium levels

59 (**a**) false (**b**) false (**c**) true (**d**) false (**e**) true

Warfarin competes with vitamin K in the production of clotting factors. Its full effect takes 2–3 days to develop and to reverse. Its effect is enhanced by drugs which displace it from protein-binding sites such as NSAIDs and sulphonamides, and reduced by drugs that cause enzyme induction such as barbiturates and so increase its rate of metabolism.

The effect is reversed over hours by vitamin K or immediately by giving clotting factors.

Paper 4 Answers

Tolbutamide is a sulphonylurea, oral hypoglycaemic agent. It is highly protein bound and so will displace warfarin and raise the plasma level, increasing the effect of warfarin.

60 (**a**) true (**b**) false (**c**) true (**d**) false (**e**) false

Sulphonylureas act by stimulating the release of insulin. The biguanides act by lowering blood glucose by suppressing gluconeogenesis in the liver and increasing glucose uptake by the tissues. They do not lower fasting blood glucose but the post-prandial rise is attenuated.

Chlorpropamide has the longest duration of action at 48 h, and a half-life of 24 h, while tolbutamide has a half-life of 6 h.

Diabetic neuropathy is a relative indication for insulin therapy.

61 (**a**) true (**b**) false (**c**) false (**d**) false (**e**) false

Physical principle

Gases that have two or more different atoms in the molecule absorb infrared radiation. If there are only two atoms, absorption only occurs if the two atoms are dissimilar. Strong infrared absorption occurs when a molecule's atoms rotate or vibrate asymmetrically. Among the respiratory and anaesthetic gases, CO_2, N_2O, and the fluorinated hydrocarbons exhibit strong absorption peaks throughout the infrared spectrum. Non-polar molecules do not, e.g. N_2 and O_2.

Measuring the energy absorbed from a single-wavelength infrared light beam passing through a gas is termed non-dispersive infrared spectroscopy (NDIR spectroscopy). The relationship between light energy absorbed and other factors are lumped together in the Beer–Lambert law, expressed mathematically as:

$$\text{Emerging light } I = \text{incident light } (I_o) \times e^{-LC\beta}$$

or, taking logs,

$$\log_e I_o/I = LC\beta$$

L = length of the light path (size of container); C = concentration of dye or chromophore, e.g. haemoglobin; β = specific absorption of dye or chromophore for a specific wavelength of light.

$$LC\beta = \text{optical density of the medium}$$

Each gas absorbs radiation at characteristic wavelengths and the absorbance peak is characteristic for a given gas.

- $CO_2 \sim 428$ nm
- $N_2O \sim 430$ nm
- Halogenated agents ~ 330 nm

As can be seen some of the absorption bands are close together and led to inaccuracies in older machines. Now N_2O is measured to correct the CO_2 reading. Another source of inaccuracy is collision broadening; this phenomenon is caused by the repeated collisions between molecules creating energy exchange. The result of this can be broadening of the absorption band.

62 (**a**) true (**b**) true (**c**) true (**d**) true (**e**) false

The standard deviation is the square root of the average squared deviation from the mean.

Standard error of the mean (SEM) is defined as standard deviation divided by square root of the number of observations.

63 (**a**) true (**b**) false (**c**) false (**d**) true (**e**) true

The oxygen fuel cell circuit consists of:

- ammeter
- gold mesh cathode
- lead anode
- compensating thermistor
- electrolyte solution (KCl) and O_2 permeable membrane
- The reaction at the cathode is

$$O_2 + 2H_2O \rightarrow 4e^- + 4OH$$

- Current flow depends upon the uptake of oxygen at the cathode
- The reaction at the anode is

$$Pb + 2(OH) \rightarrow PbO + H_2O + 2e$$

- Unlike the Clarke electrode, the fuel cell requires no external power source, acting as an oxygen-dependent battery
- Like other batteries, the fuel cell will eventually expire
- The output is affected by temperature, as is that of the Clarke electrode, however compensation may be achieved by means of a parallel thermistor
- The typical response time is ~20–30 s

64 (**a**) true (**b**) true (**c**) true (**d**) true (**e**) false

Ayre's T piece requires a high fresh gas flow to ensure normocapnia. To prevent all rebreathing the fresh gas flow will need to be equivalent to the peak inspiratory flow rate. The gas flow for intermittent positive pressure ventilation (IPPV) has been suggested at 200 ml/kg per min. Normal minute ventilation in a child is 7 ml/kg (tidal volume) ×20 (respiratory rate) or 140 ml/kg. Spontaneous breathing is said to require ×2–3 times this rate so IPPV is more economical in terms of gas flow. The length of the tube from the T piece should give a volume equal to or greater than tidal volume to act as a reservoir to prevent breathing air. It should not be too long as this will increase the resistance to expiration. When the Jackson Rees modification, of an open ended bag, is attached to the expiratory limb this is classified as a Mapleson F. The wider the expiratory limb the lower the resistance to expiration. An internal diameter of 32 mm is larger than is necessary and would be non-standard.

65 (**a**) true (**b**) true (**c**) false (**d**) false (**e**) false

A *P* value of 0.05 or 1 in 20 is often used to indicate medical significance in clinical trials. Less than 0.05, a level of say 0.01 or 1 in 100, would be more significant. At 1 in 20 the null hypothesis is normally rejected and a difference is assumed. The chances of any difference happening by chance are less than 1 in 20. The distribution of the data is given by the mean, mode and median and the scatter by the standard deviation.

66 (**a**) true (**b**) true (**c**) true (**d**) true (**e**) false

Gas cylinders are made from molybdenum steel or lighter weight aluminium. They are tested every 5 years. The body and collar of the cylinder are colour coded for the gas they contain. On the neck and valve block are etched a serial number and chemical symbol of the gas or liquid, the pressure to which the cylinder has been tested, the company supplying the cylinder and the empty or tare weight. A pin index system is on the side facing the yoke.

Details of the last test are indicated by a plastic ring that is put round the base of the valve. The ring is divided into quarters and a punch mark tells the quarter of the year it was tested. The colour of the ring gives the year of testing.

In summary the marks engraved on the cylinders are:

- test pressure
- date of test performed

- chemical formula of the cylinder's content
- tare weight (weight of the empty cylinder)

67 (a) true (b) false (c) true (d) false (e) true

Non-ionising radiation is produced by electromagnetic waves that do not have enough energy to break electron bonds. These include radio waves, infrared, visible and ultraviolet light and microwaves.

Ionising radiation disrupts an electron bond to produce alpha, beta, gamma and X-ray particles. Ionising radiation includes the electromagnetic waves from X-rays and gamma rays.

68 (a) false (b) false (c) false (d) true (e) true

A variable-orifice, constant-pressure principle is used in a rotameter and the Wright's respirometer as more vanes open up. The mass spectrometer separates molecules by molecular weight; the pneomotacograph is a fixed-orifice, variable-pressure device. The Bourdon gauge works on the principle that increasing pressure unwinds a coil that has an elliptical cross-section at low pressure but a more circular cross-section as the pressure rises.

69 (a) true (b) true (c) false (d) false (e) false

Gauge pressure = absolute pressure + atmospheric pressure (1 bar). Cylinder pressure is recorded as gauge pressure, which is the pressure above atmosphere. Some gauges (those used with hyperbaric oxygen therapy) are calibrated from absolute pressure and so would record 101 kPa or 1 atm when open to air. Most cylinder pressures are in gauge pressure and read 0 when empty and open to atmosphere.

The pressure in a full oxygen cylinder is 134.7 bar or atm, or 13650 kPa.

Absolute pressure is atmospheric pressure minus one atmosphere (gauge pressure would be 0). Biological pressures are read at gauge pressure.

70 (a) true (b) true (c) true (d) true (e) true

The Venturi oxygen mask delivers a fixed concentration which is determined by the size of the constriction in the delivery tube. The Venturi principle is based on a constant energy in the flow. At a constriction the kinetic energy or flow increases so the potential energy or pressure falls. The smaller the diameter of the constriction, the greater the flow through and so the greater the fall in pressure, which is associated with more air entrainment. A larger diameter or less constriction will entrain less air and give a higher final oxygen concentration. The oxygen concentration leaving the mask is not dependent on the flow of oxygen. The flow of oxygen is important as it determines the flow of the oxygen-enriched air coming from the mask. To prevent breathing in air from around the mask the flow coming into the mask should exceed the peak inspiratory flow rate of about 35 l/min. The holes in the side of the mask are important for expired gas to escape through. If the gas cannot escape from the mask this will cause a back pressure on the oxygen flow and will reduce the amount of air entrained. Alternatively if expired gas can only partially escape it may dilute the inspired gas.

71 (**a**) true (**b**) true (**c**) true (**d**) true (**e**) true

The vacuum-insulated evaporator (VIE) is a system for storing liquid oxygen. In order to stay in the liquid form the oxygen is kept below its critical temperature of −118°C. The pressure in the cylinder is 13,700 kPa or 1980 psi. As in cylinders that contain a proportion of liquid, the contents are measured as a weight. One volume of liquid oxygen converts to about 842 times its volume at 15°C and normal atmospheric pressure. The heat that the oxygen requires to change from liquid to a gas is used to cool the remaining oxygen and so slows the process of reheating, keeping it in a liquid state.

72 (**a**) true (**b**) true (**c**) true (**d**) true (**e**) true

If the change in pressure causes a change in pressure in the system to the correct level without under- or overshoot and without oscillations, the system is critically damped and is called D1. An overshoot with oscillations is $D<1$, or under-damped. A rise with no oscillations and no overshoot will give a slow response and is $D>1$, or over-damped.

Optimal or critical damping is a balance between obtaining a rapid response while minimising any overshoot and oscillations. This occurs at *D* 0.6–0.7. Flushing the system with a sudden high pressure and monitoring the response will give an idea of the amount of damping but each liquid will cause different amounts of damping depending on viscosity and temperature. Damping is also affected by air bubbles in the line and the configuration of the cannula. A short, rigid, parallel-walled, wide-diameter cannula causes the least oscillations.

73 (**a**) false (**b**) true (**c**) true (**d**) true (**e**) false

An aneroid gauge is a sealed bellows which changes shape as pressure is applied to the outside.

The Bourdon gauge is a coiled pipe which has been flattened and is oval in cross-section. When a pressure of gas is applied to the inside of the coil it will unwind as the shape changes to be more circular to accommodate more gas. The same effect occurs if the gas heats up and the gauge can be used as a thermometer.

Each one is labelled, colour coded and calibrated for each gas on the anaesthetic machine. The scale extends to at least 33% more than the expected full pressure at 20°C.

74 (**a**) true (**b**) true (**c**) true (**d**) true (**e**) false

A refractometer or interferometer is based on the principle that a gas or vapour will delay the passage of light passing through. The delay is a measure of the concentration of the vapour. Rubber strips absorb volatile agents and the tension falls. The degree of change in tension is proportional to the concentration of the vapour. The concentration of any substance of two or more dissimilar molecules can be measured by infrared absorption. Absorption is maximum at a particular wavelength which depends on the molecular weight of the substance. Halothane absorbs ultraviolet radiation.

The two paramagnetic gases used in anaesthetic practice are oxygen and nitric oxide.

75 (**a**) false (**b**) false (**c**) false (**d**) false (**e**) true

Measurement – non-electrical

(a) Mercury thermometers
- Accurate, reliable, cheap
- Readily made in maximum reading form
- Easily made into a thermostat
- Low coefficient of expansion and requires 2–3 minutes to reach thermal equilibrium
- Unsuitable for insertion in certain orifices

(b) Alcohol thermometers
- Cheaper than mercury
- Useful for very low temperatures, as mercury solidifies at −39°C
- Unsuitable for high temperatures as alcohol boils at 78.5°C
- Expansion also tends to be less linear than mercury

(c) Bimetallic strips

(d) Bourdon gauge

Measurement – electrical

(a) Resistance thermometer

- Electrical resistance of a metal increases linearly with temperature
- Frequently uses a platinum wire resistor, or similar
- Accuracy is improved by incorporation in a Wheatstone bridge

(b) thermistor

- Made from a small bead of metal oxide
- Unlike normal metals, the resistance falls exponentially with temperature
- May be made exceedingly small and introduced almost anywhere
- Rapid thermal equilibration
- Narrow reference range and requires different thermistors for different scales
- Accuracy improved by incorporation in a Wheatstone bridge
- Calibration may be changed by exposure to severe temperatures, e.g. sterilisation

(c) Thermocouple

- Based on the Seebeck effect
- At the junction of two dissimilar metals a small voltage is produced, the magnitude of which is determined by the temperature
- Metals such as copper and constantan, which is a copper and nickel alloy
- Requires a constant reference temperature at the second junction of the electrical circuit
- May be made exceedingly small and introduced almost anywhere

76 (**a**) true (**b**) true (**c**) true (**d**) true (**e**) true

The best way of separating the mains current from the electrical device is by using D.C. battery power. An isolated electrical supply is provided to most monitors, which use the mains to charge a battery through a transformer so there is no A.C. transmission to the monitoring circuit. D.C. thresholds for electrical effect are some 5 times greater than A.C. thresholds.

Microshock can occur with 150 μA in contact with the heart. Equipment with electrodes that may contact the heart must have a leakage current of less than 50 μA.

Equipment with direct surface contacts such as pulse oximeters and temperature probes have a leakage current of 100–500 μA. Five percent dextrose is a non-electrolyte solution and so less conductive of electricity than saline solutions.

COELCB devices compare the magnetic field created in the live and neutral wires. If the current is the same in both wires the magnetic field induced will be the same but in opposite directions and they will cancel each other out. If there is a difference in the magnetic fields produced then this new magnetic field will induce a current in a third wire, which activates a circuit breaker.

77 **(a)** true **(b)** true **(c)** true **(d)** true **(e)** false

The cycling for most ventilators is time cycled either using gated circuits and electromagnetic switches or detecting a rise in pressure with fluid dynamics.

One advantage of jet ventilation is that the lung volume is maintained above closing volume by positive end-expiratory pressure (PEEP) but the mean pressure is lower than in conventional IPPV.

The jet may sometimes acts as a Venturi to deliver a fixed concentration of oxygen. If the entrainment of air occurs in the trachea the final oxygen content may not be known. An air–oxygen mix can also be used to supply gas to the ventilator.

The frequency of ventilation ranges from 60 to 3000 cycles per minute or 1–50 cycles per second.

78 **(a)** true **(b)** true **(c)** false **(d)** true **(e)** true

Confidence intervals are the range about the sample mean that contains the unknown value with a probability which is defined for medical trials as a P value of 0.05 or 1 in 20. The limits used are 90%, 95% and 99%.

A sample mean ± 1.0 SE = 68% confidence interval or 0.68 probability. Sample mean ± 1.96 SE = 95% confidence interval or 0.95 probability. This is usually taken for medical significance at 95% if the sample means are not within ±1.95 of the reference mean. The confidence intervals are wide if the sample size is small and vice versa. Variance is the square of the standard deviation. Standard deviation is a measure of the spread of values; it includes the number of values but is not a direct indicator of sample size. The confidence interval will be wider if the standard deviation (variance) is large. The 95% confidences are ± 1.96 SEM.

79 (a) false (b) false (c) true (d) true (e) false

Core temperature is the temperature that best approximates to hypothalamic temperature. This can be obtained from the eardrum (not the external ear) and lower third of the oesophagus, away from the cooling effect of inspired gases in the trachea. Nasopharyngeal temperatures vary with respiration except in the intubated patient when they are more stable – this could be true or false depending on whether the patient is intubated or not, but note the use of the word MAY.

80 (a) true (b) false (c) true (d) true (e) true

The equation for turbulent flow is

$$\text{Flow } (\dot{Q}) = \text{radius}^2 \times \sqrt{\Delta P} \text{ divided by } \sqrt{\text{length}} \text{ times } \sqrt{\text{density}}.$$

Flow becomes turbulent when Reynold's number (R_e) is >2000.

$$R_e = \text{linear velocity} \times \text{density} \times \text{diameter/viscosity}$$

Viscosity is also important to laminar flow, rather than density which is important to turbulent flow.

81 (a) true (b) false (c) true (d) true (e) true

Specific heat capacity

- The amount of heat required to raise the temperature of 1 kg of a substance by 1 K
- SI units of specific heat capacity are J/kg per K
- Note 1 K is commensurate with 1°C
- Specific indicates that the quantity is expressed in terms of units of mass

Heat capacity

- The amount of heat required to raise the temperature of a given object by 1 K
- SI units of heat capacity are J/K
- It can be calculated from the product specific heat capacity times the mass

Specific latent heat

- Defined as the heat required to convert 1 kg of a substance from one phase to another at a given temperature
- SI units are J/kg

82 (**a**) true (**b**) false (**c**) false (**d**) true (**e**) false

The Magill is a Mapleson A breathing system. The reservoir bag is at the common gas outlet and the APL valve is at the patient end of the system. By conserving dead space gas the fresh gas flow needs to be about alveolar ventilation when breathing spontaneously. It will be used for children but it is not recommended for children under 20 kg. The T piece breathing system was designed for use in children as it has minimum dead space and minimum resistance to breathing, so we have marked this false.

83 (**a**) true (**b**) true (**c**) false (**d**) true (**e**) true

The cuff

- Should cover at least two-thirds of the upper arm
- Width should be 40% of the mid-circumference of the limb
- Middle should overlay the brachial artery

The device has a fast rate of inflation and a slow cuff deflation.

This avoids venous congestion and allows time to detect arterial pulsation.

Sources of error

- If the cuff is too small, the blood pressure over-reads
- If too large then the blood pressure under-reads (greatest error is seen with an undersized cuff)
- Systolic pressure over-reads at low pressures (<60 mmHg)
- Under-reads at high systolic pressures
- Arrhythmias such as atrial fibrillation affect accuracy
- External pressure on the cuff can cause inaccuracies

Paralysed or injured limbs may give an inaccurate blood pressure reading. This part is difficult to answer correctly but note the use of the word MAY. If the paralysis is spastic this is similar to holding the muscles in contraction and the systolic blood pressure may read high. If the paralysis is flaccid without sympathetic tone there will be vasodilatation and a lower blood pressure. The elderly have a less compliant aorta and so a higher peak systolic pressure. Smaller vessels are less compliant so less distensible than the small arteries and so the systolic pressure and pulse pressure increase towards the periphery.

84 (**a**) false (**b**) false (**c**) true (**d**) true (**e**) false

Thermistor

- Made from a small bead of metal oxide
- Unlike normal metals, the resistance falls exponentially with temperature
- May be made exceedingly small and introduced almost anywhere
- Rapid thermal equilibration
- Narrow reference range and requires a different thermistor for different scales
- Accuracy improved by incorporation in a Wheatstone bridge
- Calibration may be changed by exposure to severe temperatures, e.g. sterilisation

85 (**a**) false (**b**) false (**c**) true (**d**) false (**e**) true

(a) Hair Hygrometer
- Based on the principle that hair elongates as the humidity rises
- Very simple and cheap
- Only really accurate over the range 30%–90%

(b) Wet and dry bulb hygrometer
- The temperature of the wet bulb is reduced due to evaporation
- The lower the humidity the greater the evaporative cooling and the greater the temperature difference. Result from tables relating the two temperatures to % humidity
- Air must be flowing over the wet bulb to prevent a local rise in the humidity

(c) Regnault's Hygrometer
- Uses the principle that condensation occurs when the air is fully saturated at a given temperature = the dew point
- Air is blown through a silver test tube containing ether, reducing the temperature by evaporation
- The dew point is noted and from tables both the relative and absolute humidity can be established
- Relative humidity = saturated vapour pressure at the dew point

(d) Electrical transducers – both resistance and capacitance

(e) Mass spectrometry

If a gas is heated the:

- absolute humidity stays the same
- relative humidity decreases

Relative humidity equals vapour pressure /saturated vapour pressure.

86 (**a**) false (**b**) true (**c**) true (**d**) true (**e**) false

Damping does not alert the natural frequency but reduces the amplitude of oscillations by reducing the energy of the system. Optimum damping is $D = 0.6–0.7$. Critical damping is $D = 1$.

87 (**a**) true (**b**) false (**c**) false (**d**) false (**e**) false

SEM = SD/$\sqrt{n}$. In this example SEM = 2/$\sqrt{25}$ = 2/5 = 0.4.

The data do not indicate the precise maximum or minimum, but 3 standard deviations would contain 99.7% of the readings; 2 standard deviations would contain 95% of the readings; and 1 SD, 68% of the readings. In this case the SD is 2, so 3 × SD = ±6, which will give a spread of 4–16. Variance is the square of the SD = 4.

88 (**a**) false (**b**) false (**c**) false (**d**) false (**e**) false

Transcutaneous electrical nerve stimulation (TENS) uses frequencies usually between 50 and 100 Hz. The voltage is above 0 and driven from a 7-V battery. The pulse current is up to 50 mA, with a pulse width of 0.1–0.5 ms. The stimulation is aimed at the non-painful A sensory fibres and so closes the gate. It is not recommended for the electrodes to be placed near to the pacemaker field, but they can be used on the lower back and legs of a patient with a pacemaker. This is similar to the rule of diathermy to keep any electrical fields away from the route of the pacing impulse. It would not be effective in thalamic pain, which is of central origin and so there is no gate to close.

89 (**a**) true (**b**) false (**c**) true (**d**) false (**e**) false

Pulse oximeter probes emit two beams of light in the red spectrum. These can cause burns in patients with poor perfusion or pre-existing weakness in skin structure. Burns were reported in neonates and patients with poor blood flow but newer probes are producing less heat – this answer could be true or false.

The wavelengths used are specific for each haemoglobin. Fetal haemoglobin does not lead to inaccuracy. Inaccuracies will occur if there is a lot of other haemoglobins present, such as carboxyhaemoglobin. Methaemoglobin is read as reduced haemoglobin and the final reading for oxyhaemoglobin is low, similarly for bilirubin. Transcutaneous electrode measurement of oxygen has a slow response time and is subject to local blood flow.

90 (**a**) true (**b**) true (**c**) true (**d**) false (**e**) false

Any molecule which has two or more dissimilar molecules will absorb infrared radiation. The amount absorbed is dependent on the molecular weight, the wavelength and the amount of gas present. Oxygen and nitrogen have two molecules but they are not dissimilar.

	(a)	(b)	(c)	(d)	(e)
1	F	T	F	T	T
2	F	F	T	F	F
3	F	T	T	T	T
4	F	T	F	T	T
5	T	T	T	T	F
6	T	T	T	T	F
7	T	T	T	T	F
8	T	F	F	F	F
9	T	T	T	F	F
10	T	T	T	F	T
11	F	T	T	T	T
12	T	F	F	F	T
13	T	F	F	F	F
14	T	T	T	F	T
15	F	T	T	T	T
16	T	T	T	F	F
17	T	T	T	T	T
18	T	T	T	T	T
19	F	F	T	F	F
20	T	F	T	F	T
21	T	T	F	F	F
22	F	F	T	T	F
23	T	F	T	F	F
24	T	T	F	F	F
25	T	T	T	F	F
26	F	T	T	T	F
27	F	T	F	F	F
28	T	F	T	F	T
29	F	F	T	F	T

	(a)	(b)	(c)	(d)	(e)
30	T	F	T	T	T
31	F	F	T	T	F
32	T	F	T	T	F
33	T	F	T	F	F
34	F	F	T	F	F
35	F	F	F	T	T
36	T	T	F	F	T
37	F	F	F	F	T
38	T	F	T	T	F
39	T	F	T	T	T
40	T	F	T	F	T
41	T	F	F	F	F
42	T	F	F	T	T
43	F	F	T	T	T
44	T	T	T	T	T
45	F	F	T	T	T
46	F	F	F	T	F
47	F	T	F	F	F
48	T	T	F	T	F
49	F	T	F	F	F
50	T	F	T	T	T
51	F	T	F	T	F
52	F	F	T	T	F
53	F	T	F	T	F
54	T	T	T	T	T
55	T	F	T	F	T
56	T	T	T	F	F
57	F	T	T	F	F
58	F	T	F	T	F
59	F	F	T	F	T
60	T	F	T	F	F

	(a)	(b)	(c)	(d)	(e)
61	T	F	F	F	F
62	T	T	T	T	F
63	T	F	F	T	T
64	T	T	T	T	F
65	T	T	F	F	F
66	T	T	T	T	F
67	T	F	T	F	T
68	F	F	F	T	T
69	T	T	F	F	F
70	T	T	T	T	T
71	T	T	T	T	T
72	T	T	T	T	T
73	F	T	T	T	F
74	T	T	T	T	F
75	F	F	F	F	T
76	T	T	T	T	T
77	T	T	T	T	F
78	T	T	F	T	T
79	F	F	T	T	F
80	T	F	T	T	T
81	T	F	T	T	T
82	T	F	F	T	F
83	T	T	F	T	T
84	F	F	T	T	F
85	F	F	T	F	T
86	F	T	T	T	F
87	T	F	F	F	F
88	F	F	F	F	F
89	T	F	T	F	F
90	T	T	T	F	F

Paper 5 Answers

1 (**a**) false (**b**) true (**c**) true (**d**) true (**e**) false

Contractility describes the ability of the myocardium to contract in the absence of any changes in preload or afterload. In other words, it is the 'power' of the cardiac muscle. The most important influence on contractility is the sympathetic nervous system. Beta-adrenergic receptors are stimulated by noradrenaline released from nerve endings, and contractility increases. A similar effect is seen with circulating adrenaline and drugs such as ephedrine, digoxin and calcium. Contractility is reduced by:

- hypoxia
- acidosis
- hypercapnia
- myocardial ischaemia
- use of beta-blocking
- antiarrhythmic agents, e.g. quinidine, procainamide

As the volume at the end of diastole (end-diastolic volume) increases and stretches the muscle fibre, so the energy of contraction and stroke volume increase (Starling's Law) until a point of over-stretching when stroke volume may actually decrease, as in the failing heart.

2 (**a**) false (**b**) true (**c**) false (**d**) true (**e**) false

Standing causes pooling of blood in the lower limbs. This leads to a reduction in venous return, a fall in cardiac output and reduced firing of the baroreceptors, leading to a compensatory venoconstriction, increase in venous pressure and restoration of venous return.

In the upright position the upper portions of the lungs are above the heart. The marked pressure gradient leads to a linear decrease in pulmonary blood flow from the bases to the apices.

3 (**a**) true (**b**) false (**c**) true (**d**) true (**e**) true

Resistance in the pulmonary circulation is distributed more evenly than in the systemic circulation with approximately 50% residing in the arteries and arterioles, 30% in the capillaries and 20% in the veins. Pulmonary vascular resistance (PVR) is affected by active factors via changes in muscle tone.

(a) Systemic hypoxia increases vessel resistance by muscle constriction
(b) Hypercarbia and acidosis increase PVR
(c) Humoral control

- Vasoconstrictors
  - thromboxane A_2
  - prostaglandin F
  - histamine
  - serotonin
  - angiotensin
  - catecholamines
- Vasodilators
  - acetylcholine
  - prostaglandin E
  - prostacyclin
  - bradykinin

4 (**a**) false (**b**) false (**c**) false (**d**) false (**e**) true

Sinus arrhythmia is present during normal breathing with the heart rate (PR interval) varying approximately 5% during the various phases of the normal, resting breathing cycle. This variation may increase to 30% during deep breathing. These variations in heart rate with breathing are most effected by the baroreceptor reflex activity, which is responding to changes in the negative intrapleural pressures that elicit a waxing and waning Bainbridge reflex.

Variations in heart rate not relating to breathing (non-phasic sinus arrhythmias) are abnormal. They are a result of:

- sinoatrial node dysfunction
- aging
- digitalis intoxication

The absence of phasic changes suggests autonomic dysfunction (diabetes mellitus).

5 (**a**) true (**b**) true (**c**) false (**d**) false (**e**) true

Measured values made with a pulmonary artery flotation catheter: pressures in the right atrium, right ventricle, pulmonary artery and capillary wedge pressure, which reflects left atrial filling pressure and so left ventricular end-diastolic pressure. The left ventricular end-diastolic pressure is itself an indirect measure of left ventricular end-diastolic volume. Blood samples from these sites can be taken to determine partial pressures and so content of blood gases.

Derived values from the measurements made with a pulmonary artery flotation catheter are: cardiac output by measuring the flow of blood through the right ventricle; systemic and pulmonary vascular resistance, cardiac index and stroke volume or index. Cardiac index is cardiac output/surface area.

Other calculations

The shunt equation requires the content of oxygen in arterial blood, end-capillary blood and mixed-venous blood. These will be obtained from the pulmonary flotation catheter and an arterial catheter.

6 (**a**) true (**b**) true (**c**) false (**d**) true (**e**) true

This question is about phase one of the Valsalva manoeuvre, which represents the small rise in pressure that occurs briefly after the onset of straining. The pulse rate is steady during this short period. The sudden increase in intrathoracic pressure squeezes the intrapulmonary vessels, leading to an increased return of blood to the left side of the heart. The heart responds immediately by increasing its stroke volume.

This is an example of Starling's law of the heart. The blood pressure rises slightly. This only lasts for a few beats. The increased intrapleural pressure is also transmitted directly onto the aorta and this is a second reason for the small rise in arterial pressure.

7 (**a**) true (**b**) true (**c**) true (**d**) false (**e**) true

The passage of gastric contents from the stomach into the small intestine is influenced by many factors.

(a) Content of the meal
- The content of food material in the duodenum influences the rate of gastric emptying

- The calorific value of the food seems to be the major determinant of inhibition of gastric motility, i.e. fats are the most inhibitory
- Carbohydrates and acidic and hypertonic solutions in the duodenum inhibit gastric acid and pepsin secretion and gastric motility via gastric inhibitory peptide (GIP) and secretin and possibly via other hormones

(b) Peptides that are associated with delayed gastric emptying include
- Gastrin
- Cholecystokinin
- Vasoactive intestinal polypeptide
- Gastric inhibitory peptide

(c) Hyperglycaemia reduces vagal tone to the stomach and thus slows gastric emptying

(d) Abdominal pain and bowel distension are associated with delayed gastric emptying

(e) Vagotomy reduces gastric emptying. In this situation the gastric intrinsic nerves remain intact and still release acetylcholine in response to drugs such as metoclopramide

(f) Drugs
- Opioids
- Partial and mixed opioid agonists
- Anticholinergics
- Antihistamines
- Dopamine
- Alcohol
- Sympathomimetic, e.g. isoprenaline

8 **(a)** true **(b)** false **(c)** false **(d)** false **(e)** true

Closing volume is the lung volume above the residual volume at which the airways begin to close off because of a reduced transmural pressure, predominantly in the dependent parts of the lung.

Closing capacity is the sum of two volumes:
- residual volume
- closing volume

Paper 5 Answers

Measurement

- Single breath nitrogen curve; similar to Fowler's method for dead space
- From maximum expiration, the subject takes a maximum inspiration of pure O_2 or helium then exhales steadily; the changes in (N_2 or helium) concentration in expired gas during expiration are measured continuously
- The concentration of nitrogen or helium increases as the airways start to close
- Closing volume (CV) is the beginning of Phase IV of the washout curve to the residual volume (RV)
- Closing capacity (CC) is the difference between the onset of phase IV and zero lung volume = CV + RV

Phase I

- No marker gas
- Consists of expired dead space

Phase II

- Increase in marker gas
- Consists of mixture dead space and alveolar gas

Phase III (plateau)

- Consists of alveolar gas

Factors affecting closing volume

Increases with

- Age
    - CC = FRC at 65 years
    - CC = FRC at 40 years
- Lying flat
- Head down (Trendelenburg position)
    - when the FRC reduces, the CV may come to lie within the FRC even though the CV has not changed

Reduces with

- Anaesthesia
- Pregnancy
- Infants
- Obesity

9 **(a)** false **(b)** false **(c)** true **(d)** true **(e)** false

Surfactant is a lipoprotein, surface-tension-lowering agent.

Composition

Constituent	%
Dipalmitoyl phosphatidylcholine (DPPC)	60
Phosphatidyl glycine	5
Other phospholipids	10
Neutral lipids	13
Proteins	8
Carbohydrates	2

Synthesis

- Surfactant is produced by type II alveolar epithelial cells
- These are pneumocytes regulated by the hypothalamic–pituitary axis
- Cuboidal cells with large nuclei

Mechanism of action

The molecules of DPPC are:

- hydrophobic at one end
- hydrophilic at the other end

The hydrophilic ends align themselves in the alveolar surface. When this occurs their intermolecular forces repulse each other and oppose the normal attracting forces between the surface molecules which are responsible for surface tension.

Function

- It lowers the surface tension in the wall of alveoli; so
    - it increases the compliance of the lung
    - it reduces the work of expanding the lung
- It promotes alveolar stability
- It helps to keep the alveoli dry

Surfactant's ability to lower surface tension is directly proportional to its concentration within the alveolus.

$$\text{LaPlace's law } P = 2T/R$$

Paper 5 Answers

Where P = pressure across the wall, T = tension in the wall, R = radius of the alveolus.

Factors which *increase* the amount of surfactant produced by a fetus or neonate include:

- prolonged rupture of the membranes
- maternal hypertension and pre-eclampsia
- steroids given to the mother
- sickle cell disease in the mother
- alcohol abuse by the mother

Factors which *inhibit* surfactant production:

- bronchial obstruction
- pulmonary artery occlusion
- heavy smoking
- 100% oxygen

10 (**a**) false (**b**) true (**c**) true (**d**) true (**e**) true

Respiratory alkalosis is characterised by reduced $PaCO_2$, normal or slightly reduced serum bicarbonate and a raised pH.

A respiratory alkalosis may be pure or it may be complicated by a metabolic derangement (i.e. a mixed alkalosis). Measurement of the serum bicarbonate permits a definitive diagnosis.

Acute respiratory alkalosis

- The serum bicarbonate decreases by 2 mmol for every 1.33 kPa decrease in $PaCO_2$

Chronic respiratory alkalosis

- The serum bicarbonate decreases 5 mmol for every 1.33 kPa decrease in $PaCO_2$

Aetiology

- Stress hyperventilation – hysteria
- Hypoxic stimulation to ventilation
  - alveolar disease
  - right-to-left shunts
  - altitude
- Drug-induced stimulus to hyperventilation
  - early salicylate poisoning in adults – less likely in children

The kidneys compensate with time for loss of carbon dioxide by excreting bicarbonate ions in association with sodium and potassium ions. Tetany that accompanies alkalosis reflects hypocalcaemia due to the greater affinity of plasma proteins for calcium ions in an alkaline, compared with an acidic solution.

The pH inside the red blood cell decreases due to loss of H^+ ions in exchange for K^+ ions.

11 (**a**) true (**b**) true (**c**) true (**d**) false (**e**) false

Body water is about 45 l in the 70-kg man or two-thirds of body mass: 30 l is intracellular; 15 l, extracellular. In young men body water is about 60% and in women at the same age about 55%. Both fall with age.

The newborn has more water, nearer 80%, and a greater proportion is extracellular and less intracellular. The extracellular water exceeds intracellular in the premature baby. The elderly have less body water – 50% of total weight.

During pregnancy water is retained.

Body water is measured using a dye that will stay in one compartment and is calculated by the volume of distribution.

Plasma volume is measured using dyes attached to protein–serum albumin labelled with radioactive iodine.

Extracellular water volume is difficult to measure because its limits are ill-defined and the lymphatics form part of the ECF space. Radioactive inulin is used, as well as mannitol or sucrose.

Deuterium is heavy water, which will dilute into the total body water.

Interstitial volume is calculated by subtracting extracellular volume from total body volume.

12 (**a**) true (**b**) false (**c**) false (**d**) true (**e**) false

The renal tubules absorb large amounts of water and sodium along a concentration gradient. Sodium is moved by an active Na^+/K^+-ATPase pump. This reduces the intracellular sodium concentration and so sodium moves out of the tubular lumen and into the cell. This same mechanism is responsible for the reabsorption of glucose, amino acids, potassium and the water. Glucose is removed by secondary active transport. The energy is provided by the Na^+/K^+-ATPase pumps. All the glucose is normally reabsorbed. Transport is inhibited by phlorhizin, which competes with D-glucose for binding.

Insulin does not act on the kidney.

The intestine and kidney handle glucose in similar ways.

In the glomerulus the kidney filters glucose at 100 mg/min (80 mg/dl × 125 ml/min). Glucose appears in the urine when the mechanism for reabsorption by the tubules reaches a maximum rate. This is at about a plasma level of 10 mmol/l (180 mg/l). The amount reabsorbed is proportional to the amount filtered up to a transport maximum (T_{max}). T_{max} is about 21 mmol/min (375 mg/min) in men and 17 mmol/min (300 mg/min) in women. Tubular damage and pregnancy reduce this threshold.

13 (a) true (**b**) false (**c**) false (**d**) false (**e**) false

The barometric pressure (PB) increases by the equivalent of 1 atm for every 10 m below the surface of sea water. A person 10 m beneath the water surface is exposed to 2 atm reflecting 1 atm of pressure caused by the weight of air above the water and 1 atm caused by the weight of water. At 20 m below the water surface, the PB is equivalent to 3 atm. Below the surface of the water the gases are compressed in the lungs to smaller volumes. A high pressure produces nitrogen narcosis when the inhaled gases are air. The PN_2 at the increased PB causes sufficient absorption and deposition of nitrogen molecules in the lipid membranes of cells to produce an anaesthetic effect. Helium can be substituted for nitrogen to avoid narcosis.

14 (a) true (**b**) false (**c**) false (**d**) false (**e**) true

- The EEG trace is abnormal in hyperventilation if there is an underlying abnormality
- Eye closing gives an alpha rhythm
- Changing position does not alter the EEG
- Vasopressin is released from the posterior pituitary gland; it has three effects; to retain water in the kidney, as a vasoconstrictor and to increase the level of factor VIII

- Mental activity and arithmetic disrupt the alpha waves

15 (a) true (b) true (c) false (d) false (e) true

The somatic nervous system forms the efferent nerves to the muscles. The cell bodies of the motor neurones are located in the ventral horn. The larger diameter myelinated efferent nerves conduct at 120 m/s.

In contrast the sensory nerves have their cell bodies in ganglia outside the dorsal horn of the spinal cord. The afferent sensory nerves synapse in the dorsal horn. Afferent fibres conduct at 6–120 m/s while unmyelinated sympathetic fibres are slower at 0.5–2 m/s. Salutatory conduction is the faster conduction seen in myelinated nerves as the impulse jumps from one node of Ranvier to the next.

16 (a) false (b) false (c) false (d) false (e) true

Cerebral blood flow affects cerebral volume, oxygen delivery and removal of products of metabolism. The adult brain weighs 1500 g and receives a blood flow of 750 ml/min. This represents 15%–20% of cardiac output. Normal CBF values are:

whole brain	50 ml $100g^{-1}$ min^{-1}
grey matter	80 ml $100g^{-1}$ min^{-1}
white matter	20 ml $100g^{-1}$ min^{-1}

Regulation of cerebral blood flow

The control of cerebral blood flow (CBF) to the brain is primarily dictated by its metabolic needs and is mediated through chemical changes. Changes in arterial CO_2 produce the most marked change in CBF. Neurogenic control through the sympathetic nervous system is much less significant.

(a) Metabolic

CBF increases with an increase in metabolism. On a global basis, the highest level of CBF will be seen during epileptic seizures when brain metabolism is maximal, and low levels of CBF occur in coma. On a regional basis an increase in CBF can be demonstrated in the contralateral cortex during muscle contraction, which is coincident with an increase in oxygen demand.

(b) CO_2

CO_2 is a potent vasodilator. Cerebral blood flow increases linearly with carbon dioxide tensions between a P_a CO_2 of 2.7 and 10.7 kPa (20–80 mmHg). Cerebral blood flow increases by 2%–4% for every 0.13 kPa (1 mmHg) rise in P_a CO_2.

(c) Oxygen

Changes in PaO_2 have little effect on CBF over the normal range. Only if PaO_2 falls below 7 kPa will cerebral vasodilatation occur.

(d) Autoregulation

In the healthy brain CBF remains constant despite changes in arterial blood pressure. In normotensive subjects flow remains constant between mean arterial pressures of 50 and 150 mmHg. In chronic hypertension the autoregulatory curve is shifted to the right, protecting small capillaries from a raised perfusion pressure.

(e) Neurogenic

The cerebral vessels have a sympathetic nerve supply originating from the superior cervical ganglion and a parasympathetic supply from the facial nerve.

(f) Other factors

- Hypothermia reduces cerebral metabolism, which in turn reduces CBF. Metabolism falls approximately 5% for each degree centigrade
- Blood viscosity also affects CBF – increased viscosity reduces and decreased viscosity increases CBF
- Rapid intravenous mannitol temporarily moves fluid from the ECF space to the intravascular space and so increases CBF

17 (**a**) true (**b**) true (**c**) true (**d**) true (**e**) false

(a) **Normal** urine osmolality is 50–1200 mosmol/kg

(b) **Increased** in:

- syndrome of inappropriate ADH secretion (SIADH)
- dehydration
- *glycosuria*
- *adrenal insufficiency*
- high-protein diet

(c) **Decreased** in:

- *diabetes insipidus*
- excessive hydration (oral or intravenous)
- acute renal insufficiency
- *glomerulonephritis*

(d) Normal urine *specific gravity* values are between 1.002 and 1.028

(e) Normal value ranges may vary slightly between different laboratories

(f) **Increased urine specific gravity** may indicate:
- *dehydration*
- diarrhoea
- excessive sweating
- *glucosuria*
- *heart failure* (related to decreased blood flow to the kidneys)
- *Renal arterial stenosis*
- *SIADH*
- vomiting
- water restriction

(g) **Decreased urine specific gravity** may indicate:
- excessive fluid intake
- *diabetes insipidus – central*
- *diabetes insipidus – nephrogenic*
- *renal failure* (that is, loss of ability to reabsorb water)
- pyelonephritis

(h) Bicarbonate is reabsorbed like glucose and amino acids in the proximal tubule

(i) Ammonium ions are produced by the combination of ammonia and hydrogen ions in the distal tubule; the ammonium ions are secreted by a Na^+/NH_4^+ counter-transport pump

(j) Osmolarity is a measure of the number of moles or particles present

(k) Specific gravity is a measure of the weight of the particles. SG 1000 = 300 mosmol/l, SG 1040 = 1200 mosmol/l

18 **(a)** false **(b)** false **(c)** true **(d)** true **(e)** true

When a muscle is stretched
- Primary sensory fibres (Group Ia afferent neurones) of the muscle spindle respond to both the velocity and the degree of stretch, and send this information to the spinal cord
- Secondary sensory fibres (Group II afferent neurones) detect and send information about the degree of stretch (but not the velocity thereof) to the CNS

This information is transmitted
- Monosynaptically to an alpha efferent motor fibre, which activates extrafusal fibres of the muscle to contract, thereby reducing stretch
- Polysynaptically through an interneurone to another alpha motorneurone; this inhibits contraction in the opposing muscles

19 (**a**) true (**b**) true (**c**) true (**d**) true (**e**) false

Prothrombin is produced in the liver. Any liver enzyme activity is reduced with immaturity, seen in the newborn and in hypothermia. Vitamin K is a fat-soluble vitamin which is reliant on bile for absorption.

20 (**a**) false (**b**) true (**c**) true (**d**) true (**e**) false

Transferrin is a β1 globulin that transports iron in plasma.

Ferric iron in food is converted to ferrous iron by gastric hydrochloric acid and vitamin C. About 10% or 1–2 mg is absorbed from 10–15 mg in the diet. Absorption doubles in pregnancy.

Transferrin is produced in the liver. One molecule binds two atoms of iron in the plasma.

Iron is stored in the liver, spleen and bone marrow; 65% is stored as water-soluble ferritin and 35% as haemosiderin. Iron is required for cell respiration, in the form of iron-containing enzymes such as cytochromes, catalase and peroxidase.

21 (**a**) false (**b**) true (**c**) true (**d**) true (**e**) false

A number of hormonal changes occur in response to surgery, which influence salt and water metabolism. These changes support the preservation of adequate body fluid volumes. **Arginine vasopressin**, which is released from the posterior pituitary, promotes water retention and the production of concentrated urine by direct action on the kidney. Increased vasopressin secretion may continue for 3–5 days, depending on the severity of the surgical injury and the development of complications. **Renin** is secreted from the juxtaglomerular cells of the kidney, partly as a result of increased sympathetic efferent activation. Renin stimulates the production of **angiotensin II**. This has a number of important effects; in particular, it stimulates the release of **aldosterone** from the adrenal cortex, which in turn leads to Na^+ and water reabsorption from the distal tubules in the kidney.

22 (**a**) true (**b**) true (**c**) false (**d**) true (**e**) false

There are four parasympathetic ganglia. The ciliary on the oculomotor nerve; the pterygopalatine, also called the sphenopalatine, connected to the facial nerve but with fibres from the maxillary nerve; the submandibular, suspended from the lingual nerve; and the otic, connected to the glossopharyngeal nerve.

23 **(a)** false **(b)** false **(c)** true **(d)** false **(e)** true

To measure the volume of a compartment, one must have a substance that distributes itself only in the volume of the compartment of interest.

Volumes for compartments where no such substance exists may be determined by subtraction.

(a) Total body water (TBW)
- Deuterated water (D_2O)
- Tritiated water (^3H_2O)
- Antipyrine

(b) Extracellular fluid volume (ECFV)
- Labelled inulin
- Sucrose
- Mannitol
- Sulphate

(c) Plasma volume (PV)
- Radiolabelled albumin
- Evans Blue Dye (which binds to albumin)

(d) Intracellular fluid volume (ICFV)
- Measured by subtraction: ICFV = TBW – ECFV

(e) Interstitial fluid volume (ISFV)
- Measured by subtraction: ISFV = ECFV – PV

24 **(a)** true **(b)** false **(c)** true **(d)** true **(e)** false

The newborn prefers to nose breathe and any obstruction leads to difficulty in breathing. The tidal volume is the same/per kilogram as in an adult (7–10 ml/kg) but the respiratory rate is higher, and the dead space is 50% of tidal volume.

Maintenance fluid in the neonate is usually 100 ml/kg per 24 h except in the first week of life when it starts at 20 ml/kg on the first day and increases by 20 ml each day up to 140 ml/kg at the end of the first week.

25 **(a)** true **(b)** true **(c)** false **(d)** false **(e)** false

Gastric secretion is about 2500 ml/day. It is increased by food distending the stomach. Distension of the antrum leads to gastric secretion. Gastrin stimulates acid secretion by the release of histamine from other cells in the gastric glands binding to histamine-2 receptors and the vagus nerve.

Paper 5 Answers

Acid secretion is inhibited by high acidity through the release of somatostatin. Sympathetic activity reduces gastric activity but parasympathetic activity increases acid and gastric function.

Acid secretion is increased by gastrin, histamine, acetylcholine and food.

Acid secretion is inhibited by intestinal contents which are high in fatty acids and hydrogen ions.

26 (**a**) false (**b**) false (**c**) false (**d**) true (**e**) true

The Na^+/K^+ pump uses the energy of 3 Na^+ ions extruded from the cell to take 2 K^+ ions into the cell. This is a coupling ratio of 3/2.

It is found in many parts of the body. It does not require other ions but may affect the transport of other ions such as calcium in the heart.

The normal cell volume and osmotic pressure depend on this pump. If the pump stops Na^+ and K^+ will enter the cell and water will pass down its concentration gradient causing the cell to swell.

27 (**a**) false (**b**) false (**c**) true (**d**) false (**e**) true

Arterial and alveolar carbon dioxide tensions are decreased by the increased ventilation. An average $PaCO_2$ of 4.3 kPa and arterial oxygen tension of 13.7 kPa persist during most of gestation. The development of alkalosis is forestalled by compensatory decreases in serum bicarbonate. Only carbon dioxide tensions below 3.73 kPa will lead to a respiratory alkalosis. It is very difficult to be certain about the answers to questions (b), (c) and (e). It depends on whether the question refers to the normal physiological hyperventilation of pregnancy or additional hyperventilation.

28 (**a**) true (**b**) false (**c**) false (**d**) false (**e**) true

Parathyroid hormone (PTH)

(a) Increases movement of Ca^{2+} and HPO_4^- out of bone
(b) Increases renal tubular reabsorption of Ca^{2+}
(c) Reduces renal tubular reabsorption of HPO_4^-
(d) Stimulates production of vitamin D (indirect effect)
   - Inhibits proximal tubular H^+ secretion and HCO_3^- reabsorption
   - The decrease in plasma pH displaces Ca^{2+} from plasma protein and bone

- Increased HPO_4^- excretion aids further reabsorption from bone due to an effect on the $[HPO_4^-]\cdot[Ca^{2+}]$ solubility product

NB Hyperparathyroidism causes:

- an elevated plasma calcium with a low to normal phosphate
- enhanced bone reabsorption with cyst formation
- ectopic calcification
- renal stones – renal Ca^{2+} excretion increases, despite the elevated PTH, as the filtered mass increase is much greater than the reabsorptive increase

29 (**a**) true (**b**) false (**c**) false (**d**) true (**e**) false

Thyroid-stimulating hormone secreted from the anterior pituitary controls thyroxine secretion and the conversion of T_4 to T_3 in the peripheral tissues. There is a direct inhibitory feedback loop. Each day, 80 μg to 103 nmol of T_4 and 4 μg (7 nmol) of T_3 is secreted.

Somatostatin inhibits growth hormone and the production of insulin and glucagons. As a neural transmitter it may be part of the nociceptive pathway.

30 (**a**) false (**b**) true (**c**) true (**d**) true (**e**) true

Aldosterone is released for the adrenal cortex, stimulated by angiotensin II, increased plasma potassium and adrenocorticotrophin or ACTH. It acts on the renal collecting ducts to stimulate sodium reabsorption and potassium and hydrogen excretion. Aldosterone is responsible for the reabsorption of sodium in the kidney, intestine, sweat and salivary glands.

31 (**a**) true (**b**) false (**c**) true (**d**) false (**e**) false

Total clearance represents the volume of blood or plasma from which a drug is completely eliminated in unit time, measured in ml/min. This is the rate of drug elimination (mg/ml) per unit of blood or plasma concentration (mg/ml). The total clearance is made up of renal + hepatic + non-organ clearance of drugs. When a drug is eliminated by the kidney the clearance is the amount of the substance excreted in the urine per unit time divided by the plasma concentration of the substance. Clearance is not just dependent on glomerular filtration: it may depend on enzyme action in the tissues and the liver. Rarely the enzyme action is rate or capacity limited, e.g. with alcohol. Clearance of creatinine, which is produced by muscle breakdown, is used to determine renal glomerular filtration rate, which is a function of renal blood flow. When clearance is less than glomerular filtration rate, there is another path of elimination in addition to the kidney. Most drugs are eliminated by more than one route not just the kidney.

Volume of distribution = clearance × half-life/0.693.

The rate constant is the reciprocal of the time constant. Time constant is the time in which the process would have been completed had it continued at the original rate of change.

The rate of elimination is proportional to the plasma concentration. The time constant is another way of expressing the half-life. The half-life is the time it takes for the initial concentration to fall to half. So clearance is inversely proportional to the half-life, which is proportional to the time constant, which is inversely proportional to the rate constant. Or, the clearance is proportional to the reciprocal of the rate constant.

Drugs with a small volume of distribution are easily cleared from the plasma.

32 (**a**) false (**b**) false (**c**) true (**d**) false (**e**) false

Sodium nitroprusside is a potent short-acting vasodilator used as an antihypertensive agent but it has been replaced by glycerol trinitrate, which is safer.

It acts through nitric oxide to reduce systemic vascular resistance. It increases coronary, renal and cerebral blood flows. Pulmonary vascular resistance is reduced due to vasodilatation. Heart rate may rise to compensate for the hypotension. Raised intracranial pressure may occur.

Various factors may lead to acidosis with larger doses. It is metabolised in red cells to produce cyanide ions, which inhibit the cytochrome oxidase system and other enzymes involved in cell respiration. A small amount binds with haemoglobin to form methaemoglobin so (e) has been marked false.

33 (**a**) true (**b**) true (**c**) true (**d**) true (**e**) true

Allopurinol is used in gout to inhibit xanthine oxidase. This inhibits the conversion of hypoxanthine to xanthine, which converts to uric acid.

Ibuprofen is a cyclo-oxygenase inhibitor. Enalapril is an angiotensin-converting enzyme inhibitor. Enoximone is a phosphodiesterase inhibitor.

Lansoprazole inhibits H^+/K^+-ATPase enzyme on the luminal surface of gastric parietal cells. It inhibits this proton pump to stop gastric acid secretion.

34 (**a**) true (**b**) false (**c**) false (**d**) true (**e**) true

Morphine increases the tone of smooth muscle in the gut and the visceral sphincters but not bronchial tone. Ketamine increases sympathetic tone by central sympathetic stimulation and acts to block the reuptake of noradrenaline at sympathetic nerve endings. PGE_2 causes bronchodilatation. $PGF_{2\alpha}$ causes bronchoconstriction.

Cyclo-oxygenase inhibitors block the conversion of arachadonic acid to prostaglandin, which is a smooth muscle relaxant. They are associated with bronchospasm in patients with asthma and nasal polyps.

35 (**a**) true (**b**) true (**c**) false (**d**) false (**e**) false

- Amitriptyline causes a dry mouth
- Trimetaphan is a short-acting ganglion blocker, metabolised by plasma cholinesterase
- Metoclopramide causes an increase in gastric emptying and pressure in the lower oesophageal sphincter through cholinergic receptors
- Clonidine is a centrally acting alpha-2 adrenergic receptor agonist
- Cisapride is similar to metoclopramide but does not have the antiemetic central antidopaminergic properties
- Morphine causes tonic contraction of bowel smooth muscle by a direct action on Mu receptors

36 (**a**) true (**b**) false (**c**) true (**d**) false (**e**) false

Isoflurane reduces myocardial contractility. It causes vasodilatation and hypotension, which may lead to a compensatory tachycardia. Intracranial pressure is increased due to an increase in cerebral blood flow. Peripheral blood flow is increased with the general vasodilatation. Skeletal and uterine muscles are relaxed.

Paper 5 Answers

37 (**a**) true (**b**) true (**c**) true (**d**) true (**e**) true

The volume of distribution is a measure of the total amount of drug in the body. It is calculated from a graph which plots the plasma drug concentration against time after an intravenous bolus. The plasma contains a concentration which reflects the water phase. For drugs that are lipid soluble this is a large water volume, far greater than the body weight – often in the region of 10–15 l/kg.

Drugs with a small volume of distribution have a rapid onset of action and are quickly cleared from the body. Those with a large volume of distribution may be slow in onset and are slowly cleared from the body.

The volume of distribution is affected by p*K*a, which reflects the amount of free drug, which in turn will affect binding to phospholipid and to plasma proteins.

38 (**a**) true (**b**) true (**c**) true (**d**) true (**e**) false

Inorganic fluoride is produced, in different amounts, by the metabolism of most of the fluorinated volatile anaesthetic agents.

Halothane and desflurane produce only very small amounts. Enflurane can produce 30 μmol/l after hours of use. Isoflurane produces <5 μmol/l with prolonged use and higher amounts after use for days in ITU.

39 (**a**) false (**b**) true (**c**) false (**d**) true (**e**) true

Desflurane is a methylethyl ether. The structure is very similar to that of isoflurane. The ether molecule gives stability; the fluoridation gives a non-irritant anaesthetic. It boils at 23°C, which means it has a high s.v.p. of 88 kPa. It has a blood/gas coefficient of 0.42, so it rapidly reaches equilibrium between alveolar gas and blood, giving rapid induction of anaesthesia. All volatile agents react with soda lime but the products are not usually toxic.

40 (**a**) false (**b**) false (**c**) true (**d**) false (**e**) true

The action of local anaesthetics is affected by the amount given, lipid solubility, the rate of elimination through metabolism or excretion and binding to receptor sites for the duration of action. These factors are related to molecular weight and the size of the molecule. It is the lipid-soluble, non-ionised local anaesthetic that passes through the nerve membrane. Local anaesthetics have a p*K*a of 7.5–9.0. The further the p*K*a is from the body pH of 7.4 the more ionised it will be in the body. They are presented as acid solutions at pH 5 to make them water soluble for injection. At the body pH of 7.4 more of the drug dissociates to produce more free base, which is lipid soluble. This lipid soluble form passes through the cell membrane to the interior of the axon. In the axon, the re-ionised form blocks the sodium channels from within. Acidosis increases the amount of ionised drug and therefore less unionised drug crosses the cell membrane, hence the reduced effect seen in inflamed tissues.

Duration of action is dependent on the binding to the sodium channels not to proteins. Toxicity is dependent on the dose, speed of injection, distribution and rate of elimination, not protein binding.

41 (**a**) false (**b**) false (**c**) true (**d**) false (**e**) false

A eutectic mixture is a mixture in which the melting point of each substance is lowered by being in the mixture. This happens with lidocaine and prilocaine. Other local anaesthetic mixtures are made to increase speed of onset and duration of action, but they are not necessarily eutectic mixtures. EMLA contain 2.5% lidocaine and 2.5% prilocaine. EMLA is used as a cream, relying on skin absorption which would be reduced by the presence of adrenaline.

Carbonated salts have been produced to try to improve the speed of onset of local anaesthetics. Once the local anaesthetic has passed through the cell membrane into the axon, the body pH causes release of carbon dioxide. This lowers the pH, which favours the formation of the ionised form that blocks the sodium channels.

42 (**a**) false (**b**) false (**c**) false (**d**) true (**e**) true

Pethidine was discovered by the Germans in the 1940s when looking for an anticholinergic drug. It acts at μ (mu) and κ (kappa) receptors and has atropine-like action. Some 90% is metabolised and one breakdown product is norpethidine, which is an analgesic, but it can also produce convulsions and hallucinations. As with all opioids the respiratory drive becomes less sensitive to carbon dioxide, requiring a higher $Pa\text{CO}_2$ to stimulate respiration. The level of CO_2 plateaus at a new level with a slower deeper tidal volume.

43 (**a**) false (**b**) true (**c**) true (**d**) true (**e**) false

Naloxone is related to oxymorphone. It is a competitive antagonist to opioid analgesics. It reverses the respiratory effect and the analgesic effect. It does not affect other types of analgesics or sedatives drugs. It does not reverse the effect of the partial agonist buprenorphine, which produces a respiratory depression that reaches a maximum effect that is not exceeded by higher doses. It reverses the agonist-antagonist pentazocine. Pentazocine acts at κ–kappa and sigma receptors but is an antagonist at the μ-mu receptor and so pentazocine can be used to antagonise the respiratory effects of morphine while keeping some analgesic effect. Dextropropoxyphene is a less potent form of methadone.

44 (**a**) true (**b**) true (**c**) true (**d**) true (**e**) false

Esterases exist in the plasma, red cells and other organs. When involved in drug metabolism it usually means that the drug is short acting. They are involved in the hydrolysis of acetylcholine at the neuromuscular junction: procaine in the tissues, suxamethonium in the plasma, up to 50% of atracurium is hydrolysed by esters in plasma and tissue fluids and esmolol is metabolised in the red cells and tissue fluid. Edrophonium binds to acetylcholinesterase.

45 (**a**) false (**b**) true (**c**) true (**d**) true (**e**) true

Atracurium is a biquaternary benzyl-isoquinolinium, pH 3.5, which is stable under refrigeration at 5°C for 2 years. Degradation is proportional to the temperature. Monoquaternary non-depolarising blockers at body pH are curare, vecuronium and rocuronium. The cis-isomer of atracurium is five times more potent with almost no histamine release.

46 (**a**) true (b) true (**c**) false (**d**) true (**e**) true

Obstructive jaundice is caused by erythromycin, sulphonylureas and testosterone.

Drugs that can cause jaundice due to impaired liver enzyme function include paracetamol, tricyclic antidepressants and NSAIDs.

Contraceptive drugs can cause enzyme derangement giving a hepatitis picture and also induce biliary cirrhosis.

Rifampicin induces liver enzymes and so accelerates the metabolism of oestrogens, corticosteroids, phenytoin, sulphonylureas and anticoagulants.

Drugs which can cause cholestasis include:

- oral contraceptives
- sensitivity reaction to phenothiazines – commonly chlorpromazine, erythromycin, sulphonamides, sulphonylureas, tricyclic antidepressants, penicillamine and gold
- dose-related cholestasis – complicates 17-alkylated steroid therapy

47 (**a**) false (**b**) true (**c**) true (**d**) false (**e**) false

Salbutamol is a beta$_2$-adrenergic agonist. It inhibits uterine contractions in premature labour. Beta-adrenergic agonists cause pulmonary vascular vasodilatation. Hypokalaemia has been reported after long usage. It may produce a tachycardia and so increases cardiac output.

Catecholamines tend to increase blood glucose levels.

48 (**a**) true (**b**) false (**c**) true (**d**) true (**e**) false

Antibiotics potentiate the non-depolarising muscle relaxants in two ways. Neomycin is an aminoglycoside antibiotic that impairs neuromuscular function producing a myasthenic-like condition if given in large doses.

Aminoglycercides and tetracycline reduce acetylcholine release from nerves. Neostigmine improves the abnormal neuromuscular function as it does in myasthenia gravis. Calcium will only have an effect if there is a deficiency. Polymyxins, lincomycin and clindomycin interfere with the action of the ion channels opened by acetylcholine on the postjunctional membrane. Enflurane produces more neuromuscular blockade and relaxation of skeletal muscle than most other volatile agents.

Other drugs that affect ion channels at other sites may affect the acetylcholine receptor-operated channels on the postjunctional membrane and potentiate neuromuscular blockers. These include local anaesthetics, quinidine and dispyramide-like antiarrythmics and calcium channel blockers.

Trimethoprim potentiates the effect of sulphonamides.

Non-depolarising muscle relaxants are potentiated by:

(a) Volatile agents by CNS depression and reduced muscle tone – dose dependent
(b) Aminoglycosides especially streptomycin and neomycin

(c) Local anaesthetics by
- decreased prejunctional ACh release
- stabilised postsynaptic membrane
- direct depolarising of skeletal muscle

(d) Antiarrhythmic – lidocaine, quinidine
(e) Diuretics – frusemide
(f) Magnesium, lithium, phenytoin, steroids, ciclosporins
(g) Hypothermia – slows enzymatic activity, decreases clearance
(h) Electrolyte disturbance
- Hypokalaemia, hyperkalaemia, hypocalcaemia

(i) Acid–base disturbance
- Acidosis, hypocapnia

49 (**a**) true (**b**) true (**c**) false (**d**) false (**e**) true

A neurotransmitter is any substance which is released from a presynaptic nerve ending and activates a receptor on the postsynaptic nerve or other cell receptor.

A drug which competes with a neurotransmitter will reduce its effect and act as an antagonist. Morphine and tramadol are agonists.

50 (**a**) true (**b**) true (**c**) true (**d**) true (**e**) true

Isomers (or chirality) are compounds that have the same molecular structure in the same order but their three-dimensional configurations are different due to rotation in different directions between bonds. Most drugs are racemic mixtures of two or more isomers. One isomer usually is more clinically active while the other is responsible for more of the side-effects.

Some drugs have been produced as the isomer. Isoflurane and enflurane are isomers, as are promazine and promethazine. Ropivacaine and etomidate are single isomers. Other specific isomers are L-hyoscine, L-bupivaine, D-tubocurare, (*S*+)-ketamine, D-ketoprofen and *cis*-atracurium.

There are a number of ways of defining isomers.

Some molecules are mirror images of each other and deflect light to the left or to the right. These take the Latin terms dextro (+, d or D), or laevo (–, L or l). The configuration of the chiral centre is also described by the Latin rectus right (*R*–) and sinister left (S+) depending on whether the atoms are arranged clockwise or anticlockwise.

Cis and *trans* describe whether the atoms are on the same side (*cis*) of a double bond or on different sides (*trans*).

51 (**a**) true (**b**) false (**c**) true (**d**) true (**e**) false

Adenylate cyclase is an enzyme on the inner surface of the cell membrane. It is activated by surface receptors. This process is modulated by neurotransmitters and hormones through guanine nucleotide regulatory protein (Gs and Gi proteins). Adenyl cyclase potentiates the conversion of adenosine triphosphate (ATP) to the second messenger cAMP.

The other important enzyme to produce a second messenger is phosphodiesterase, acting on phosphatidylinositol. Membrane phosphodiesterase converts phosphatidylinositol to give inositol triphosphate, which opens calcium channels, and diacylglycerol, which stimulates membrane protein kinase to control calcium, potassium and chloride channels.

Beta-receptors are linked to adenyl cyclase. Aminophylline is a phosphodiesterase inhibitor that increases levels of cAMP.

52 (**a**) true (**b**) true (**c**) true (**d**) true (**e**) true

The hepatic artery has α and β adrenergic receptors while the portal vein only has α receptors. Propranolol is a β-antagonist and a smooth muscle relaxant used in systemic and portal hypertension.

Splanchnic blood flow is increased by dopexamine, which is used to improve mesenteric blood flow, and glucagon, which vasodilates to increase hepatic blood flow.

Vasopressin is a vasoconstrictor due to a direct effect on smooth muscle. Somatostatin has been used to constrict oesophageal varices.

Splanchnic blood flow is reduced with exercise, hypocapnia, volatile anaesthetic agents, intravenous induction agents and catecholamines.

53 (**a**) true (**b**) true (**c**) false (**d**) true (**e**) false

Aprotinin is a proteolytic enzyme inhibitor. It blocks the formation of plasmin from plasminogen. Plasmin clears fibrin and fibrinogen from the blood. It inhibits kallikreins, which are produced by the conversion of kininogens to kinins and renin from pro-renin. It blocks trypsin, an endopeptidase which breaks peptide links to form dipeptides and other small chains that can be absorbed through the intestinal wall.

Its main use is as an antifibrinolytic and haemostatic agent.

54 (**a**) true (**b**) true (**c**) true (**d**) false (**e**) false

The mechanisms of action of insulin are initiated through binding to cell membrane insulin receptors in muscle, liver and adipose tissue. This stimulates a cascade of events which is dependent on the synthesis and transfer of the glucose transport protein GLUT 4 to the cell membrane. GLUT 4 is an insulin-responsive transporter located in adipose, skeletal and cardiac muscle. Insulin is metabolised by the liver insulinase, this causes a first-pass effect.

The plasma half-life of insulin is 4–6 min with a clearance of 8–18 ml/min per kg.

The actions of insulin promote the uptake of glucose into cells. This leads to the synthesis of glycogen, protein and fat. With the uptake of glucose, potassium moves into the cell. Insulin inhibits the breakdown of glycogen, fat and protein.

55 (**a**) true (**b**) true (**c**) true (**d**) false (**e**) true

Non-steroidal anti-inflammatory drugs inhibit cyclo-oxygenase, which normally facilitates the conversion of arachidonic acid to prostaglandin. They cause a reduced production of prostaglandin, prostacyclin and thromboxane. The prostaglandin sensitises the nociceptors to reduce their threshold for firing to a painful stimulus.

Most effects are due to this reduced prostaglandin: in the gastric mucosa to give peptic ulceration; in the renal vasculature leading to vasoconstriction; in the lung leading to bronchospasm. Clotting is impaired and platelet aggregation is reduced. Other side-effects include derangement of liver enzymes and diarrhoea.

56 (**a**) true (**b**) false (**c**) false (**d**) true (**e**) true

Heparin is a mucopolysaccharide (a glycosaminoglycan) which binds to amines and protein. It is stored in secretory granules within mast cells. It acts as an antithrombotic agent by the binding ATIII to a pentasaccharide sequence on the heparin. This complex then inhibits factor Xa and thrombin as well as other parts of the intrinsic coagulation pathway. Heparin in larger doses inhibits clot-bound thrombin, which may be important in extracorporeal circulation. The external pathway is also inhibited as heparin promotes the release of tissue factor pathway inhibitor. Unfractionated heparin may inhibit or activate platelets, affect endothelial function or vessel wall permeability. It may also potentiate the inhibition of fibrinolysis by plasminogen activator inhibitor I.

Molecules up to 600 Da molecular weight, depending on their lipid solubility, will pass to the placenta. Heparin preparations: low-molecular-weight starts at 2000 Da and other forms are up to a molecular weight of 40 000 Da.

Side-effects include bleeding and thrombocytopenia. It inhibits aldosterone, leading to a loss of sodium and retention of potassium, osteoporosis and hypersensitivity.

57 (**a**) false (**b**) true (**c**) true (**d**) false (**e**) true

Omeprazole is a proton pump inhibitor that reduces gastric acid production but it is irreversible. It is a pro-drug which acts for 24 h. It is a weak base (p*K*a 4). It ionises in the parietal cells where it is trapped. The proton pump is a H^+/K^+-ATPase enzyme. Gastric acid converts the drug to a non-absorbable protonated form, so it is given as an enteric-coated tablet to be absorbed in the small intestine. As the gastric acid is reduced, less is affected by gastric acid and so more is available to be absorbed. It has a short half-life of 60 min in dogs but a long duration of action, and the acid-inhibiting effects increase with repeated dosing. It is a very safe drug with a therapeutic index of 1000. Side-effects include liver enzyme and haematological derangement.

Once the maximum inhibitory effect is reached, on 30 mg after 3 days, raising the dose has no more effect. The plasma level does not relate to the effect on gastric acid secretion. Side-effects include increased secretion of gastrin.

It is eliminated by cytochrome P450 in the liver. This is a part of the cytochrome oxidase system which might be expected to give drug interactions but these are rare. A slight reduction in the metabolism of diazepam, phenytoin and *R*-warfarin are seen in in vivo studies. Profound acid suppression may reduce the absorption of iron, ketoconazole and ampicillin esters. It crosses the blood–brain barrier.

58 (**a**) true (**b**) true (**c**) false (**d**) true (**e**) true

Central administration of a short-acting drug is indicated if the effect is on the myocardium and titration of the dose to effect is important as a bolus or for a continuous infusion. Digoxin is a drug of slow onset and long duration of action so there is no indication for intravenous administration, which may precipitate arrhythmias.

Phenytoin is used as an anticonvulsant or as an antiarrhythmic. It is an alkaline solution which is irritant and so should be given slowly through a central line over 1 h with ECG monitoring.

59 (**a**) false (**b**) true (**c**) false (**d**) false (**e**) false

Intraocular pressure (IOP) is 1.3–2 kPa

Methohexitone is a short-acting barbiturate for induction of anaesthesia. It produces global depression of the CNS but may cause hyperexcitable phenomena and convulsions. All intravenous induction drugs reduce IOP.

Suxamethonium may increase the pressure during the fasciculation phase.

Ecothiopate is an organophosphorus compound used to reduce plasma cholinesterase and reduce IOP in glaucoma.

Atracurium and all non-depolarising muscle relaxants reduce IOP. All volatile agents reduce IOP. Atropine, if given as drops in glaucoma-prone eyes, increases IOP.

Acetazolomide inhibits carbonic anhydrase which leads to a reduction in the amount of aqueous humour produced in the eye to relieve glaucoma.

60 (**a**) false (**b**) false (**c**) true (**d**) false (**e**) true

Benzylpenicillin or penicillin G is used for Gram-positive cocci; it is particularly used in meningococcal disease (as it crosses the blood–brain barrier), gas gangrene and tetanus.

It is a beta-lactam and acts on the cell wall to inhibit synthesis.

In recent years resistance has developed, particularly due to inactivation by bacterial beta-lactamase.

61 (**a**) true (**b**) true (**c**) false (**d**) true (**e**) false

The Mapleson E system performs in a similar way to the Mapleson D, but because there are no valves and there is very little resistance to breathing it has proved very suitable for use with children. It was originally introduced in 1937 by P. Ayre and is known as the Ayre's T piece. The version most commonly used is the Jackson-Rees modification which has an open bag (not a closed bag) attached to the expiratory limb (classified as a Mapleson F system although it was not included in the original description by Professor Mapleson). Movement of the bag can be seen during spontaneous breathing, and the bag can be compressed to provide manual ventilation. As in the Bain circuit, the bag may be replaced by a mechanical ventilator designed for use with children. The volume of the tubing should be at least the tidal volume to prevent rebreathing. This system is suitable for children under 20 kg. Fresh gas flows of 2–3 times minute volume should be used to prevent rebreathing during spontaneous ventilation, with a minimum flow of 3 l/min, e.g. a 4-year-old child weighing 20 kg has a normal minute volume of 3 l/min and would require a fresh gas flow of 6–9 l/min. During controlled ventilation in children normocapnia can be maintained with a fresh gas flow of 1000 ml + 100 ml/kg. e.g. a 4-year-old weighing 20 kg would need a total fresh gas flow of around 3 l/min.

62 (**a**) true (**b**) false (**c**) true (**d**) false (**e**) true

The causes of fires are combustible material, such as plastic, and a source of fire, such as sparks from static electricity.

The build up of static charge is reduced by having an electrically conductive theatre floor. Too low a resistance increases the risk of electrocution while too high a resistance will allow static charges to build up. Resistance between two electrodes 60 cm apart should be over 20 000 Ω and less than 5 000 000 Ω.

Battery-operated equipment and transformers reduce the risk of electrocution.

Mains electricity switches are the potential source of sparks. In 1956 a group suggested that the fire risk extends to a height of 1.4 m and a distance of 1.2 m from any anaesthetic apparatus. Since that time these distances have been reduced to 40 cm high and 25 cm from anaesthetic apparatus.

63 (**a**) true (**b**) true (**c**) false (**d**) false (**e**) true

An earth fault detector or a current-operated earth leakage circuit breaker consists of the live and the neutral wires wound around a core of a transformer with exactly the same number of turns. A third winding is connected to the coil of a relay, which operates the circuit breaker. When the currents in the live and in neutral wires are the same and there is no earth leak the magnetic fields induced in each winding will cancel each other out. If current is leaking to earth then the current in the live wire will not be equal to the current in the neutral and the magnetic fields will not be equal. This will create a magnetic field in the third winding, which will trip the relay and break the circuit. The device is sensitive to a current difference as little as 30 mA and cuts the current within 0.03 s.

An earth fault detector is affected by A.C. current, not static. It does not detect a broken earth, only a difference between the current in the live and neutral wires. The leak current may be taking another path, not necessarily the earth wire. It detects a leakage current of 30 mA; so it is not strictly true to say an excessive leakage current, as it is sensitive to very small currents.

64 (**a**) false (**b**) false (**c**) true (**d**) true (**e**) true

The Seebeck effect is the principle behind the thermocouple, where two dissimilar metals produce a voltage where they are joined.

The thermistor resistance increases exponentially as temperature falls, not in a linear fashion.

Calibration changes with severe changes in temperature.

Hysteresis means a lag between the change and the effect in the device. The response time of the thermistor is very short.

The temperature coefficient of resistance is the degree by which the temperature depends on the resistance. If the resistance increases with temperature it is positive, due to the thermal vibrations impeding electron flow. If the resistance falls with temperature then the coefficient is negative. This occurs in pure semiconductors such as the thermistor, due to thermal vibration producing a greatly increasing number of charged carriers.

65 (**a**) false (**b**) false (**c**) false (**d**) true (**e**) true

The length of the Bain tubing adds resistance to the expiratory limb. It is a limited fresh gas flow that leads to rebreathing and hypercarbia. Increased dead space may lead to the rebreathing of carbon dioxide.

Low fresh gas flows in a circle do not lead to hypercarbia if the soda lime is effective.

Lack of unidirectional valves and functioning soda lime will lead to an accumulation of carbon dioxide in the circle.

An increased expiratory time will reduce the time for inspiration, which may reduce tidal volume, slow rate and reduce tidal volume. If these fall below a critical level there will be hypercarbia.

66 (**a**) false (**b**) true (**c**) false (**d**) true (**e**) false

Table 5.66 Pin index safety system

Gas	Pin index
Air	1 and 5
Oxygen	2 and 5
N_2O	3 and 5
CO_2	1 and 6
Entonox	3
He-O_2 (less than 80%)	2 and 4
He-O_2 (more than 80%)	4 and 6

67 (**a**) false (**b**) true (**c**) true (**d**) true (**e**) false

Types of blood filters include

(a) Screen filters
- Function as sieves
- Usually constructed from a woven mesh
- Have a regular pore size (40 μm)
- Less damage to the red cells
- Efficacy increases progressively with each unit of blood passed as the pore size tends to decrease progressively down to 20 μm

(b) Depth filters
- The mechanism of action is by adsorption of unwanted material down to a size of about 10 μm
- Synthetic Dacron
- The adsorption is probably due to electrical charge differences between the particles and the fibres

- Efficacy decreases with each unit of blood probably due to channelling in the pack of fibres

(c) Leukocyte filter

- Used to prevent the contamination of the components with the white cells, if filtered during collection process or before storage
- The individual component is filtered before being administered to the patient to avoid non-haemolytic febrile transfusion reactions, the refractoriness or the alloimmunisation with HLA antigens, transmission of leukocyte-associated disease such as cytomegalovirus, or graft-versus-host disease

Features

- Mechanical and adhesive filtration principle
- Biocompatible
- The percentage of recovery is almost 95% for the red cells and platelets
- Saline priming is not required
- Both bedside and the laboratory varieties are available
- Tubes are compatible with the sterile connecting device
- The filters are gamma-ray sterilised

68 **(a)** false **(b)** false **(c)** true **(d)** false **(e)** false

Laser stands for Light amplification by stimulated emission of radiation.

Types of laser

(a) **Carbon dioxide laser**

- Light wavelength: far infrared (10 600 nm)
- Laser beam is absorbed within 0.1–0.2 mm of the tissue

(b) **Nd-YAG laser** (neodymium-yttrium aluminium garnet laser)

- Light wavelength: near infrared (1064 nm)
- Laser beam is absorbed within 2–6 mm of the tissue

(c) **Argon laser**

- Light wavelength: blue/green (500 nm)
- Laser beam is absorbed within 0.5–2 mm of the tissue

Properties of the laser beam

- Monochromatic – all waves are of the same *wavelength*
- Coherence – all waves are in *phase* in both time and space
- Collimated – all waves are travelling in a *parallel* direction

Problems of using lasers

(a) To the staff
- The main danger is to the eyes especially with Nd-YAG laser

(b) To the patient
- Airway: risk of fire and explosion in the airway following ignition of PVC tracheal tube and anaesthetic gases or by the laser
- Burns
- Eye: irreversible retinal damage

Safety precautions

The following must be taken in the operating theatre when using lasers:

(a) Low inspired oxygen concentrations
- Nitrogen, air, or helium should be used to reduce the oxygen concentration to the lowest level that will provide satisfactory patient oxygenation (because some tubes which ignite at high oxygen concentrations are safer at low concentration)
- Nitrous oxide supports combustion and should not be used as the diluent gas

(b) Limiting laser power density and duration: laser should always be kept in stand-by mode except when ready to use

(c) Filling the cuff with water or saline
- The cuff is not laser resistant; if a beam penetrates an air-filled cuff, airway gas can leak into the operative field and if the O_2 or NO_2 content is high this increases the risk of fire
- Fluid in a cuff acts as a heat sink, which prevents heat build-up and makes the cuff less likely to perforate

(d) Use a technique not requiring intubation

(e) Use of protective wrappings

(f) Use of special burn-resistant tubes

69 **(a)** false **(b)** true **(c)** true **(d)** false **(e)** false

The following are useful to remember:

- Voltage = current × resistance ($V = IR$)
- Charge = capacitance × voltage ($Q = CV$)
- Energy (joules) = (charge × voltage)/2 ($E = 0.5QV$)
- **Therefore, $E = 0.5CV^2$**
- Power (watts) = voltage × current ($P = VI$)

- Also, power (watts) = energy/time (J/s) ($P = E/t$)
- Current = charge per secound ($I = Q/t$)

Therefore

- **Power (watts) = voltage × charge per secound ($P = VQ/t$)**

This shows how the voltage and charge are important

A typical profile is 2500 V to produce 50 A into 50 Ω over 4 ms, with a charge of 80 μF. So, remembering $E = 0.5CV^2$

$$E = 0.5 \times 80 \times 10^{-6} \times 2500^2$$
$$= 250\ J.$$

When the defibrillator discharges the inductor absorbs some energy and energy is lost into the chest wall, particularly in obese and muscular people. If a lot of energy is lost, burning would occur so a good electrical contact with the skin is essential.

AC current is not used.

The maximum energy starts with 200 J followed by 360 J in an adult.

70 (**a**) false (**b**) false (**c**) false (**d**) false (**e**) true

Audible sound waves are in the region up to 20 kHz. Ultrasound frequencies are much higher at 2–7 MHz. Ultrasound is not audible to the human ear. The structures are visualised by passing a beam of ultrasound through the tissues. When the beam meets an interface some of the waves are reflected back to the detectors. It is these reflections that are computed to build up a picture of the tissues. Doppler shift is used to detect and show movement. Structures are shown by the sound wave being reflected back onto the detector.

Ultrasound is poorly transmitted through air and bone. It is well transmitted through water and most body tissues including muscle, intra-abdominal and intra-thoracic organs, but not the lungs containing air.

The frequency is higher so the wavelength is shorter.

71 (**a**) true (**b**) true (**c**) true (**d**) true (**e**) true

Different parts of the equipment should function at similar voltage, current and frequency.

72 (**a**) false (**b**) true (**c**) false (**d**) false (**e**) false

A step-down transformer steps the voltage down from a high voltage to a low voltage. The number of turns on the secondary coil is less than the number on the primary coil so the output voltage is smaller than the input voltage. In an ideal transformer the power out is the same as the power in. In reality, the power out is slightly less, due to heat loss.

73 (**a**) true (**b**) true (**c**) true (**d**) false (**e**) true

The cell membrane has a positive charge of about 90 mV on the exterior, compared to the interior. Much of this potential is absorbed as it passes through the tissues and the ECG signal only detects 1000 μV to 2 mV at the skin and not the initial 90 mV of the potential. The signal is increased due to the large bulk of muscle contracting at one time. The waveform is complicated with frequencies of 1–100 Hz.

The EMG detects a range of voltages from muscle of 10 μV to 100 μV, but of short duration, 5–10 ms. Frequencies 1–>1000 Hz.

The EEG potentials are smaller at 1–50 μV. The waves are called, from lowest frequency, delta, theta, alpha, beta. The frequencies range from 1 to 50 Hz.

When two waves interact interference occurs. Interference is least when one of the waves is of a relatively low voltage.

74 (**a**) true (**b**) false (**c**) false (**d**) true (**e**) false

French gauge sizes are used for urinary catheters and nasogastric tubes. The size is the circumference in millimetres.

SWG or wire gauge is used for cannulae and needles. The smaller the diameter the larger the number, so 21 gauge has a larger diameter than 23 gauge.

A 14-gauge cannula allows flow of 270 ml/min, or 1.3 l in 5 min. (This is a difficult one to be certain of the answer as the question specifies maximum flow and a short cannula. It will allow much more than 1 litre so we have marked the answer false.)

The size of endotracheal tubes is the internal diameter. The thickness of the wall increases as the diameter increases. Different manufacturers make tubes of different thickness.

The standard connector sizes are 15 mm for male and 22 mm for female and 30 mm for scavenging.

Table 5.74 Gauges and flow rates

Gauge of cannula	Flow rate (ml/min)
18	80
17	125
16	180
14	270

75 (**a**) true (**b**) true (**c**) false (**d**) true (**e**) false

The use of a condenser–humidifier will conserve expired water loss and enable inspired air to be warmer and moister than dry anaesthetic gases.

The soda lime reaction with carbon dioxide is exothermic. It generates heat by its reaction with carbon dioxide, but it is likely that heat is lost by the time it reaches the patient due to the low thermal capacity of air.

Laminar flow air conditioning will lead to cooling and volatile cleaning agents will evaporate, taking some of their heat of vaporisation from the patient.

76 (**a**) true (**b**) true (**c**) true (**d**) true (**e**) true

Computers have two forms of memory: random access memory (RAM) and read only memory (ROM). RAM changes as the computer is used and is lost when it is switched off. This is known as volatile memory. ROM retains its contents, which cannot be easily changed and is known as non-volatile memory.

Computers use the binary systems of 0 or 1 for storing data. Each binary digit is known as a bit. Eight binary bits are put together to form a byte, which represents an alphanumeric character. The decimal system has ten values from 0 to 9.

77 (**a**) true (**b**) false (**c**) false (**d**) true (**e**) false

Cylinders are made of molybdenum steel or chromium steel, which are high-strength alloys. Aluminium cylinders are an alternative lighter weight.

The plastic disc round the neck has a specific colour and four straight sides. The colour and shape denote the year of the last test. On the disc is stamped the year of the last test and a hole is punched into one of the four segments to say which quarter of the year the test took place in. Tests are made every 5 years.

Cylinders are filled to a ratio of the weight of gas in the cylinder to the weight of water the cylinder could hold. In the UK the ratio is 0.75 or 75%. In tropical climates the ratio is reduced to 0.67. The problems of expansion with temperature are a particular concern for gases such as carbon dioxide (critical temperature 31°C) and nitrous oxide (critical temperature 36.5°C) which are liquid at room temperatures below their critical temperatures. Cylinders containing a gas are filled to pressures of 43.5 atm (N_2O) and 49.2 atm (CO_2) whereas cylinders filled with a gas mix of O_2 and Entonox are filled at a pressure of 134.7 atm.

Gas-filled cylinders are filled to a pressure of 137 bar but are tested to tolerate 200–250 bar. This is an extra 60%–70% over the filled pressure. The thread connections on the large bull-nosed cylinders are gas specific, just as the pin index system is gas specific for smaller cylinders.

78 (**a**) false (**b**) true (**c**) false (**d**) false (**e**) true

Nuclei within atoms are charged and so act as if they were a small magnet.

The MRI unit creates a large external magnetic field, which lines up these nuclei. A short pulse of another magnetic field at right angles to the first is then applied. This pulse changes the direction in which the nuclei are spinning and the resulting magnetic field is measured and used to form an image of the body.

The commonest element used for imaging the body is hydrogen, which is a common ion in the body, in water and so in all organs. Hydrogen has a strong response to a magnetic field.

The magnets are 0.1–4 tesla. It may be said that the atoms line up. In reality they spin, like tops, about an axis.

Electromagnetics are used. The coils of the magnetic resonance unit are cooled by immersion in liquid helium. Liquid helium is expensive so liquid nitrogen is used to slow the rate at which helium boils by lowering the environmental temperature.

The strong magnetic fields will attract any ferrous material, and may induce currents in metallic objects which will heat them up. No metallic object should come near a MRI scanner, especially iron-based objects.

79 (**a**) false (**b**) true (**c**) false (**d**) false (**e**) true

An amplifier is a device for increasing a signal. The ratio of the output to the input voltage is known as the gain. The simplest amplifier increases all signals, which would mean that the mains signal would over-ride the weaker ECG signal. One solution is the differential amplifier. The commonest form of amplifier is a transistor made of a semiconductor sandwich. They have three wires, each connected to a different layer. The layers or terminals are called collector, base and emitter. In operation a small change in the base current produces a large change in the collector current.

A differential amplifier measures the difference between the potential from two sources. In the latter case any interference that is common to both sources, such as mains frequency, is reduced. This ability to ignore interference is essential when the signal is small or weak as in the ECG or EEG signals.

A transducer changes one form of energy to another.

Interference may be a problem when the initial signal is weak. A form of interference will occur if the amplifier is made from a semiconductor, which is affected by temperature. This is known as drift.

80 (**a**) false (**b**) true (**c**) false (**d**) true (**e**) true

In laminar flow the flow at the centre is twice the mean flow. Flow at the periphery falls to virtually zero where the fluid contacts the wall.

Laminar flow is proportional to the fourth power of the radius or varies by a factor of 16. So if the diameter is halved the flow will fall by a factor of 16. The flow is inversely proportional to length. Flow is proportional to the pressure change and inversely related to resistance. Resistance is proportional to viscosity times length divided by radius for laminar flow and proportional to density divided by radius for turbulent flow.

81 (**a**) true (**b**) true (**c**) true (**d**) false (**e**) true

When a study is undertaken it is necessary to define whether the population studied is representative of the whole population. The confidence intervals are a measure of the difference between the group studied and the whole population. They are of value in assessing the importance of a difference. A statistic may be reported as a significant result but the actual difference may be so small as to mean it has little clinical relevance.

It is usual practice in medicine to use 95% confidence intervals. Confidence intervals are large or wide if the size of the sample is small or the standard deviation is large.

82 (**a**) false (**b**) true (**c**) false (**d**) true (**e**) true

Categorical variables are results such as Yes/No, sometimes referred to as non-parametric data as compared to parametric or numerical data.

The statistical tests for nominal data are chi-squared and Fisher's exact test. For ordinal data rank order, tests such as Spearman's and Mann Whitney are used.

83 (**a**) true (**b**) false (**c**) true (**d**) true (**e**) false

Cardiac output assessment must be made with a steady injection into the right atrium. In the past cold solutions were used but solutions at room temperature are used now. Cardiac output varies slightly with respiration and the changes in intrathoracic pressure. The temperature of the air in the oesophagus may affect the measurements. Tricuspid incompetence allows blood, and with it dye, to back flow into the right atrium from the right ventricle during systole. Atrial fibrillation does not affect the measurements.

84 (**a**) true (**b**) true (**c**) false (**d**) true (**e**) false

Specific heat capacity is the amount of heat required to raise the temperature of unit mass by 1 K or units of joules/kg per K.

Heat capacity is the heat required to raise the temperature of a mass by 1 K or joules/K.

Latent heat is the amount of heat required to change a substance from one form to another without a change in temperature, e.g. water to ice at 0°C or water to steam at 100°C.

Gases have very low heat capacity. Metals, and copper in particular, have a high specific heat or heat capacity.

85 (**a**) true (**b**) true (**c**) true (**d**) false (**e**) false

Electrical burns occur when there is a high current density, or a fault with the connection between the skin and the negative electrode plate. Any leakage current may lead to a burn.

The ECG and defibrillator are protected from current passing back through the wires. This is the meaning of the symbol of a heart with two pad symbols on either side.

86 (**a**) true (**b**) false (**c**) true (**d**) true (**e**) true

Humidity can be assessed from tables knowing the room temperature and the dew point, which is the temperature at which the air is fully saturated.

The mass spectrometer will measure the amount of water vapour in air but it needs to be calibrated. A simple means of measuring humidity is by the shortening of biological tissue, for instance a hair, as it dries.

87 (**a**) false (**b**) false (**c**) true (**d**) false (**e**) false

A constant-pressure ventilator generates a pressure in the physiological range up to about 25 cmH_2O. The tidal volume is a function of time and pressure during inspiration. A leak is only compensated for if the ventilator is pressure cycled and it allows a longer time to reach the cycling pressure. If it is time cycled the tidal volume will be reduced due to the volume lost by the leak. The tidal volume will be affected by changes in airway pressure. Compliance varies with the size of the lung.

The peak inspiratory pressure is fixed in a constant-pressure ventilator so it does not indicate airway resistance. Tidal volume is an indirect measure of resistance, as it will be reduced when airway resistance increases.

88 (**a**) true (**b**) false (**c**) false (**d**) false (**e**) false

The Doppler effect is the change in wavelength in sound waves when they are reflected off a moving surface. If the surface is moving towards the source of the waves then the reflected waves have a shorter wavelength and vice versa. Hence a train coming towards the observer makes an increasingly high-pitched noise but as it goes away the pitch falls.

89 (**a**) true (**b**) true (**c**) true (**d**) true (**e**) true

The Venturi principle is based on the concept of a system having a constant energy. Gas flow has two energies: kinetic or flow energy and potential or pressure energy. When the gas flow comes to a constriction the flow increases and the pressure decreases. If that pressure decrease beyond the constriction is negative then air is sucked into the stream. The constriction orifice is fixed so the entrainment ratio is the same whatever the flow of oxygen. The total flow of oxygen and air mix into the mask should be equal to or above the peak inspiratory flow rate to ensure that only the oxygen mixture from the mask is inspired to give the prescribed percentage of oxygen. Less than the peak inspiratory flow rate will mean air is drawn into the mask.

The side holes are for expired gas to escape through. Plugging them will mean the expired gas and the Venturi oxygen will mix in the mask. If the diameter of the Venturi is increased the flow rate will not increase as much and so the pressure drop will be less and so less air will be entrained resulting in a higher oxygen concentration.

90 (**a**) false (**b**) false (**c**) true (**d**) true (**e**) false

Paramagnetic gases are those that are attracted into a magnetic field. In clinical practice there are two, oxygen and nitric oxide.

The paramagnetic analyser for oxygen needs calibration. The advantages are a rapid response, accuracy, there is no interference from other gases, and it has a long life. The main disadvantage is the initial cost.

MCQ answers primary paper 5

	(a)	(b)	(c)	(d)	(e)
1	F	T	T	T	F
2	F	T	F	T	F
3	T	F	T	T	T
4	F	F	F	F	T
5	T	T	F	F	T
6	T	T	F	T	T
7	T	T	T	F	T
8	T	F	F	F	T
9	F	F	T	T	F
10	F	T	T	T	T
11	T	T	T	F	F
12	T	F	F	T	F
13	T	F	F	F	F
14	T	F	F	F	T
15	T	T	F	F	T
16	F	F	F	F	T
17	T	T	T	T	F
18	F	F	T	T	T
19	T	T	T	T	F
20	F	T	T	T	F
21	F	T	T	T	F
22	T	T	F	T	F
23	F	F	T	F	T
24	T	F	T	T	F
25	T	T	F	F	F
26	F	F	F	T	T
27	F	F	T	F	T
28	T	F	F	F	T
29	T	F	F	T	F

	(a)	(b)	(c)	(d)	(e)
30	F	T	T	T	T
31	T	F	T	F	F
32	F	F	T	F	F
33	T	T	T	T	T
34	T	F	F	T	T
35	T	T	F	F	F
36	T	F	T	F	F
37	T	T	T	T	T
38	T	T	T	T	F
39	F	T	F	T	T
40	F	F	T	F	T
41	F	F	T	F	F
42	F	F	F	T	T
43	F	T	T	T	F
44	T	T	T	T	F
45	F	T	T	T	T
46	T	T	F	T	T
47	F	T	T	F	F
48	T	F	T	T	F
49	T	T	F	F	T
50	T	T	T	T	T
51	T	F	T	T	F
52	T	T	T	T	T
53	T	T	F	T	F
54	T	T	T	F	F
55	T	T	T	F	T
56	T	F	F	T	T
57	F	T	T	F	T
58	T	T	F	T	T
59	F	T	F	F	F
60	F	F	T	F	T

	(a)	(b)	(c)	(d)	(e)
61	T	T	F	T	F
62	T	F	T	F	T
63	T	T	F	F	T
64	F	F	T	T	T
65	F	F	F	T	T
66	F	T	F	T	F
67	F	T	T	T	F
68	F	F	T	F	F
69	F	T	T	F	F
70	F	F	F	F	T
71	T	T	T	T	T
72	F	T	F	F	F
73	T	T	T	F	T
74	T	F	F	T	F
75	T	T	F	T	F
76	T	T	T	T	T
77	T	F	F	T	F
78	F	T	F	F	T
79	F	T	F	F	T
80	F	T	F	T	T
81	T	T	T	F	T
82	F	T	F	T	T
83	T	F	T	T	F
84	T	T	F	T	F
85	T	T	T	F	F
86	T	F	T	T	T
87	F	F	T	F	F
88	T	F	F	F	F
89	T	T	T	T	T
90	F	F	T	T	F

Paper 6 Answers

1 (**a**) false (**b**) false (**c**) true (**d**) true (**e**) true

Hyperventilation will reduce the $PaCO_2$ but it will not lead to a 50% reduction with twice the minute ventilation.

Hyperventilation reduces sympathetic activity and hence reduces cardiac output and systolic blood pressure. Cerebral blood flow increases by 2%–4% for every 1 mmHg or 0.13 kPa increase in $PaCO_2$. Other effects of a reduced carbon dioxide tension include a reduction in awareness and eventually a form of anaesthesia, a shift of the oxygen dissociation curve to the left and a respiratory alkalosis.

2 (**a**) true (**b**) true (**c**) true (**d**) false (**e**) true

Interruption of the cervical sympathetic chain causes Horner's syndrome of miosis, ptosis, enophthalmos and anhidrosis. Nasal stuffiness also occurs due to an excess of sympathetic activity but this was not described as part of the syndrome.

3 (**a**) false (**b**) false (**c**) true (**d**) false (**e**) true

The hypothalamus directly controls the posterior pituitary. It controls the anterior pituitary through releasing or inhibitory factors.

The hypothalamus synthesises and secretes ADH and oxytocin, which it releases through the posterior pituitary gland. Acetylcholine increases release and noradrenaline inhibits release.

The anterior pituitary granular secretory cells are either acidophils, producing prolactin and somatotropin, or basophils, producing the trophic glycoproteins ACTH, TSH, LH and FSH and beta-lipotrophin (LPH). The anterior pituitary neurones are postganglionic sympathetic nerves.

- From the basophils:
  - TSH (thyrotrophin) is a glycoprotein acting on the thyroid gland

    - ACTH (adrenocorticotrophin) is a 39-amino-acid polypeptide acting on the adrenal cortex
    - Growth hormone is a 191-amino-acid polypeptide controlled by somatotrophin releasing factor
- From the acidophils
    - Prolactin is a polypeptide promoting milk production

4 (**a**) false (**b**) true (**c**) false (**d**) false (**e**) false

Absorption is from the proximal small intestine involving an active carrier mechanism promoted by vitamin D and parathyroid hormone. Vitamin D acts on bone, kidneys and the small intestine to raise plasma calcium levels.

Parathyroid hormone acts to raise plasma calcium levels by bone resorption and to reduce renal tubular loss of calcium in the distal tubules and collecting ducts. Calcitonin reduces plasma calcium by increasing renal excretion, inhibiting bone reabsorption and inhibiting jejunal reabsorption.

Deficiencies of vitamin D and cholecalciferol will lead to poor calcium absorption.

The fat-soluble vitamins are A, D, E and K.

5 (**a**) false (**b**) true (**c**) false (**d**) true (**e**) false

The diaphragm is the main muscle of inspiration, innervated by the phrenic nerve. The phrenic nerve includes nerve roots from C 3, 4 and 5. In the past a unilateral phrenic nerve crush was performed to rest a lung with tuberculosis. Loss of one diaphragm will reduce vital capacity but does not reduce minute ventilation.

6 (**a**) true (**b**) true (**c**) false (**d**) false (**e**) false

CSF is formed by secretory cells in the choroid plexus as an ultrafiltrate of plasma with secretion of specific ions such as glucose by facilitated transport.

Reabsorption is into the venous blood through the arachnoid villi in the dural sacs of the sagittal and sigmoid sinuses. The CSF is carried across the endothelium by pinocytosis. The rate of production is dependent on CSF pressure. CSF is produced at 20–30 ml/h. There is 70 ml in the spinal canal and 70 ml within the skull with 40 ml in the ventricles.

7 (**a**) true (**b**) false (**c**) true (**d**) false (**e**) true

The A–a gradient is normally increased with age and with an increase in the inspired oxygen tension. It will increase with diseases that thicken the alveolar capillary membrane such as pulmonary oedema, infection and increases in shunt due to hypotension or hypoventilation.

8 (**a**) true (**b**) false (**c**) false (**d**) false (**e**) true

Arterialised blood flows in the umbilical vein through the ductus venosus to bypass the liver and enter the right atrium. Most of this blood then bypasses the lung by passing through the foramen ovale to the left atrium and then to the aorta and brain.

Deoxygenated blood from the brain also enters the right atrium but passes into the pulmonary artery. From here it bypasses the left side of the heart by passing via the ductus arteriosus into the aorta but beyond the carotid arteries and so most of the better oxygenated blood from the inferior vena cava (IVC) flows to the brain. Some of the blood from the SVC will also pass this way.

Blood flows back to the placenta through two umbilical arteries which are branches of the internal iliac arteries.

9 (**a**) true (**b**) true (**c**) true (**d**) true (**e**) true

- Glomerular filtration rate is related to the surface area, permeability and the net filtration pressure $= P_{GC} - P_{BS} - \pi_{GC}$, where P_{GC} is glomerular capillary hydrostatic pressure, P_{BS} is Bowman's capsule hydrostatic pressure and π_{GC} is glomerular oncotic pressure
- Obstruction to urine flow increases the Bowman's capsule pressure
- Angiotensin II reduces the surface area by contracting the mesangial cells
- At high concentrations ADH is a vasoconstrictor and will reduce renal blood flow and thence the filtration rate
- Renin is an enzyme which facilitates the formation of angiotensin I from the larger molecule angiotensinogen; renin is produced in response to low intrarenal vascular pressures

10 (**a**) true (**b**) false (**c**) false (**d**) false (**e**) true

Cardiac output is usually measured using a technique based on the Fick principle. This is that the blood flowing through an organ equals the amount of a substance taken out by or put in by an organ divided by the difference between the concentration going in and the concentration coming out.

So the carbon dioxide exhaled from the lungs divided by the difference between venous and arterial carbon dioxide contents will give the cardiac output. Similarly, cardiac output can be determined by injecting dye into the right atrium and measuring its concentration in the pulmonary artery, assuming there is no dye in the vena cava.

11 (**a**) true (**b**) true (**c**) true (**d**) true (**e**) true

- Basal metabolic rate is the energy output when the body is mentally and physically at rest
- It is measured as watts = joules /s or $W.m^2$
- It is increased by thyroxine and adrenaline, pregnancy and after a meal
- It is higher in the newborn and lower with old age
- It is lower in a hot climate than in a cold climate
- A calorimeter is used to measure the total heat production: as heat production is related to the oxygen consumption it is the latter that is often measured (the assumption is made that 1 l of oxygen is used to produce 4.8 kcal of energy)

12 (**a**) true (**b**) true (**c**) false (**d**) false (**e**) true

- Fat is in the diet as triglycerides which are broken down by lipases
- Bile salts are required to emulsify the fat to form micelles, which are spheres of lipid and bile salt
- The micelles enter the enterocytes to be formed into chylomicrons
- These chylomicrons diffuse into the lacteals
- Both glucose and fatty acids are broken down into acetyl CoA, which enters the citric acid cycle; excess fat is converted back into acetyl
- CoA in the liver and adipose tissue
- RQ of carbohydrate is 1; protein, 0.8; fat, 0.7

13 (**a**) true (**b**) false (**c**) false (**d**) false (**e**) false

- Functional residual capacity (FRC) is the residual volume and the expiratory reserve volume
- It is total lung capacity minus the inspiratory capacity; total lung capacity would still need to be measured

- FRC is measured using helium dilution, nitrogen washout or body plethysmography
- FRC is reduced in obesity, pregnancy or the presence of any intra-abdominal mass, and anaesthesia, including IPPV
- FRC is increased by PEEP, CPAP, asthma and exercise

14 (**a**) true (**b**) false (**c**) false (**d**) false (**e**) false

Baroreceptors are found in the carotid sinus, as well as the atria, aorta and pulmonary circulation. They are stretch receptors that detect low pressures.

With stretch due to an increase in blood pressure the afferent discharge increases, leading to reduced sympathetic discharge, reduced vasoconstriction and bradycardia; cardiac output falls, as does peripheral vascular resistance. At normal blood pressure the baroreceptors fire slowly. A fall in discharge would increase renin production. Chemoreceptors in the carotid sinus respond to hypoxaemia by increasing sympathetic activity.

15 (**a**) true (**b**) false (**c**) false (**d**) true (**e**) false

On changing from the erect position to being supine, more blood returns from the lower limbs and cardiac output increases. The venous pressure will reduce due to a smaller gravitational effect. Heart rate will fall due to the increased venous return.

16 (**a**) true (**b**) false (**c**) true (**d**) false (**e**) true

A cough is like a Valsalva manoeuvre with an increase in intrathoracic pressure against a closed glottis and then a rapid release of pressure.

The intrathoracic pressure increases up to 40 kPa, airways widen, and alveoli are distended. The diaphragm contracts on inspiration and will relax on expiration. The venous return will fall until the intrathoracic pressure falls. Repeated coughing can lead to syncope due to a low cardiac output. Cerebral perfusion will be reduced but jugular venous pressure will increase.

17 (**a**) true (**b**) true (**c**) false (**d**) true (**e**) true

Pulse pressure reflects the intermittent ejection of blood into the aorta by the heart. The difference between systolic and diastolic blood pressure is the pulse pressure.

The principle factors that alter pulse pressure in the arteries are:

(a) *Left ventricular stroke volume*: the larger the stroke volume the greater is the volume of blood that must be accommodated in the arterial vessels with each contraction, resulting in an increased pulse pressure.

(b) *Velocity of blood flow*: pulse pressure increases when the flow of blood from arteries to veins is accelerated. i.e.:
   - patent ductus arteriosus (reflecting rapid run off of blood into the pulmonary circulation or left ventricle)
   - aortic regurgitation (reflection of run off of blood into the left ventricle)
   - pulse pressure increase when systemic vascular resistance decreases
   - an increase in heart rate while the cardiac output remains constant causes the stroke volume and pulse pressure to decrease.

(c) *Compliance of arterial tree*: pulse pressure is inversely proportional to compliance (distensibility) of the arterial system; for example, with aging the distensibility of the arterial walls often decrease and pulse pressure increases.

18 (**a**) false (**b**) false (**c**) true (**d**) true (**e**) false

The pathway for non-painful sensations such as touch ascends in the dorsal columns where they synapse in the gracile and cuneate nuclei. The second-order neurones from these nuclei cross the midline and ascend in the medial lemniscus to the sensory relay nuclei of the thalamus. This ascending system is called the dorsal column or lemniscal system.

Pain afferents are carried by small-diameter C and A delta afferents, with cell bodies in the dorsal ganglia, to the dorsal horn. The nerves synapse in substantia gelatinosa, lamina II of the dorsal grey matter. The second-order neurones cross to the contralateral spinothalamic and spinoreticular tracts forming the anterolateral funiculus to terminate in various brainstem nuclei of the thalamus.

The hippocampus forms part of the limbic system. Stimulation leads to somatovisceral responses to do with the emotions and arousal. It may be the site of action of the benzodiazepines and some anaesthetic drugs.

19 (**a**) true (**b**) false (**c**) true (**d**) false (**e**) false

- Insulin is a polypeptide, molecular weight 5734, synthesised in the beta cells of the pancreas; it has an alpha and a beta chain

- In general it promotes cellular uptake, increased storage and decreased breakdown of carbohydrates, fat and protein
- *Carbohydrate*: plasma glucose is actively taken up into the tissues except cells that are permeable to glucose such as the renal tubules, erythrocytes, intestinal mucosa and brain. Insulin increases glycogen synthesis, reduces glycogenolysis and gluconeogenesis, and leads to reduced release of glucose from the liver
- *Proteins*: increased protein stores, synthesis and reduced breakdown
- *Fat*: increases fat synthesis from glucose, clearance of fat from the blood
- Insulin decreases the cell membrane permeability to sodium, which allows potassium to enter the cell, particularly into muscle and hepatic cells
- Insulin stimulates the uptake of glucagon by muscle and fat

20 (**a**) true (**b**) false (**c**) true (**d**) false (**e**) false

The carbon dioxide response curve is obtained by measuring the minute ventilation at different $PaCO_2$ levels.

A parallel shift to the right indicates a reduced respiratory drive. A shallower slope indicates that the respiratory centre is less sensitive to changes in carbon dioxide. Both occur with anaesthetics and opioids. Hypoxaemia directly depresses the respiratory centre but increases the chemoreceptor activity.

Anaesthesia and hypoxaemia reduce the respiratory drive.

Pain has an arousal effect causing the patient to hyperventilate.

The curve is shifted to the left with exercise as the minute ventilation is increased at a lower $PaCO_2$ and in pregnancy.

21 (**a**) true (**b**) true (**c**) true (**d**) true (**e**) false

The many functions of the liver are carried out by two cell types: the parenchymal cells or hepatocytes (60%), which release substances into the bile canaliculi and into blood and lymph channels; and the Kupffer cells, which form part of the lining of blood and lymph channels and have a macrophage function. The rest of the sinusoidal lining consists of squamous cells which constitute a discontinuous endothelium. The parenchymal cells are organised into plates which are one or two cells thick. These plates are arranged in a radial pattern originating around the central veins. They form a continuous network through many lobules at the areas around the portal vessels.

- Parenchymal cell liver functions include
  - metabolic activity of carbohydrates, proteins and lipids
  - storage of vitamins A, D, E and K, iron, copper and glycogen
  - synthesis of clotting factors and immunoglobulins
  - degradation and elimination of drugs, waste products and hormones
- Kupffer cell liver functions include
  - macrophage, phagocytosis, activation of cytokines

22 (**a**) false (**b**) true (**c**) false (**d**) false (**e**) false

Gamma motor fibres innervate the contractile ends of the muscle spindles in skeletal muscles. Muscle spindles are capsules of specialised muscle fibres within the muscle which detect muscle length and movement. The tension is detected by tendon organs.

The gamma efferents are stimulated by the extrapyramidal system, which produces contraction of intrafusal fibres which leads, through stimulation of spindle afferents and alpha activation, to contraction of the skeletal muscle. The tendon reflex is the only monosynaptic reflex in the body. It involves the stretching of the muscle which activates the spindle afferents Ia, excitation of the motor neurone and a muscle contraction.

23 (**a**) true (**b**) false (**c**) false (**d**) true (**e**) true

The accurate measurement of total body water is difficult because it requires a dilution technique with an agent that stays in the total body water without selectively concentrating in the intracellular or extracellular water.

Red cell volume is more easily measured by the packed cell volume.

Neonates are 80% water. The proportion of water falls with age to about 60% in adult males and 55% in adult females.

Body water increases in pregnancy.

24 (**a**) false (**b**) false (**c**) false (**d**) true (**e**) false

$\dot{V}/\dot{Q}$ mismatch is of two types:

(a) Wasted ventilation, which is assessed by measuring the physiological dead space using the Bohr equation. The Bohr equation uses the volume of carbon dioxide in ideal alveolar gas multiplied by alveolar ventilation and the amount of carbon dioxide in mixed expired times minute ventilation.

(b) Areas of lung which are under ventilated and lead to an increase in venous admixture. These are assessed by using the shunt equation, which uses cardiac output, oxygen content in arterial blood, in mixed-venous blood and pulmonary end-capillary blood.

Intrapulmonary shunt is the small amount of blood passing from the bronchial circulation into the pulmonary veins and thebesian myocardial vessels draining into the left ventricle.

Venous admixture is increased in right-to-left cardiac defects, pulmonary cancers and infection and lung collapse.

Carbon monoxide transfer factor assesses the diffusing capacity of the alveoli-capillary membrane, normally 17–25 ml/min per mmHg. It is reduced when the capillary–alveolar membrane is thickened or the area of the membrane is reduced. The overall result given by a transfer gas test may be affected by ventilation, perfusion and diffusion.

Helium has been used to assess the lung volumes and the resistance to flow in the smaller airways. A flow–volume loop when breathing air and then when breathing helium with air are compared.

The arterio-venous oxygen difference is increased when tissue oxygen usage is high or cardiac output is low. It is decreased with arterio-venous shunting or if oxygen usage is reduced.

The difference between inspired or alveolar oxygen tensions compared to the inspired oxygen is a measure of $\dot{V}/\dot{Q}$ mismatch. It also increases with higher inspired oxygen tensions and age.

Giving 100% oxygen makes little difference to correcting the venous admixture due to intrapleural shunt.

A–a carbon dioxide difference is little affected by venous admixture or $\dot{V}/\dot{Q}$ mismatch due to the steeper haemoglobin dissociation curve of carbon dioxide and the response to alter ventilation to changes in carbon dioxide partial pressure.

25 (**a**) true (**b**) false (**c**) true (**d**) true (**e**) true

The emptying time of the stomach is prolonged or increased by: high acidity; food, carbohydrate less than by fat; increased sympathetic activity such as anxiety, fear and pain; and drugs such as opioids, anticholinergics, alcohol and catecholamines.

Secretin is released from the duodenum in response to acid, and inhibits gastric smooth muscle. Secretin and cholecystokinin stimulate pancreatic secretion in response to a meal.

26 (**a**) true (**b**) false (**c**) true (**d**) true (**e**) false

The liver is the second largest organ in the body (the skin is the largest). The liver receives 20%–30% of the cardiac output of 5 l or about 1–1.5 l/min. Of the blood flow, 70% is from the portal vein, which has passed through the gut but provides the liver with 50%–60% of its oxygen requirement. This blood is normally 85% saturated but the saturation falls when the gut activity increases. The hepatic artery carries arterial blood but only supplies 40%–50% of the oxygen requirements of the liver.

27 (**a**) false (**b**) true (**c**) false (**d**) false (**e**) false

Compliance is volume per unit pressure. Lung compliance in an adult with a tidal volume of 7 ml/kg is 200 ml/cm/H_2O. Chest wall compliance is 200 ml/cmH_2O. The total compliance is 100 ml/cmH_2O. In a child the tidal volume remains the same at 7 ml/kg but the respiratory rate is increased. The inflation pressures remain the same. So the compliance in a 15-kg child will be 105 ml/5 cmH_2O or 21 ml/cmH_2O.

Dynamic compliance is measured by plotting a pressure-volume loop during breathing. Dynamic compliance is usually less than static compliance.

Tidal volume depends on compliance, airway resistance and the time for inspiration.

The $\dot{V}/\dot{Q}$ ratio tends to get wider in situations such as pulmonary oedema, chest infection and asthma, when the compliance is getting less.

28 (**a**) false (**b**) false (**c**) false (**d**) true (**e**) false

The main stimulus to normal respiration is the carbon dioxide drive on peripheral and central chemoreceptors. Chemoreceptors are situated in the carotid and aortic bodies. The carotid sinus has baroreceptors, which monitor blood pressure, pulse pressure and heart rate.

Oxygen levels have their effect on respiration through the peripheral chemoreceptors. A lack of oxygen causes central nervous depression, not specific to respiration.

29 (**a**) false (**b**) false (**c**) true (**d**) true (**e**) false

The velocity in nerve conduction is increased by myelination and a larger diameter. The motor nerves have larger diameters than the sensory nerves.

Pressure and cold slow conduction have been used in the past as a poor substitute for local anaesthesia.

30 (**a**) false (**b**) true (**c**) true (**d**) true (**e**) false

Shivering is controlled by the hypothalamus through the sympathetic nervous system. Beta 3 receptors are responsible for uncoupling oxidative phosphorylation in brown fat and in skeletal muscle. Within the hypothalamus noradrenaline, 5-hydroxytryptamine, dopamine and prostaglandins are important transmitters.

Prostaglandins cause an increase in body temperature, hence the use of non-steroidal anti-inflammatory drugs in the control of pyrexia.

Higher centres play a vital role in the gross changes in body heat such as a change in clothing while the sympathetic system provides the fine control.

31 (**a**) false (**b**) true (**c**) true (**d**) false (**e**) true

Half-life is the time taken for the concentration to fall to half (50%) of its original concentration. This focuses on the elimination from the whole body. One time constant is the time it would have taken to eliminate the drug if the rate of elimination had continued at the original rate. The reciprocal of the time constant is the rate constant. The concentration of a drug depends on its clearance from the plasma. Clearance (Cl) focuses on the effectiveness of an organ to eliminate the drug from the blood. The rate of clearance varies, depending on the drug and the organ through which it passes. For many drugs cleared by renal excretion the half-life is dependent on glomerular filtration rate. The elimination rate constant K_e is defined as the fraction of drug eliminated per unit time.

The elimination half-life is the time required for the amount of drug (or concentration) in the body to decrease by half.

Clearance (Cl), elimination rate constant (K_e), volume of distribution (V_d) and half-life are related as follows:

$$K_e = \text{Cl}/V_d \quad [\text{fraction/hour} = (\text{l/h})/\text{l}]$$
$$\text{Half life} = 0.693/K_e$$

Note the use of the word 'only' in 31 part(a).

32 (**a**) false (**b**) false (**c**) false (**d**) true (**e**) false

- Ringer's lactate: pH 6.5; saline: pH 5.0; glucose 5%: pH 4.0; suxamethonium 2% solution: pH 2–3
- Propofol: pH 7.4, p*K*a 11.0
- Thiopentone 2.5%: pH 10.5, p*K*a 7.6
- Lidocaine: p*K*a 7.9

33 (**a**) false (**b**) true (**c**) true (**d**) false (**e**) true

Heparin is a mucopolysaccharide with a molecular weight ranging from 2000 to 40 000 Da.

It is metabolised by desulphonation in the reticular endothelial system.

Its main actions are to bind to antithrombin III (ATIII); to inhibit factors XII, XI, X and IX, and thrombin; and to inhibit platelet aggregation.

Neither heparin nor low-molecular-weight heparin crosses the placenta, and both are considered the anticoagulant drugs of choice in pregnancy, in contrast to warfarin, which does cross the placenta.

34 (**a**) false (**b**) false (**c**) true (**d**) false (**e**) false

Buprenorphine is a strong partial agonist at the mu receptor, a weak antagonist at the kappa receptor and has no effect at the sigma receptor.

Potency is a comparison of doses that produce a similar effect: 400 μg buprenorphine is said to be equivalent to 10 mg morphine. It causes respiratory depression but this reaches a maximum which is not increased by increasing the dose. This respiratory depression is only partly reversed by large doses (5 mg) of naloxone and the maximum effect takes up to 3 h.

Buprenorphine can reverse the respiratory depression effect of high-dose fentanyl.

The duration of action is up to 8 h and 72 h with the transdermal patch.

35 (**a**) false (**b**) true (**c**) false (**d**) false (**e**) true

Flumazenil is a benzodiazepine antagonist specific to the GABA receptors. It can cause excitation and convulsions, particularly in patients who are receiving benzodiazepines to control epilepsy. After an intravenous dose its effect is apparent in 1–2 min with a maximum effect after 10 min. It has a short half-life of 1 h and so its effect will pass off before the action of the longer-acting benzodiazepine.

Flumazenil is hydrolysed by hepatic microsomal enzymes to a number of inactive metabolites.

36 (**a**) true (**b**) true (**c**) true (**d**) false (**e**) true

Hoffmann degradation to produce laudanosine is temperature dependent. About 50% of atracurium is metabolised by ester hydrolysis. The *cis* isomer is active with less histamine release. *Cis* means the molecules are on the same side of the double bond; *trans* means the molecules are on opposite sides.

37 (**a**) false (**b**) true (**c**) false (**d**) true (**e**) false

Histamine is attached to the mast cells and can be displaced by a number of drugs, particularly when given quickly in high concentrations. Histamine release is associated with most opioids, d-tubocurare and atracurium, and some antibiotics such as ampicillin.

Histamine release is not associated with etomidate.

38 (**a**) false (**b**) false (**c**) true (**d**) true (**e**) false

- Bradycardia is associated with vagotonic drugs such as neostigmine
- Atracurium has little effect on heart rate
- Nifedipine is a calcium channel blocker with a mildly negative inotropic effect but any fall in cardiac output is compensated by a tachycardia
- Verapamil slows conduction through the atrioventricular node
- Desflurane, like isoflurane, causes vasodilatation and hypotension with a compensatory tachycardia

39 (**a**) true (**b**) false (**c**) true (**d**) true (**e**) false

Warfarin therapy should be avoided in pregnancy. If warfarin is essential it should be avoided in the first trimester because of teratogenicity and at 2–4 weeks before delivery to reduce bleeding complications. Unfractionated or low-molecular-weight heparin can be substituted as these agents do not cross the placenta and are the anticoagulants of choice.

Suxamethonium crosses the placenta in small amounts. Residual neuromuscular blockade has been seen in the neonate after repeated, high doses of suxamethonium given to the mother delivered by caesarean section. Pancuronium has been found to cross the placenta in small amounts.

40 (**a**) false (**b**) true (**c**) true (**d**) true (**e**) true

Spironolactone antagonises aldosterone. It favours the retention of potassium and hydrogen ions with loss of sodium in the distal tubule.

Amiloride is potassium sparing.

Acetazolomide inhibits the enzyme carbonic anhydrase and the formation of bicarbonate and hydrogen ions from carbon dioxide and water. Hydrogen ion excretion is reduced leading to a metabolic acidosis.

41 (**a**) true (**b**) true (**c**) false (**d**) true (**e**) false

Caffeine is a non-specific phosphodiesterase (PDE) inhibitor. PDE has many isoenzymes; one, PDE1, is stimulated by calcium.

Calcium channel blockers such as nifedipine, verapamil and diltiazem work through calcium ions.

Flecainide is a class IC drug used to treat arrhythmias. It acts as a sodium channel blocker.

42 (**a**) true (**b**) true (**c**) true (**d**) false (**e**) true

Monoamine oxidase (MAO) is an enzyme that speeds the deactivation of amines including catecholamines.

MAO inhibitors are only rarely given now for depression to increase the brain store of catchecholamines.

Opioids inhibit the production of catecholamine by inhibiting cGMP.

There are a number of interactions between MAOIs and opioids: hypertension and convulsions are the most common. Pethidine in particular causes hypertension due to the inhibition of 5-HT re-uptake into nerve endings. Morphine has been used but needs to be given carefully and is not entirely without effects, so we have suggested true.

43 (**a**) false (**b**) false (**c**) false (**d**) true (**e**) true

Methaemoglobin contains ferric ions that are unable to bind oxygen. It is associated with drugs such as prilocaine, sulphonamides and nitrites. Sodium nitroprusside produces cyanide ions.

44 (**a**) false (**b**) false (**c**) false (**d**) false (**e**) true

Depolarising (phase 1 block) is associated with suxamethonium. The characteristics of the block are fasciculations, except in children and at term in pregnancy. No fade or post-tetanic fasciculation is seen with a non-depolarising block. Small doses of non-depolarising muscle relaxants given to prevent muscle pains tend to antagonise the block. The block is potentiated by hyperkalaemia, hypermagnesaemia, hypothermia and alkalosis. Large doses of suxamethonium and acetylcholine potentiate the block, as do acetylcholine esterase inhibitors.

45 (**a**) false (**b**) false (**c**) true (**d**) false (**e**) true

Gentamycin has been reported as causing otic nerve damage, particularly if given by rapid IV. Cefotaxime is a third-generation cephalosporin that is metabolised in the liver to produce an inactive metabolite which is excreted in the urine. The BNF recommends that if the creatinine clearance is $<$5 ml/min give 1 g as the initial dose, then use half the normal dose. Flucloxacillin is a penicillinase-resistant penicillin. Rifampicin causes enzyme induction, which will reduce the effectiveness of anticoagulants, phenytoin and oral contraceptives. The action of sulphonamides to inhibit dihydrofolate synthesis is potentiated by trimethoprim which inhibits tetrahydrofolate synthesis.

46 (**a**) true (**b**) true (**c**) false (**d**) true (**e**) false

The cytochrome system is a series of enzymes responsible for oxidising foreign compounds. The system is induced by phenobarbitone and most of the barbiturates, phenylbutazone, griseofulvin and rifampicin.

Carbamazepine, phenytoin, benzodiazepines and other anticonvulsants can induce hepatic enzyme function.

The system is inhibited and so drug action is prolonged by cimetidine, chloramphenicol, cyclophosphamide, indomethacine, isoniazid, methadone, various cholinesterases such as neostigmine, physostigmine and ecothiopate, and monoamine oxidase inhibitors affecting the catecholamines.

47 (**a**) false (**b**) true (**c**) true (**d**) false (**e**) true

Methaemoglobin contains iron in the ferric form within the haemoglobin molecule. It may be caused by a congenital deficiency of reducing enzymes, or be due to drugs and aniline dyes.

It is treated with a reducing agent, such as methylene blue, starting with 1 mg/kg. Cyanosis occurs at 1.5 g/100 ml or 10% of the haemoglobin; symptoms of headache and dyspnoea come at 3 g/100ml (20%).

48 (**a**) true (**b**) true (**c**) true (**d**) true (**e**) true

Most drugs cross the placenta. A molecular weight of less that 600 Da passes easily and this includes most of the drugs used in anaesthetic practice. Transfer is facilitated by unionised molecules, high lipid solubility and high placental blood flow.

Warfarin is especially teratogenic in the first trimester and may cause haemorrhage in the third trimester.

The d-isomer of glucose is actively transported.

49 (**a**) false (**b**) false (**c**) false (**d**) true (**e**) true

The normal ECG changes with digoxin include prolonged PR interval, ST segment depression, sign of a reverse tick, T wave inversion and shortened QT interval. These are not signs of toxicity.

Toxicity is likely above 2 ng/ml and almost certain over 3 ng/ml. The features of toxicity include:

- *arrhythmias*: the most common arrhythmias are ventricular extrasystoles, ventricular bigeminy/trigeminy and atrial tachycardia with complete heart block
- anorexia, nausea and vomiting and, occasionally, diarrhoea
- confusion, especially in the elderly
- yellow vision (xanthopsia), blurred vision and photophobia

Cardiac glycosides should be used with caution in:

- recent myocardial infarction and constrictive pericarditis, for similar reasons
- hypothyroidism – decreased efficacy and increased risk of toxicity
- chronic cor pulmonale – decreased efficacy and increased risk of toxicity
- elderly – smaller doses needed
- renal impairment – smaller doses needed

Also note to:

- avoid hypokalaemia
- avoid rapid intravenous administration

Contraindications include:

- arrhythmias associated with accessory conduction pathways (e.g. Wolff–Parkinson–White syndrome) – these drugs should not be used to treat these sorts of arrhythmia because they will impair conduction through the normal conducting pathway without affecting the accessory pathways
- intermittent complete heart block, second-degree AV block
- left ventricular outflow obstruction (e.g. hypertrophic cardiac myopathy, aortic stenosis) or increased force of contraction against an obstruction – occasionally digoxin may be used if there is concomitant atrial fibrillation and heart failure (consult expert advice on management in this situation)

Management of toxicity

(a) Conservative management is indicated if
  - The patient is nauseated but not vomiting
  - There are only occasional ventricular ectopics
    - discontinue the digoxin for 2–3 days
    - give 20–40 mmol/day potassium orally, when the serum potassium is known

(b) First-line treatment for serious toxicity
  - The indications for a more energetic approach to digoxin toxicity include:
    - persistent nausea with vomiting
    - heart block

    - heart failure
    - cardiac arrhythmia
- The management includes:
    - intravenous potassium
        - 40 mmol potassium in 5% dextrose over 1 h
        - ECG monitoring throughout
        - potassium is stopped if sinus rhythm returns or there are signs of hyperkalaemia, e.g. peaked T waves
        - a total of 120 mmol may be given
        - if initial potassium levels were normal, then the risk of hyperkalaemia is reduced if the potassium is infused in 250 ml of 20% dextrose with 30 U of soluble insulin
    - intravenous magnesium:
        - magnesium protects the myocardium
        - give 50 ml of 2% magnesium sulphate over 1 h
        - repeat infusion as required
- Activated charcoal orally

(c) Second-line treatment for serious toxicity

If first-line treatment for digoxin toxicity fails, the intervention of choice is digoxin-specific fab (DSFab) therapy:

- DSFabs are biologically active fragments of digoxin-neutralising antibodies
- Patients respond within 30 min, with full effect seen in 3–4 h
- The dose of DSFab is calculated by multiplying the amount of digoxin ingested by 60, e.g. 5 mg of digoxin is neutralised by 300 mg of DSFab
- Other treatments:
    - propranolol: 1–2 mg intravenously slowly to control ectopics and tachyarrhythmias
    - atropine: 0.6 mg intravenously may control bradycardia
    - temporary pacing if there is persistent heart block
    - DC cardioversion: risks of inducing heart block or tachycardia; indicated in cases of life-threatening arrhythmia where DSFab is not considered appropriate
    - cardioversion should begin with low energies, e.g. 10 J

50 **(a)** false **(b)** true **(c)** true **(d)** true **(e)** true

Clopidogrel is an antiplatelet drug indicated for use in patients at risk from coronary artery occlusion.

Mechanism of action

Its action is to inhibit ADP-induced platelet aggregation by directly inhibiting the bonding of ADP to its receptor and the subsequent ADP mediated activation of the glycoprotein GP IIb/IIIa complex.

Pharmacokinetics

- It is insoluble in water at pH 7 but soluble at pH 1
- A tablet contains 97.875 mg of clopidogrel bisulphate, giving 75 mg of clopidogrel base
- Molecular weight 419.9

Pharmacodynamics

- The first dose affects clotting within 2 h and subsequent doses have an accumulative effect
- On stopping it may take up to 5 days before the bleeding time returns to normal

Side-effects

- Tiredness
- Headache
- Dizziness, stomach pain
- Diarrhoea
- Constipation
- Bleeding

It does not inhibit phosphodiesterase activity.

51 (**a**) false (**b**) true (**c**) true (**d**) true (**e**) false

Cocaine is an ester local anaesthetic with marked vasoconstrictor activity.

Uses

- Its use is limited to the nasal passages due to corneal and cardiac toxicity

Preparations

- Solutions of 4% and 10% are used

Paper 6 Answers

Dose

- The maximum dose should be limited to 1.5 mg/kg

Mechanism of action

- Action is by blocking the fast sodium channels in nerve membranes
- It causes vasoconstriction by blocking catecholamine neuronal uptake-1 and inhibiting monoamine oxidase
- This increases synaptic levels of dopamine and noradrenaline

Overdose

- Overdose initially leads to central nervous excitation with euphoria and convulsions but then central inhibition with sedation and respiratory depression
- Nausea and vomiting, arrhythmias and cardiac failure may occur
- It is not used in the eye due to corneal damage
- Hypersensitivity is very rare with all local anaesthetic agents
- Liver metabolism produces inactive metabolites, which are excreted in the urine

52 (**a**) true (**b**) false (**c**) false (**d**) true (**e**) true

Enoximone acts by selectively inhibiting phosphodiesterase III iso-enzyme in the cell. This leads to a reduction in the degradation of cAMP. By increasing cAMP in the myocardium it increases the slow calcium ion inward current. By altering the calcium ion flux into smooth muscle it produces vasodilatation.

It increases inotropic activity and vasodilates coronary vessels.

The non-specific methylxanthines such as theophylline inhibit the five iso-enzymes.

There are two types of specific PDE III inhibitors, bipyridines, e.g. milarone, and imidazolines, e.g. enoximone.

Enoximone undergoes metabolism in the liver to active and inactive metabolites. The dose should be reduced in liver failure.

53 (**a**) true (**b**) false (**c**) true (**d**) false (**e**) false

(a) Alpha adrenergic agonists (phenylephedrine)
  - Contract the iris dilator muscles and the smooth muscle of the conjunctival arterioles

(b) Beta-blockers
  - Have little or no effect on pupil size

(c) Carbonic anhydrase inhibitors
  - Decrease the production of intraocular fluid
  - Since the eye-drop form of this medication is relatively new, long-term studies are yet to be completed
  - Current effects of the eye-drops include stinging, burning and other eye discomfort

(d) Cholinergic (miotic)
  - Increase drainage of intraocular fluid
  - Miotics increase drainage of intraocular fluid by making the pupil size smaller (miosis), thereby increasing the flow of intraocular fluid from the eye

(e) Cholinesterase inhibitor (pilocarpine)
  - Acetyl cholinesterase inhibitors when applied to the conjunctiva produce: constriction of the pupillary sphincter muscle (miosis) and contraction of the ciliary muscle (paralysis of accommodation or loss of far vision)

54 (**a**) true (**b**) false (**c**) false (**d**) true (**e**) true

Theophylline is the active ingredient in aminophylline. It is a non-selective inhibitor of the five phosphodiesterase iso-enzymes.

Its actions are inotropic, chronotropic and relaxation of coronary vessel smooth muscle. It can lead to ventricular dysrrhythmias.

It inhibits tubular reabsorption of sodium, leading to a weak diuresis.

It relaxes bronchial smooth muscle, which will increase anatomical dead space but not alveolar dead space.

It increases central nervous stimulation leading to agitation and convulsions.

55 (**a**) true (**b**) false (**c**) true (**d**) false (**e**) false

Alfentanil is a synthetic phenylpiperidine derivative of fentanyl. Compared to fentanyl (4.0 l/kg), alfentanil has a much smaller volume of distribution (0.6 l/kg). It is more protein bound than fentanyl.

The lipid solubility of alfentanil is lower than that of fentanyl, but the unionised fraction is much larger (89%) due to a lower pK_a at body pH.

Both midazolam and alfentanil are metabolized by hepatic enzymes (CYP3A3/4). Concurrent administration will prolong the half-lives of both drugs.

Alfentanil is metabolised by non-specific plasma esterases. It is not affected by cholinesterase deficiency or anticholinesterase drugs.

56 (**a**) false (**b**) false (**c**) true (**d**) true (**e**) true

Benzodiazepines act at the $GABA_A$ receptor complex of five subunits. They increase the frequency of opening of chloride channels.

They are lipid soluble and bound to plasma albumin.

Equipotent doses range from clonazepam 500 (μg), to lorazepam (1 mg), to diazepam (5–10 mg), up to tempazepam (20–40 mg).

Warfarin's effect is potentiated by drugs competing for protein binding such as NSAIDs and inhibition of metabolism by cimetidine, alcohol, erthythromycin and ciprofloxacin.

The effects of warfarin are reduced by drugs that induce liver enzymes, such as rifampicin and carbamazepine.

57 (**a**) false (**b**) false (**c**) true (**d**) true (**e**) false

The following drugs are given through the nasal mucosa: diamorphine, midazolam, GTN.

Local anaesthetics and cocaine are used to give surface anaesthesia for examinations of the oral and nasal passages. Some of the local anaesthetic will be absorbed. The reliable route for therapeutic lidocaine in cardiac dysrrhythmias is through the bronchial mucosa.

58 (**a**) true (**b**) true (**c**) true (**d**) true (**e**) true

Ropivacaine is the *S*-enantiomer of the propyl (C_3 H_7) derivative of *N*-alkyl pipecoloxylidine.

Compared with bupivacaine, ropivacaine:

- is a pure *S* (I) enantiomer
- has similar
  - p*K*a
  - protein binding
- has an equivalent duration of sensory block

- is less lipid soluble and therefore less potent
- has a smaller volume of distribution
- has a faster clearance
- has a shorter terminal half-life
- blocks C fibres as bupivacaine but A fibres less
- gives less motor block
- is less toxic

59 **(a)** false **(b)** false **(c)** true **(d)** true **(e)** true

Mode of action

A local anaesthetic agent is a weak base.
It is injected as a hydrochloride salt in an acidic solution. The tertiary amine group becomes quaternary and dissolves in solution.

$$\underset{\text{(Ionised drug)}}{\mathrm{BH}+} \rightleftharpoons \underset{\text{(Freebase)}}{\mathrm{B}+\mathrm{H}^+}$$

Following injection at the extracellular pH 7.4, the drug dissociates to a degree that depends on p*K*a and free base is released. The free base is relatively lipophilic (non-ionised), and passes passively down its concentration gradient through the membrane into the axon. Inside the axon the pH is lower (because the environment is more acidic) and re-ionisation takes place.

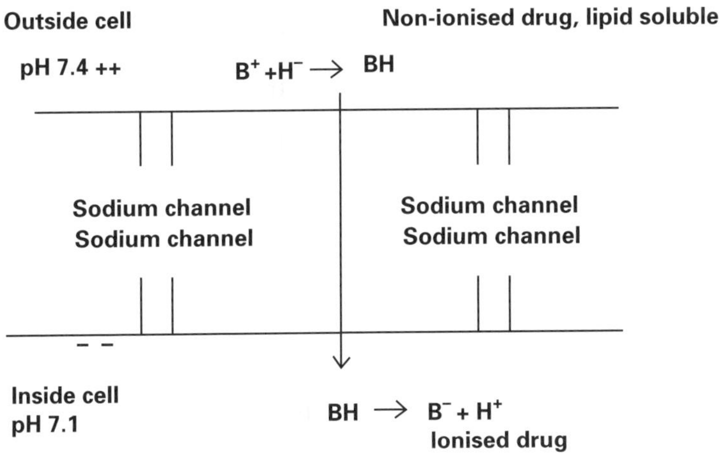

The ionised portion is attracted by the negative charge of the membrane protein, and then passes into the open ion channel, which remains open but is blocked to further transmission of sodium. Blockade is use dependent, because the ionophore is only blocked while open.

60 (**a**) true (**b**) true (**c**) true (**d**) true (**e**) false

Phosphodiesterase inactivates cAMP (3′,5′-adenosine monophosphate) by conversion to 5′-AMP. Inhibition of phosphodiesterase causes an increase in cAMP and cGMP.

Their main effects are to be positively ionotropic and chronotropic, and to induce vasodilatation and bronchodilatation.

61 (**a**) false (**b**) true (**c**) false (**d**) false (**e**) true

Gas chromatography works by separating the gases as they pass through an oil-coated column. Gases are held back depending on their oil solubility.

62 (**a**) false (**b**) false (**c**) false (**d**) false (**e**) true

Any current over 1 mA is painful and at 15 mA muscle spasm makes it impossible to release the source. A current of 80–100 mA causes arrhythmias. Class I equipment has a mains supply with three leads, live, neutral and earth; class II has no earth; and class III has a low voltage power supply.

To prevent static charges building up, the floor of the operating theatre has a high resistance of 240 kΩ and the resistance of shoes are 75–100 kΩ to slow the passage of charge to earth. A high humidity also reduces static charge.

63 (**a**) false (**b**) false (**c**) true (**d**) true (**e**) true

Gauge pressure is the pressure of gas in a cylinder counting atmospheric pressure as zero.

Cylinders that contain part gas and part liquid will show a constant pressure until all the liquid is in the gas form. These gases are nitrous oxide and carbon dioxide, which are below their critical temperatures of 36.5°C and 31°C at room temperature.

64 (**a**) false (**b**) true (**c**) false (**d**) true (**e**) false

The pneumotachograph detects flow by measuring the pressure drop as gas passes through one or more openings. In laminar flow the flow rate is proportional to the pressure drop. The size and number of openings are chosen to ensure laminar flow. The pressure gradient is affected by the density and viscosity of the gas, which in turn are affected by temperature.

65 (**a**) true (**b**) false (**c**) false (**d**) false (**e**) false

Heat is lost by conduction (passing heat directly to a touching object), convection (removing heat into an air stream) and radiation.

Air in contact with the body is warmed by conduction. This air is now less dense and so rises, and colder, denser air moves in to replace the lighter air.

Water vapour in expired gas is trapped in the HME. This water vapour has taken heat from the body by the heat of vaporisation.

Blankets will reduce any convection currents. Spirit takes the heat of evaporation from the skin and so cools the skin.

66 (**a**) true (**b**) true (**c**) true (**d**) false (**e**) true

Damping occurs because the fluid does not move freely and quickly in the tubing. Any obstacles such as bubbles, kinking or clots in the tubing increase damping.

Ideally the catheter should be wide, short and stiff without connections.

If the flushing system malfunctions then clotting may occur.

67 (**a**) true (**b**) false (**c**) true (**d**) true (**e**) false

The Doppler effect is the change in frequency in a sound wave when it is reflected off a surface that is moving towards or away from the origin of the sound wave.

The Doppler effect is used to detect blood flow. The time it takes for a sound wave to return to the transmitter is used to measure the distance a wave has travelled, hence the depth of a structure.

Compliance is the reciprocal of resistance. Systemic vascular resistance can be calculated from cardiac output and blood pressure. The Doppler effect is used to calculate cardiac output.

68 (a) false (b) true (c) true (d) false (e) false

BiS is a specific Fourier form of mathematical analysis of the frequency of waveforms in specific sections of an ongoing pulsatile biological activity. It has been used to analyse the EEG, R–R intervals and blood pressure variability. The BiS from the EEG records a state of the brain and not the effect of a particular drug. BiS gives a numerical value between 0 and 100 and data are generated over 30 EEG recordings, with the average updated every 2–5 s. A low BiS value indicates hypnosis. BiS decreases during natural sleep though not to the level produced by anaesthesia. The opioids do not affect the BiS value at clinical concentrations. A BiS value of 100 indicates a patient is wide awake. A lower number is not drug specific but indicates a level of sedation whatever means are used to produce it. An index of EEG activity below 70 gives a measure of anaesthetic depth; below 60 implies that the patient is unaware.

69 (a) true (b) false (c) false (d) true (e) false

Critical pressure is the vapour pressure at the critical temperature or the pressure at which the gas can be liquefied at the critical temperature. The boiling point is lower than the critical temperature. It is defined as the temperature at which the saturated vapour pressure equals atmospheric pressure.

70 (a) true (b) true (c) true (d) true (e) false

A transducer changes one form of energy to another form of energy. The photodetector is a semiconductor that changes light radiation energy into electrical current. An ammeter is a measuring device. A measuring device is not a transducer, but transducers may be used in a measuring device.

71 (a) false (b) false (c) false (d) false (e) true

The average (mean) is the total 24 divided by the number 8 = 3. The most frequently occurring (mode) number is 1 and the middle (median) number is 2. The sample is not normally distributed to form a bell shaped curve. It is positively skewed to the left with a mean at a higher value than the mode.

The data are not normally distributed, therefore the tests used for normally distributed data will give erroneous results.

72 (a) false (b) false (c) false (d) false (e) false

Positively skewed data are not normally distributed. There are more readings to the left and a long tail to the right. The mean occurs at a higher value than the mode. The lower the *P* value the more likely it is that the difference has not occurred by chance and there is a significant difference between the groups.

SEM is standard deviation divided by the root of the number of results.

Variance is the square of the standard deviation.

73 (**a**) true (**b**) true (**c**) true (**d**) false (**e**) false

Normal adult peak expiratory flow rate is 450–600 l/min.
The Wright peak flow meter is a constant-pressure, variable-orifice meter. The flow of gas moves a vane which rotates about a central axis. As the vane rotates it opens up slots for the gas to escape through. The amount of rotation is a measure of the gas flow.

The Wright respirometer is used for measuring gas volumes. Gas flow is passed into a circular chamber, which has flange like vanes with slits around the edge, and a vane, which rotates about a central axis. The flanges make the flow unidirectional. The flow of gas causes the vane to rotate and the amount of rotation is proportional to the volume of gas that has passed. It is calibrated for tidal volume. It is inaccurate if used to measure flow rates.

74 (**a**) true (**b**) true (**c**) true (**d**) false (**e**) true

Henry's law states that the quantity of gas dissolved in a liquid is proportional to the pressure.

Carbon dioxide and oxygen combine with haemoglobin to increase the amount held in blood.

75 (**a**) false (**b**) false (**c**) true (**d**) false (**e**) false

Interference is a problem because the ECG signal is a small voltage of 0.1–6 V. The detection is affected by electrode contact and skin movement. Drift is a slow change in the signal over time. This was commoner in older oscilloscopes. The trace would rise or fall noticeably as it passed across the screen. Heating of the transducer components can lead to drift. The drift in the trace is usually corrected after the QRS complex to give an artificial shift in the ST segment. Mains interference is reduced by good electrode contact and a high common mode rejection ratio (CMRR). CMRR is the capacity of an amplifier to reject mains frequencies and only amplify the signal such as the ECG. Filters are used to remove mains frequency and can be used to remove other frequencies but may distort the ECG signal.

Gain is the amplitude of the display.

76 (**a**) false (**b**) false (**c**) false (**d**) true (**e**) true

Infrared radiation energy is absorbed by any molecule with two or more dissimilar atoms. It will not analyse oxygen or nitrogen. Water vapour causes interference either because the vapour condenses in the piping to form droplets, which will obstruct the gas flow, or the water vapour absorbs infrared radiation.

Glass will absorb or reflect electromagnetic energy. Collision broadening is due to the infrared radiation being absorbed by molecules, which increases their energy and rate of movement. The rate of collision is increased.

The measuring chamber is kept small to avoid dilutional effects.

77 (**a**) true (**b**) true (**c**) false (**d**) true (**e**) true

In laminar flow resistance is proportional to the pressure gradient and inversely proportional to the flow rate. Resistance is made up of viscosity and length (laminar flow) or density (turbulent flow) divided by radius. Curves, kinks and other obstructions will change laminar flow to turbulent flow.

78 (**a**) true (**b**) false (**c**) false (**d**) false (**e**) false

Laminar flow of a substance can be considered to be in layers, fastest at the centre and slowest at the periphery, where it is near to zero on the wall. The flow at the centre is about twice the mean flow. Newton stated that the frictional force in any region is proportional to the velocity gradient and the area parallel to the fluid flow. The unit of viscosity is the poise (after Poiseuille). The resistance equals the pressure drop divided by the flow rate. Resistance equals viscosity times length (laminar flow) or density (turbulent flow) divided by the radius.

79 (**a**) false (**b**) true (**c**) false (**d**) false (**e**) true

The train of four pulses is at 2 Hz. The double-burst stimulus is two sets of three pulses of 50 Hz separated by 750 ms. Sustained head lift indicates less than 30% residual blockade.

80 (**a**) true (**b**) false (**c**) true (**d**) true (**e**) true

The field strength is usually up to 4 tesla. The MRI scanner exerts large forces on all iron-containing objects. The A.C. field can induce a current in all metal and conducting materials. Hydrogen is the commonest element in the body water and is very responsive to an external magnetic force.

81 (a) false (b) false (c) true (d) true (e) true

Gas flowing through a tube is passed through a constriction or narrowing formed in the tube. The gas increases speed to pass through the narrowing and therefore gains kinetic energy because of increased velocity. The total energy of a gas is the pressure it exerts, therefore if there is a fall in potential energy there will be a fall in pressure at that point.

A second gas can be sucked in or entrained through a side arm into the area of low pressure.

82 (a) false (b) false (c) false (d) true (e) true

Alveolar vapour pressure is dependent on:

- respiration, and increases as minute ventilation increases
- the inspired partial pressure
- blood/gas solubility coefficient: a low value will mean low blood solubility and so a quicker equilibrium between the alveolar tension and the blood
- cardiac output: increased cardiac output increases uptake and so lowers the alveolar concentration

83 (a) false (b) false (c) true (d) false (e) true

Table 6.83 SI units and derived units

Unit	Unit of	Definition
Newton	Force	Force = mass × acceleration 1 newton is the force required to accelerate a mass of 1 kg by 1 m/s^2
Pascal	Pressure	Pressure is force/area 1 Pa is 1 N/m^2
Joule	Energy Work	Potential energy is the energy possessed by a body by virtue of its position Kinetic energy is the energy of the body due to its motion 1 J is the work done (energy used) when a force of 1 N moves 1 m.
Watt	Power	Power is the rate of doing work. This is work/time: 1 W = 1 J/s
Hertz	Frequency	1 Hertz = 1 cycle/s

84 (**a**) false (**b**) true (**c**) true (**d**) true (**e**) true

Interference is reduced by the use of good electrodes which make good contact with the skin. Amplification will increase extraneous noise as well as the ECG signal.

85 (**a**) true (**b**) true (**c**) true (**d**) true (**e**) true

Isolating capacitors are used in diathermy equipment. Capacitors have a high impedance to low-frequency (50 Hz) current, but a low impedance to high-frequency (1 MHz) current, so the damaging effects of all stray low-frequency mains currents are minimised.

Isolating transformer: the design of the circuit prevents the flow of current to earth by any alternative earth-linked path.

Circuit breakers (current-operated earth-leakage circuit breakers) cut the mains power if there is a difference in current between the live and neutral wires. The simplest safety device is a fuse which melts to cut the live current when a high current flows.

The risk of ventricular fibrillation is negligible above 1 MHz used in diathermy.

86 (**a**) true (**b**) false (**c**) true (**d**) true (**e**) true

The Bain circuit is a Mapleson D. Alveolar gas will be rebreathed from the expiratory limb. One advantage of the Bain breathing circuit is that the tubing can be several metres long. It can be used for children but the T piece is preferred for children under 20 kg. The Bain circuit is effectively a T piece with resistance on the expiratory limb. Mapleson calculated a fresh gas flow of 2–3 times the minute ventilation to prevent rebreathing. Since then lower values of 70–100 ml/kg have been suggested as sufficient to prevent a rise in arterial carbon dioxide.

If the inner tube becomes detached from the patient connection then the whole of the tubing becomes dead space.

87 (**a**) true (**b**) false (**c**) false (**d**) true (**e**) true

The pressure reducing valve reduces the very high cylinder pressure to about 400 kPa or 4 bar, which is the working pressure for the anaesthetic machine. The valve not only reduces the cylinder pressure but also ensures that the lower pressure is constant despite a falling cylinder pressure.

88 (**a**) true (**b**) false (**c**) true (**d**) false (**e**) false

The cylinder should be brought into a warm environment before use and inverted several times to ensure mixing. It should be used in the upright position. The pseudocritical temperature is dependent on the gas ratio. The 50:50 ratio has a pseudocritical temperature of −7°C.

The cylinder is filled to 137 bar at room temperature. This will rise as the ambient temperature rises.

89 (**a**) false (**b**) false (**c**) true (**d**) false (**e**) true

The molecules are closer together when the pressure increases, the temperate falls and there are molecules in solution reflected by the osmotic pressure.

The presence of a solute decreases the vapour pressure, makes the solvent less volatile, and so the boiling point is raised.

Depression of freezing point, depression of vapour pressure and elevation of boiling point are all related to osmolarity. The term colligative properties of a solution literally refers to the binding together or the closeness of the molecules.

90 (**a**) true (**b**) false (**c**) true (**d**) true (**e**) false

The frequency of audible sound is 20–20 000 Hz. Medical ultrasound is 1 000 000–30 000 000 Hz.

Piezoelectric transducers are polarised materials which alter shape when a voltage is applied, and also when pressure is applied to them they cause a change in voltage. So they act as both emitters and receivers of ultrasound.

MCQ answers primary paper 6

	(a)	(b)	(c)	(d)	(e)
1	F	F	T	T	T
2	T	T	T	F	T
3	F	F	T	F	T
4	F	T	F	F	F
5	F	T	F	T	F
6	T	T	F	F	F
7	T	F	T	F	T
8	T	F	F	F	T
9	T	T	T	T	T
10	T	F	F	F	T
11	T	T	T	T	T
12	T	T	F	F	T
13	T	F	F	F	F
14	T	F	F	F	F
15	T	F	F	T	F
16	T	F	T	F	T
17	T	T	F	T	T
18	F	F	T	T	F
19	T	F	T	F	F
20	T	F	T	F	F
21	T	T	T	T	F
22	F	T	F	F	F
23	T	F	F	T	T
24	F	F	F	T	F
25	T	F	T	T	T
26	T	F	T	T	F
27	F	T	F	F	F
28	F	F	F	T	F
29	F	F	T	T	F

	(a)	(b)	(c)	(d)	(e)
30	F	T	T	T	F
31	F	T	T	F	T
32	F	F	F	T	F
33	F	T	T	F	T
34	F	F	T	F	F
35	F	T	F	F	T
36	T	T	T	F	T
37	F	T	F	T	F
38	F	F	T	T	F
39	T	F	T	T	F
40	F	T	T	T	T
41	T	T	F	T	F
42	T	T	T	F	T
43	F	F	F	T	T
44	F	F	F	F	T
45	F	F	T	F	T
46	T	T	F	T	F
47	F	T	T	F	T
48	T	T	T	T	T
49	F	F	F	T	T
50	F	T	T	T	T
51	F	T	T	T	F
52	T	F	F	T	T
53	T	F	T	F	F
54	T	F	F	T	T
55	T	F	T	F	F
56	F	F	T	T	T
57	F	F	T	T	F
58	T	T	T	T	T
59	F	F	T	T	T
60	T	T	T	T	F

	(a)	(b)	(c)	(d)	(e)
61	F	T	F	F	T
62	F	F	F	F	T
63	F	F	T	T	T
64	F	T	F	T	F
65	T	F	F	F	F
66	T	T	T	F	T
67	T	F	T	T	F
68	F	T	T	F	F
69	T	F	F	T	F
70	T	T	T	T	F
71	F	F	F	F	T
72	F	F	F	F	F
73	T	T	T	F	F
74	T	T	T	F	T
75	F	F	T	F	F
76	F	F	F	T	T
77	T	T	F	T	T
78	T	F	F	F	F
79	F	T	F	F	T
80	T	F	T	T	T
81	F	F	T	T	T
82	F	F	F	T	T
83	F	F	T	F	T
84	F	T	T	T	T
85	T	T	T	T	T
86	T	F	T	T	T
87	T	F	F	T	T
88	T	F	T	F	F
89	F	F	T	F	T
90	T	F	T	T	F

Bibliography

Physiology

Power, I. and Kam, P. *Principles of Physiology for Anaesthetists*. London: Arnold, 2001.

Ganong, F. M. D. *Review of Medical Physiology*, 22nd edn. New York: McGraw-Hill, 2005.

Lumb, A. B. *Nunn's Applied Respiratory Physiology*, 6th edn. London: Butterworth-Heinemann, 2005.

West, J. B. *Respiratory Physiology: The Essentials*, 7th edn. Baltimore: Lippincott, Williams & Wilkins, 2005.

Klabunde, R. E. *Cardiovascular Physiology Concepts*. Baltimore: Lippincott, Williams and Wilkins, 2005.

Pharmacology

British National Formulary. London: BMJ Publishing.

Peck, T. E., Hill, S. A. and Williams, M. *Pharmacology for Anaesthesia and Intensive Care*, 2nd edn. London: Greenwich Medical Media, 2003.

Sasada, M. and Smith, S. *Drugs in Anaesthesia and Intensive Care*, 3rd edn. Oxford: Oxford University Press, 2003.

Calvey, T. N. and Williams, N. E. *Principles and Practice of Pharmacology for Anaesthetists*, 4th edn. London: Blackwell Science, 2001.

Physics, measurement and statistics

Davies, P. D. and Kenny, G., *Basic Physics and Measurements in Anaesthesia*, 5th edn. New York: Butterworth Heinmann, 2003.

Moyle, J. T. B., Davey, A. and Ward, C. C. *Ward's Anaesthesia Equipment*, 4th edn. Philadelphia: WB Saunders, 1998.

Dorsch, J. A. and Dorsch, S. *Understanding Anaesthesia Equipment*. Baltimore: Williams and Wilkins, 1998.

Hutton, P. and Prys-Roberts, C. *Monitoring in Anaesthesia and Intensive Care*. Philadelphia: WB Saunders, 1994.

Magee, P. and Tooley, M. *Physics, Clinical Measurement and Equipment in Anaesthetic Practice*, Oxford: Oxford University Press, 2005.

Al-Shaikh, B. and Stacey, S. *Essentials of Anaesthetic Equipment*, 2nd edn. London: Churchill Livingstone, 2002.

Bonner, S. and Dodds, C. *Clinical Data Interpretation in Anaesthesia and Intensive Care.* London: Churchill Livingstone, 2002.

Books covering several sections

Aitkenhead, A. R., Smith, C. and Rowbottom, D. *Textbook of Anaesthesia*, 4th edn. London: Churchill Livingstone, 2001.

Yentis, S. M., Hirsch, N. P. and Smith, G. B. *Anaesthesia and Intensive Care A to Z*, 3rd edn. New York: Elsevier Butterworth Heinemann, 2004.

Pinnock, C., Lin, T. and Smith, T. *Fundamentals of Anaesthesia*, 2nd edn. London: Greenwich Medical Media, 2003.

Scarr, C. and Feldman, S. *Scientific Foundations of Anaesthesia*, 4th edn. New York: Butterworth Heinmann, 1990.

Morgan, M. *Short Practice of Anaesthesia.* London: Chapman and Hall Medical, 1998.

Bissonnette, B. *Pediatric Anesthesia, Principles and Practice*, 1st edn. New York: McGraw-Hill, 2002.

Baskett, P. J. F., Bow, A., Nolan, J. and Maull, K. *Practical Procedures in Anaesthesia and Critical Care.* New York: Mosby, 1995.

Morton, N. S. *Paediatric Intensive Care*, 1st edn. Oxford: Oxford University Press, 1997.

Gwinnutt, C. *Lecture Notes on Clinical Anaesthesia*, 2nd edn. Oxford: Blackwell Science, 2004.

Morgan, G. E., Maged, S. and Mikhail, S. *Clinical Anaesthesiology*, 3rd edn. New York: McGraw-Hill, 2002.

Stoelting, R. K. *Pharmacology and Physiology in Anaesthetic Practice*, 3rd edn. New York: Lippincott-Raven, 1999.

Robinson, N. and Hall, G. *How to Survive in Anaesthesia*, 2nd edn. London: BMJ, 2002.

Deakin, C. D. *Clinical Notes for the FRCA*, 2nd edn. New York: Churchill Livingstone, 2000.

Mills, S. J., Maguire, S. L. and Baker, J. M. *The Clinical Anaesthesia VIVA Book.* London: Greenwich Medical Media, 2002.

Cartwright, P. *The Royal College of Anaesthetists Guide to the FRCA Examination. The Primary.* London: The Royal College of Anaesthetists, 2001.

Journals

British Journal of Anaesthesia, Journal of the Royal College of Anaesthetists. Look particularly at editorials, review articles and supplements.

Continuing Education in Anaesthesia, Critical Care & Pain. A BJA Publication

Current Anaesthesia and Critical Care. Churchill Livingstone
Anaesthesia and Intensive Care Medicine. The Medicine Publishing Company Ltd.
Anaesthesia. Journal of the Association of Anaesthetists of Current Britain and Ireland. Blackwell Publishing. Look particularly at editorials and review articles.

Websites

For specific drugs – search by name of drug
www.rcoa.co.uk
www.frca.co.uk